Hybrid healing

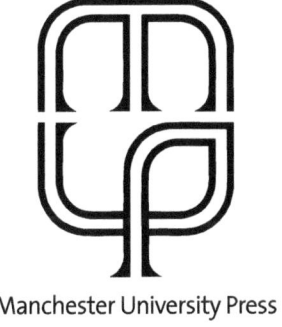
Manchester University Press

MANCHESTER MEDIEVAL LITERATURE AND CULTURE

Series editors: Anke Bernau, David Matthews and James Paz
Series founded by: J. J. Anderson and Gail Ashton
Advisory board: Ruth Evans, Patricia C. Ingham, Andrew James Johnston, Chris Jones, Catherine Karkov, Nicola McDonald, Haruko Momma, Susan Phillips, Sarah Salih, Larry Scanlon, Stephanie Trigg and Matthew Vernon

Manchester Medieval Literature and Culture publishes monographs and essay collections comprising new research informed by current critical methodologies on the literary cultures of the global Middle Ages. We are interested in all periods, from the early Middle Ages through to the late, and we include post-medieval engagements with and representations of the medieval period (or 'medievalism'). 'Literature' is taken in a broad sense, to include the many different medieval genres: imaginative, historical, political, scientific and religious.

Titles available in the series

23. *The politics of Middle English parables: Fiction, theology, and social practice* Mary Raschko

24. *Contemporary Chaucer across the centuries* Helen M. Hickey, Anne McKendry and Melissa Raine (eds)

25. *Borrowed objects and the art of poetry:* Spolia *in Old English verse* Denis Ferhatović

26. *Rebel angels: Space and sovereignty in Anglo-Saxon England* Jill Fitzgerald

27. *A landscape of words: Ireland, Britain and the poetics of space, 700–1250* Amy Mulligan

28. *Household knowledges in late-medieval England and France* Glenn D. Burger and Rory G. Critten (eds)

29. *Practising shame: Female honour in later medieval England* Mary C. Flannery

30. *Dating Beowulf: Studies in intimacy* Daniel C. Remein and Erica Weaver (eds)

31. *Enacting the Bible in medieval and early modern drama* Eva von Contzen and Chanita Goodblatt (eds)

32. *Riddles at work in the early medieval tradition: Words, ideas, interactions* Megan Cavell and Jennifer Neville (eds)

33. *From Iceland to the Americas: Vinland and historical imagination* Tim William Machan and Jón Karl Helgason (eds)

34. *Northern memories and the English Middle Ages* Tim William Machan

35. *Harley manuscript geographies: Literary history and the medieval miscellany* Daniel Birkholz

36. *Play time: Gender, anti-Semitism and temporality in medieval biblical drama* Daisy Black

37. *Transfiguring medievalism: Poetry, attention and the mysteries of the body* Cary Howie

38. *Objects of affection: The book and the household in late medieval England* Myra Seaman

39. *The gift of narrative in medieval England* Nicholas Perkins

40. *Sleep and its spaces in Middle English literature: Emotions, ethics, dreams* Megan G. Leitch

41. *Encountering* The Book of Margery Kempe Laura Kalas and Laura Varnam (eds)

42. *The narrative grotesque in medieval Scottish poetry* Caitlin Flynn

43. *Painful pleasures: Sadomasochism in medieval cultures* Christopher Vaccaro (ed.)

44. *Bestsellers and masterpieces: The changing medieval canon* Heather Blurton and Dwight F. Reynolds (eds)

45. *Medieval literary voices: Embodiment, materiality and performance* Louise D'Arcens and Sif Ríkharðsdóttir (eds)

Hybrid healing

Old English remedies and medical texts

Lori Ann Garner

MANCHESTER UNIVERSITY PRESS

Copyright © Lori Ann Garner 2022

The right of Lori Ann Garner to be identified as the author of this work has been asserted in accordance with the Copyright, Designs and Patents Act 1988.

Published by Manchester University Press
Oxford Road, Manchester M13 9PL

www.manchesteruniversitypress.co.uk

British Library Cataloguing-in-Publication Data
A catalogue record for this book is available from the British Library

ISBN 978 1 5261 5849 9 hardback

First published 2022

The publisher has no responsibility for the persistence or accuracy of URLs for any external or third-party internet websites referred to in this book, and does not guarantee that any content on such websites is, or will remain, accurate or appropriate.

Typeset
by Cheshire Typesetting Ltd, Cuddington, Cheshire

Contents

List of figures	page vi
List of tables	vii
Preface and dedication	viii
Acknowledgments	xvi
Introduction: an Old English poetics of health and healing	1
1 With hope and humility: hybridity as theoretical framework	22
2 Of swords and status: hybridity of metaphor in *Ic me on þisse gyrde beluce*	48
3 When healers are heroes: hybridity of battle in *Wið færstice*	97
4 To persuade a plant: hybridity of rhetoric in Harley 585	129
5 Of mandrakes and manuscripts: hybridity of being in Harley 6258B	160
6 On health and hearing: hybridity of environment in *Bald's Leechbook*	206
7 From remedies to riddles: hybridity of genre in an Exeter Book riddle	248
Conclusion: with empathy and imagination—hybridity in the field	272
Bibliography	288
Index	310

List of figures

2.1 *Herbarium* entry for yarrow, *millefolium*, British Library MS Cotton Vitellius C.iii, f. 46r (© The British Library Board)   50
2.2 *Herbarium* entry for woodruff, *astula regia*, British Library MS Cotton Vitellius C.iii, f. 32r (© The British Library Board)   59
2.3 Leaf-shaped spear-head, early medieval England (Museum number: 1964,0702.491 © Trustees of the British Museum)   59
3.1 *Lacnunga* entry, British Library MS Harley 585, f. 175v (© The British Library Board)   104
4.1 Entry for *ricinum*, British Library MS Harley 585, f. 94r (© The British Library Board)   135
4.2 Entry for periwinkle, British Library MS Harley 585, f. 96 v (© The British Library Board)   135
4.3 Entry for periwinkle, British Library MS Cotton Vitellius C.iii, f. 72v (© The British Library Board)   136
5.1 Entry for *mandragora*, British Library MS Harley 6258B, f. 20v (© The British Library Board)   161
5.2 Entry for *mandragora*, British Library MS Cotton Vitellius C.iii, f. 57v (© The British Library Board)   163
5.3 Entry for *gorgonion*, British Library MS Cotton Vitellius C.iii, f. 73v (© The British Library Board)   175
6.1 *Bald's Leechbook* (I.iii), British Library MS Royal 12 D.xvii, f. 14v–15r (© The British Library Board)   220

List of tables

3.1 Rhetorical structure of *Wið færstice*   110
6.1 Rhetorical structure of *Bald's Leechbook* (I.iii)   218

Preface and dedication

In Memory of John Miles Foley

Potential avenues for discovery and cocreation are everywhere.
(John Miles Foley, *Oral Tradition and the Internet: Pathways of the Mind*)[1]

At its core, this book is about the multivalence of traditional language and ritual, about the power of tradition to heal and make whole, and—most importantly—about the potential of genuinely interdisciplinary methodologies to unlock this meaning and power. While the focus here will ultimately be on texts of healing, I want first to pause briefly and consider the project's most significant influence and inspiration.

I have dedicated this work to the memory of John Miles Foley, not only because he was a teacher beloved by all his students, and was a dear friend and mentor to me, my husband, and son, but also because the book's fundamental structure and methodology are framed by a concept of hybridity that was central to John's work throughout his scholarship, from his very earliest articles, through his final posthumously published book. In many important ways, it was his unwavering interest in what he saw as the 'hybrid' nature of oral and oral-derived texts that forged the most productive path in the comparative field he pioneered, and the impact of his work across disciplines has been profound.[2] While some early scholars of what was originally known as oral-formulaic theory were devising quantitative tests for orality in hopes of objectively distinguishing manuscript poems that were written down as records of performances from those that were actively composed in writing, John

Foley gently but persistently advocated a very different model, one that not only acknowledged but embraced the interface of these largely hypothetical extremes. In explaining the relationship of oral tradition to literate culture in early medieval verse, the metaphor to which he returned most consistently was biological hybridity.

For instance, as early as 1980, he pushed back against descriptors of single half-lines in Old English verse as failed or, at best, irregular verse forms with his own theory of 'hybrid prosody', grounded in comparative work with living oral poetries. The Old English poetic line is most typically understood as 'a balance of two half-lines, notionally equal in prosody',[3] wherein alliteration links one or more stressed syllables in the first half-line with one or more stressed syllables in the second half-line. But through his characteristically comparative approach, which demonstrated 'the functional similarity between the Serbo-Croatian octosyllable and the Old English alliterative line', Foley noted in both 'a two-level, hybrid prosody and a resultant potential for modulation from whole-line to half-line rhythm'.[4] In his line of thinking, far from mistakes, the so-called single 'half' lines sometimes work in tandem with 'whole' lines to produce distinct patterns of metrics and meaning.

Having exonerated numerous anonymous Old English poets previously dismissed on grounds of failed and incomplete verses, Foley then extended the notion of hybridity in 1983 from prosody to diction in 'Genre(s) in the Making'. This compelling analysis of the *Seafarer*, a poem he loved well, alleviated the need to reduce the poem to any single, definitive reading, positing instead 'an audience which corresponds in preparation and expectation to the hybrid nature of the text, in particular to its hybrid diction', a poetics deriving meaning from both Latin learning and Germanic tradition, at once both 'traditional and nontraditional'.[5] Given his bachelor's degree with majors in math, physics, and chemistry, it is perhaps unsurprising that he would seek scientific models and metaphors for understanding the synthesis of learned Latinate conventions and traditional Germanic poetics for the diverse audience(s) to which the poem clearly spoke: 'The chemistry of the reading process will involve both audiences, or more accurately both aspects of a single real or rhetorical group, each in the mode suited to its imaginative reconstruction'.[6] He later expanded this concept to accommodate even more layers of complexity.

In *Traditional Oral Epic*, he returned to the metaphor from biology to describe the *Seafarer* in terms of a 'hybrid phraseology, rhetorical structure, and Christian sophistication', the composite resulting in a powerful hybridity of genre.[7] Ever resisting the pressure to take sides in the so-called 'Great Divide', Foley stressed that 'the presence of two kinds of forms for articulating meaning need not prompt an accusation of interference between the two. Rather, we may understand the traditional and non-traditional as simply two different and complementary ways of evoking meaning'.[8] In *Singer of Tales in Performance*, he then drew again on the model to explain his bringing together of Receptionalism and Performance Theory in what he described as a 'hybrid theory' that probed the intersections of literary theory and anthropological study.[9]

While he dropped much of his earlier theoretical language for *How to Read an Oral Poem*, a book designed explicitly to 'speak to the nonspecialist in a straightforward, uncomplicated way',[10] the metaphor of hybridity remained a constant. Here the dual layers of Scyld Scefing's funeral that opens *Beowulf* (especially lines 50b–52) are described in terms of a 'hybrid poetics', the localized meaning conveying a funerary ship burial like that of the ship found at Sutton Hoo, while the backdrop of the larger tradition infuses this already poignant scene with the elements from the traditional theme of a ship voyage, in this instance a voyage never completed.[11] Expanding the notion to include other genres and cultural traditions as well, he then went on to explain that 'oral poetry thrives on its ability to vary within limits', that 'every instance of a "classic" situation or incident is somehow different from all others; every context is unprecedented as well as generic; each poet and poem and performance is in some fashion unique'.[12] This situation thus means that all successful oral poetry is inherently 'hybrid'. In John Foley's view, 'if we fail to take realistic account of these aspects of uniqueness, we falsify the hybrid nature of oral poetry as both traditional and particular. We lose half of every poem's expressive force. Put more positively, it's precisely at the intersection of traditional and particular, of idiomatic and literal [...] that the art of oral poetry lives'.[13]

In his 2003 contribution to *Unlocking the Wordhord* (edited by Katherine O'Brien O'Keeffe and Mark Amodio), 'How Genres Leak in Traditional Verse', he took the metaphor even more literally, pushing further the point begun twenty years earlier that hybridity is the means by which traditional verbal art thrives: 'I will be maintaining, perhaps surprisingly, that cross-species fertilization is a fact of systemic life in an oral poetry, that it occurs as a matter of course. Traditional genres leak not by accident but regularly, predictably, and productively. While any poetic strategy can suffer from inept usage, in the hands of a talented poet generic exchange can produce a brilliant hybrid'.[14]

It was, however, the elegies to which Foley most regularly returned for developing his model of hybridity. When seen as the result of hybrid vigor, the interpretive problems presented in such poems as the *Seafarer* became, for Foley, not flaws but rather channels for rich meaning: 'The text is, in modern critical terms, "active"—that is, it calls for a complex, multi-leveled response on the part of the reader, and it offers an aesthetic experience which takes shape along two distinct phenomenological axes'.[15] This model of hybridity across multiple axes, which became especially foundational in his later work, is the construct that will be employed most directly in the chapters that follow.

John Foley had long envisioned a book-length work, which he eventually gave the working title *Hybrid Vigor: Reading the Old English Elegies.*[16] He referenced this project on hybridity and the elegies as early as a 2004 conference presentation on performance theory, where he described it as 'part of a larger project aimed at the hybrid vigor engendered' by such pairs of concepts as textuality/orality and individuality/tradition, concepts better understood 'as fruitful syncreses than opposing binaries'. In applying a model of hybridity, he intended to demonstrate that 'a full share of the elegies' artistry and rhetorical power stems from the idiomatic language of oral performance, which resonates even in the textual medium'.[17] While the book he had planned never had the chance to materialize, Foley did continue to more thoroughly and creatively exploit the concept of hybridity—in particular the generative potential of 'hybrid vigor'—for understanding Old English oral-connected texts. For instance, in his final, posthumously published volume, *Oral Tradition and the Internet: Pathways of the Mind*, he described the interaction between oral and written technologies in terms of 'a distinctive hybrid vigor' and applied the model specifically to the lovely and playful *Moððe* riddle, which enacts the paradox of a new hybrid communication with the capacity to render song as physical object through the image of a bookworm who, rather tragically, is none the wiser for having swallowed words.[18]

While hybridity served as a central concept from the beginning of John Foley's scholarly career, this particular aspect of a resultant 'vigor' became increasingly explicit through the years, and in this final book he thus offered his most direct challenge to any reductive or polarizing interpretations that risk missing the vibrancy of 'mixed' works:

> when a poem is informed by *both* a traditional *and* a non-traditional, learned aesthetic, there is very often a tendency on the part of critics to eliminate either the one or the other aspect. In an effort to make its poetics more straightforward, these critics would dismiss the vigor of such a hybrid text by miscasting its real nature or by characterizing it pejoratively as a 'mixed' work.[19]

He urged scholars instead to embrace the variation characterizing works produced at the interface of oral tradition and literate culture.

As this brief overview of even a single concept from John Foley's work demonstrates, he was always far more interested in opening up dialogue than in closing discussion with definitive final answers.[20] Ultimately, all of these notions of 'hybrid prosody', 'hybrid diction', and 'hybrid poetics' underscore the need for inherently flexible interpretive models, for more attention to how we approach the seemingly oxymoronic phenomenon of 'oral' texts, and even the activity of study and interpretation was described as a 'hybrid experience'.[21] His work reminds us that reading allows us only a limited perspective on what he termed 'voices from the past', a reality that holds especially true in the case of the medical texts, which so frequently call upon oral performance as part of their healing ritual. Read with this openness to discovery inherent in hybridity, long-textualized Old English poems can become vibrant and alive—fixed in form but ever-changing and new in our perceptions.

Another term that appears throughout Foley's work with increasing frequency is 'discovery', the usage in the epigraph only one of many in his final book alone.[22] As his student at the University of Missouri from 1995 until 2000 and in all the years that followed, I learned quickly not to expect direct answers to questions about how I might pursue projects. Infinitely more valuable than directives, what he offered was a space to enter the conversation, and an exciting one at that: 'That's the discovery', he said. It is this continuing spirit of exploration and discovery, inspired by—and, in its early stages, encouraged by—John Foley that has driven the present work. *Hybrid Healing* takes as its starting point the premise that textualized traditions deriving from oral traditions, but now long removed from their performance and cultural contexts, require frames of reference sensitive to their infinite complexities—a situation that is especially relevant for analyzing the Old English healing remedies. Both in the moment of performance and across oral and literary networks of transmission, these essentially hybrid medical texts survive as witness to a deep rootedness in traditional poetics and an indebtedness to diverse beliefs, rituals, and practices.

As I hope to show, Old English remedies seldom if ever provide anything as wholly straightforward as the ailment and cure that modern medicine might lead us to expect. Modern categories sharply delineating superstition from science, ritual from recipe, and even person from plant quickly become devoid of meaning when we engage closely with these vibrant and often enigmatic texts. The remedies and medical texts from early medieval England attest to a fundamentally different—and perhaps more empathetic—way of thinking about health and healing than is often seen in modern medical discourse. Early remedies and medicinal texts depend upon a complex network of relationships—relationships with pain, with each other, with healers, and with the very process of healing itself. For me, in this project, that has been the discovery. But as John Foley's work has shown, there is always more to be discovered.

Notes

1 John Miles Foley, *Oral Tradition and the Internet: Pathways of the Mind* (Urbana, IL: University of Illinois Press, 2012), p. 83.
2 As but one example illustrating the range of his impact, see *John Miles Foley's World of Oralities: Text, Tradition, and Contemporary Oral Theory*, edited by Mark Amodio (Leeds: ARC Humanities Press, 2020), a collection published in 2020 that brings together work influenced by Foley, with studies on Old English and Old Norse literature, the Hebrew Bible, medieval music, and Greek epic, among others. See, too, a special issue of *Oral Tradition* 26.2 (2011) presented by his students.
3 Alexander, Michael, *A History of Old English Literature* (Peterborough, ON: Broadview Press, 2002), p. 62.
4 John Miles Foley, 'Hybrid Prosody and Single Half-lines in Old English and Serbo-Croatian Poetry', *Neophilologus* 64 (1990), 284–289, at 287. Foley later returned to this idea of 'hybrid prosody', clarifying that his concept of both half- and whole-line phraseological units 'does not amount to a contradictory hypothesis; rather it recognizes the hybrid character of the meter and anticipates its reflection in the poetic diction', *Traditional Oral Epic: The* Odyssey, Beowulf, *and the Serbo-Croatian Return Song* (Berkeley, CA: University of California Press, 1993), p. 205.
5 John Miles Foley, 'Genre(s) in the Making: Diction, Audience, and Text in the Old English *Seafarer*', *Poetics Today*, 4.4 (1983), 683–706, at 697, 700.
6 Ibid., 697.
7 Foley, *Traditional*, p. 19.
8 Ibid., p. 196.
9 John Miles Foley, *The Singer of Tales in Performance* (Bloomington, IN: Indiana University Press, 1995), p. 41.
10 John Miles Foley, *How to Read an Oral Poem* (Urbana, IL: University of Illinois Press, 2002), p. xi.
11 Ibid., pp. 106–107.
12 Ibid., p. 140.
13 Ibid.
14 John Miles Foley, 'How Genres Leak in Traditional Verse', in Mark C. Amodio and Katherine O'Brien O'Keeffe (eds), *Unlocking the Wordhord* (Toronto: University of Toronto Press, 2003), 76–108, at 79.
15 Foley, *Traditional*, p. 19.

16 One of my first tasks as his graduate research assistant at the University of Missouri in 1995 involved compiling and annotating scholarship on the Old English elegies.
17 The presentation itself was shared at the Midwest Modern Language Association Annual Meeting in St. Louis, and the abstract appeared in *The Old English Newsletter* 38.3 (2005), 80. The panel was organized by Heather Maring, also a student of John Foley. Heather's own innovative work on oral-traditional, written, and liturgical hybridity in early medieval England can be found in *Signs that Sing: Hybrid Poetics in Old English Verse* (Gainesville, FL: University of Florida Press, 2017).
18 Foley, *Oral Tradition and the Internet*, p. 117.
19 Foley, *Traditional*, p. 6.
20 The sheer volume of work that he produced is staggering—eight single-authored books, eleven edited collections, and almost two hundred articles and shorter pieces, which together provide methodologies for analysis that have been applied across countless cultural and linguistic traditions. See R. Scott Garner, 'Annotated Bibliography of Works by John Miles Foley', Special Issue: Festschrift for John Miles Foley, *Oral Tradition*, 26.2 (2011), 677–724.
21 Foley, *How to Read an Oral Poem*, p. 21.
22 A quick search of the digital edition displays no fewer than 39 instances of *discover* or *discovery*.

Acknowledgments

The multidisciplinary nature of this book has drawn me into much new and unfamiliar terrain. I have needed a great deal of help, and I am beyond fortunate to be surrounded by tremendously knowledgeable and generous friends, colleagues, and family. Their support enabled me to take on the risks of this endeavor with better frames of reference and—I hope—with greater sensitivity and awareness than I might have had otherwise. I am delighted to express publicly my deep gratitude, and my heart is full.

One of the most wonderful things about teaching at a small liberal arts college is the ease of conversation across departments and fields of inquiry. Among the many individuals at Rhodes College who have shared generative insights, I am especially grateful to Elaine Frawley and Rob Laport (Biology) for sources and stimulating conversation on plant hybridity, to Jason Richards and Marshall Boswell (English) for discussions of cultural hybridity, to David Sick and Susan Satterfield (Ancient Mediterranean Studies) for insights into Roman ritual and medieval Latin. I am thankful also for my wonderful writing group: Judy Haas, Hannah Barker (now at ASU), Stephanie Elsky, Laura Loth, and Clara Pascual-Argentes. Thank you to Scott Newstok for much-needed encouragement and for always keeping an eye out for sources and resources I might need. I am most fortunate to have a home department that truly feels like a home with colleagues Amy Benson, Leslie Petty, Rashna Richards, Brian Shaffer, Rebecca Finlayson, Caki Wilkinson, Seth Rudy, Tim Lem-Smith, Marilyn Koester, and Gordon Bigelow. I am deeply grateful also to my many students at Rhodes College, whose excitement and curiosity about medieval literature keep these texts alive for me. I owe thanks to the entire library staff, but I am especially indebted to ILL librarian Kenan Padgett. Without her help acquiring research materials—especially during the period of COVID-19 restrictions limiting physical access to research libraries—there is no way I could have completed this work. Many thanks also to Lorie Yearwood in English.

In addition to this amazing community of faculty, staff, and students, Rhodes College has been generous in providing both time and funding to help see this book through completion. I was fortunate to receive a Faculty Development summer grant when the project was still nascent. Generous support from the Connie Abston Chair in Literature fund supported travel and provided invaluable resources over six years, and a sabbatical leave in Fall 2021 allowed me to keep pace with the publication schedule.

Beyond the gates of Rhodes, I want to thank my circle of Memphis friends for providing a healing balance to my own life, in particular Marjean Liggett for long walks and tai chi, Gretchen Stroud for countless forest runs and an always open door, and Ardelle Walters for a lifetime of friendship and—more to the point—weekly working lunches. I am grateful, too, for the support of family, especially my brothers and sisters—Kyle Peterson, Christopher Peterson, Sarah Vraneza, and Gretchen Maguire—and all their families as well as my cousin Nethery Wylie, whose interest in medieval history inspired me long before I entered the field myself.

For helping me at least begin to understand the field of Deaf studies, though I still have much to learn, I am thankful to graduate-school friend Kristen Harmon (now at Gallaudet University) and to Sonia Howley and Connie Robinson (former directors of Deaf Family Literacy-Midsouth) and to the participants in the 2013 AALAC Deaf Across the Curriculum workshop hosted by Donna Jo Napoli (Swarthmore). For my ventures into medieval rhetoric, I am especially grateful for the chance to have participated in the festschrift celebrating Martin Camargo, an incredible teacher I am honored to have worked with at the University of Missouri. Conversations with that project's authors and editors—most especially Denise Stodola, Jory Wood, and James Murphy—led to what eventually became Chapter 4.

While working on this book, I have been inspired by and learned much from amazing friends and colleagues in the fields of medieval studies and oral theory, including Lindy Brady, Mary Hayes, Donna Beth Ellard, Mark Amodio, Jack Niles, Jonathan Hsy, Dana Oswald, Andrew Rabin, Marijane Osborn, Irina Dumitrescu, Renée Trilling, Charlie Wright, Erin Sweany, Melissa Elmes, Tarren Andrews, Eliza Buhrer, Lea Olsan, Chao Gejin, Jan-Peer Hartmann, and so many more. I have found dear friends and inspiring colleagues in the fellow students of John Foley, most especially Rebecca Mouser, Justin Arft, Heather Maring, and Aaron Tate. I remain grateful also to Anne-Marie Foley for years of friendship and support.

Shelby Seese offered invaluable assistance with the formatting of the bibliography and notes, and Laura Helper gave me feedback and courage when I needed it most. I am thankful to Marylaura Papalas for her daily encouragement and to the National Center for Faculty Development and Diversity (NCFDD) for pairing us as writing partners. Thanks beyond what I can ever hope to repay go to Tiffany Beechy, who has attended talks related to almost every chapter and who read the entire manuscript at a point when I was too close to see many of its flaws and inconsistencies.

At Manchester University Press, I deeply appreciate the expertise, patience, and imagination of Meredith Carroll. I feel so fortunate that she and the series editors (Anke Bernau, David Matthews, and James Paz) believed in this project. I am also grateful to the anonymous readers for their support of the project and for their time and generosity in sharing substantive critiques and invaluable correctives for revisions, and to Alun Richards, Lianne Slavin, Laura Swift, Jen Mellor, and Rachel Evans for seeing it through production.

I thank the British Museum and the British Library (especially Bruna Lago-Fazolo) for permission to reproduce images from their collections and the staff at the Bodleian Library for the opportunity to consult manuscripts and books in the special collections in Oxford.

Earlier versions of some analyses appeared in the following publications, and I am grateful to the editors for permission to publish portions in revised form: 'Weapons of Healing: Materiality and

Oral Poetics in Old English Remedies and Medicinal Charms', in *Material Remains: Reading the Past in Medieval and Early Modern British Literature*, edited by Jan-Peer Hartmann and Andrew James Johnston (Columbus, OH: Ohio State University Press, 2021); 'Deaf Studies, Oral Tradition, and Old English Texts', *Exemplaria*, 29 (2017), 21–40; 'Rhetoric and Remedies; or, How to Persuade a Plant in Anglo-Saxon England', in *Public Declamations: Essays on Medieval Rhetoric, Education, and Letters in Honor of Martin Camargo*, edited by Georgiana Donovan and Denise Stodola (Turnhout: Brepols, 2015), 155–168.

I feel drawn also to express gratitude to the healers, compilers, and scribes whose work over 1000 years ago connects us to these otherwise ephemeral healing traditions.

Now for those closest. I'm grateful for the calming presence of my sweet Nana (dog, not grandmother), who slept at my feet for the writing of almost every word. My dear Nathaniel, who sometimes plays through his medieval fantasy games as a healer just so I can watch, left for his first semester of college the very same week the first full manuscript of this book left for the press. As he has grown into an adult, he has become a wonderful sounding board for new ideas. And last, of course, is Scott, whom I met at the Center for Studies in Oral Tradition through John Foley over 25 years ago (perhaps the greatest reason I am grateful to John!). He has been the most supportive, generous, loving partner I could imagine in every possible way. But right now, I am glad most of all that his love at times takes form in proof-reading and indexing and that he edits as hard as he runs.

Perhaps most important, I want to express thanks to those not included here due to the limits of space and the deficiencies of my own memory. To those I have inadvertently omitted here, please know I am grateful and that when I remember later I will be deeply sorry. Thank you, all. And may you be well!

Introduction: an Old English poetics of health and healing

            Næfre læcecynn
on folcstede   findan meahte,
þara þe mid wyrtum   wunde gehælde.

[Never healer-kind
could I find in the dwelling place,
one of those who healed a wound with herbs.]

                                                (Exeter Book riddle)[1]

The enigma of Old English remedies

Modern readers seeking to understand healing practices of early medieval England[2] can at least partly relate to the frustration expressed by the speaker of the riddle in the lines above. After earlier describing fierce and unrelenting military attacks, the speaker now laments that no healers can be found. But this tragic speaker does not require actual medical attention to a physical body, the persona of the solitary warrior under attack having been cleverly projected, in typical riddlic fashion, onto a material object instead. Various solutions for the identity of this object have been proposed (most notably *shield*, *cutting board* or *chopping block*, and *whetstone*)— all of which would have profound implications for the riddle and its cultural context, as will be discussed at length in Chapter 7. However, it is worth pausing here early on to consider first how much we as readers have in common with the unfortunate speaker in the lines above, as we struggle to understand the often cryptic remedies that survive in the early medieval medical texts without the insights of the healers themselves, a challenge that at times feels wholly insurmountable. As in the riddle tradition, however, there are clues to be found in paradox, in beings and spaces and texts that embody combinations of traits so seemingly antithetical that they prove difficult to recognize. Hybridity obscures, even as it points the way towards clarity.

Though the articulation of absence in this riddle arguably offers the only explicit reference to herbal healers in surviving Old English poetry outside of the medical texts themselves, its enigmatic hybrid speaker—a paradoxical crossing of human warrior and utilitarian object—can suggest a good deal about notions of health and healing. The complaint of being unable to find an herbal healer in the dwelling place to tend its wounds tells us that ordinarily one *would* seek out a healer for battle wounds, that such wounds would probably be treated with herbs, and that healers could, under ideal circumstances, reliably be found in the *folcstede* or, literally, 'people-place'. The reference to *læcecynne*, 'healer-kind', reinforces the sense that healers should not be understood as rare individuals, but rather as members of a collective *cynn*, a *kind* of person one could typically expect to find in the *folcstede*, wherever people dwell in groups.[3]

This riddle's plaintive speaker thus invites us to think deeply about the role of healers and healing even when firm evidence of their existence as a distinct category is quite limited. This text further reminds us that even the most silent of objects can nonetheless find enduring modes of expression, provided we can find the means to engage them. Most of all, this riddle implies that healers and healing occupy a potentially important, albeit enigmatic, space in the often paradoxical world presented in Old English texts. This book attempts to show ways that healing and hybridity can be viewed productively as deeply intertwined concepts within the context of early medieval English culture. As a first step, I want to establish here at the outset that 'hybridity' is—and always has been—a deeply fraught construct.

Rethinking hybridity

By late 2020, the mere mention of a 'hybrid classroom' was enough to spark intense debate, as administrators, teachers, parents, and students around the world struggled with varying degrees of success in adapting to the challenging environment of the pandemic through various attempts to cross online with in-person learning.[4] Though the COVID-19 pandemic has been, as many of us have heard countless times, 'unprecedented', the mixed response of energy, anxiety, loathing, and hope surrounding 'hybridity' is far from new. As even the most cursory look at the primary definitions and attestations of *hybrid* in English language history reveals, hybridity has always been a complicated concept, the term itself having 'a mixed character', hybridity itself hybrid, at once literal and metaphorical, natural and at the same time socially constructed. The amorphous nature of 'hybridity' might even suggest that we should retire the notion as too imprecise to be meaningful. However, I would argue that it is precisely its multivalence and dynamism that makes *hybridity* an especially apt model for the study of Old English healing remedies. Unlike related concepts of *syncretism* or *fusion*—which also certainly play important roles in early medieval textual production generally and in the medical texts more specifically—*hybridity* centers our awareness on the fundamental aliveness of the texts that survive to us. Where syncretism and fusion by definition emphasize the *act* of merging, *hybridity* refocuses our attention on the *product* of such fusions and the ongoing process by which new hybrids endlessly emerge.[5]

The use of hybridity as a metaphor for cross-cultural and multigeneric literature is of course far from new, and hybridity has long proven a compelling model for understanding Old English poetry and culture in particular. While a comprehensive treatment of hybridity as it has been employed within Old English studies is far beyond the scope of what any single chapter can provide, a few particular applications have been especially helpful for my own thinking in connection with Old English remedies and medical texts. First, and perhaps most important, is scholarship, such as that of Elaine Treharne, which insists upon an understanding of hybridity as more than a simple 'assimilative impulse' and rather as a 'complex, processual, and separate state-of-being', a new existence created specifically within 'contested space'.[6] As will be discussed further in Chapter 1, biological hybridity as it relates to new species creation does indeed involve contest and conquest, as newly emerged hybrids thrive or fail in their surrounding landscapes.

The destabilization inherent in this process is a second aspect of hybridity that underpins the thinking of *Hybrid Healing*. For instance, the merging of Christian content with vernacular form is not a process of simple supplantation, as Renée Trilling has observed: 'instead a hybrid form results, with elements both similar to and different from the traditions that spawned it'.[7] As a result, 'what begins as the imposition of authoritative discourses of colonial power gradually becomes a site of reassertion for those supposedly inferior subjects'.[8] Focusing on Bede's choice to present *Caedmon's Hymn* as a prose paraphrase rather than in a Latin verse translation, Trilling argues that 'hybridity destabilizes the simple binary opposition between colonizer and colonized and refutes identity at either pole. It becomes a site for the reformulation of power, and the hybrid reflects back to authority its own ideological ambivalences'.[9] Through this same type of cultural hybridity, the so-called 'Nine Herbs Charm', with its dual references to both Woden and Christ,[10] in effect reformulates competing power structures and in so doing activates a fundamentally new source of healing.[11] Such is the potential of hybridity.

The role of mediation is a third aspect of hybridity crucial to the chapters that follow. Old English medical texts frequently offer highly condensed examples of cultural hybridity, with multiple traditions—Latin and Old English, Christian and Germanic, heroic and elegiac—often sharing the same verbal and ritual space. Such a concentrated site of cultural exchange is quite potent. Noting the 'intermingling of medicine, liturgy, and folklore' in medieval healing lore, Karen Louise Jolly suggests that 'elf charms in particular are a hybrid of these diverse, intertwining contexts and constitute middle practices that reveal negotiated territory between popular and formal religion in the process of cultural conversion'.[12] As such, the medical texts operating on such principles must be understood as far more than simplistic harmonious exchanges. Remedies implicitly pit healer against ailment, and, in the battle for the 'negotiated' territory of the body itself, competing influences are thrust together, erupting in an even more powerful manifestation of power.

Lastly, my work in this volume understands hybridity as reflecting sometimes overlooked modes of difference and as having the potential to effect subtle change. As Nicole Guenther Discenza reminds us in her discussion of spaces and hybridity, 'the most obvious hybrids are not the only hybrids'.[13] While Discenza is here focusing on the portrayal of monsters in such texts as *Wonders of the East*, this reminder is equally important in the study of medical texts, which provide fairly obvious hybrids such as the mandrake, a plant described as having hands and feet ('hyre handa 7 hyre fet')[14] and illustrated in the Cotton Vitellius C.iii with a correspondingly humanoid body, but also more subtle hybrids, such as plants with the capacity to hear and to remember, as we see in the 'Nine Herbs Charm', and plants in the *Herbarium* such as periwinkle and *ricinum*, which are the actual recipients of invocations. Focusing more specifically on matters of orality and literacy, Daniel Donoghue argues that the 'actual emergence of literacy from orality' is 'the least interesting part. What is of more interest is that relatively rare condition (from the modern literate point of view) when the two retain a functioning vigor in an ongoing negotiation, resulting in a poetics of hybridity'.[15] This nuanced model of hybridity productively frustrates simple binaries polarizing orality and literacy and will be especially helpful in investigating medical texts that are simultaneously textual and performative.

In developing these views, I am inspired by applications of hybridity that have been employed to explore the rich, multivalent, and often transgressive nature of medieval texts, such as Dana Oswald's insightful discussion of Grendel's mother in the context of monsters whose bodies are 'hybrid in terms of their physical form and their sex and gender characteristics', as beings that 'transgress codes of gender' and thus establish such bodies as 'threats to established patterns of sex, gender, and sexuality';[16] Alf Siewers' ecocritical analysis of human interactions in the natural world, which describes the speaking tree in *Dream of the Rood* as 'dynamically hybridized with the body of the Creator-God';[17] or—perhaps most of all—Heather Maring's view of 'hybrid signification' as a mode employed by poets 'to celebrate' unconventional yet meaningful connections.[18] The often transgressive connections in medicinal texts do in fact offer much to celebrate.

The remedies found in extant manuscripts not only draw from and connect multiple traditions in order to free individuals from the constraints of physical ailments, but also become new healing entities in the process, with their own capacity to mediate and effect change. Linguistic hybridity perhaps illustrates the phenomenon in the most obvious way, as in a remedy for lost cattle that includes incantations in Latin as well as the vernacular Old English; even at the level of individual words and morphemes, this remedy exhibits a revealing hybridity. An incantation beginning 'Crux Christi' is repeated four times, once for each of the cardinal directions, 'May the cross of Christ bring it back from the east/west/south/north'. In the first instance, however, the inflection of the verb *reducat* is changed to a distinctively Old English ending: 'Crux Christi ab oriente reduca<u>ð</u>' (emphasis added).[19] While on one hand the 'mistake' can simply be written off as a scribal slip, this kind of linguistic merging reflects a much broader tendency toward hybridization, one that is fundamental to healing in the Old English tradition. New words, new phrases, new combinations all hold the promise of new healing power.

While this confluence of traditions, languages, and modes of expression is quite common throughout Old English poetry and has been well noted, the phenomenon is arguably more dramatic within the specific corpus of medical texts and remedies. Unprecedented and sometimes extreme measures—innovations or adaptations sometimes accompanied by serious risks—are, even today, quite natural responses to serious illness and adversity, and it is thus to be expected that the record reflects a relatively high degree of hybridity. Yet incorporation of multiple religious or cultural traditions has often been simplistically ascribed to a fear-induced hedging of bets, assuming that the individuals involved believed one religion or mode of thinking must have been 'right' but that they were simply incapable of ascertaining with absolutely certainty which one. While such reductive phrasing is quite common in academic as well as popular discussions of early medieval religion,[20] these assessments are fundamentally anachronistic. Replacing this model from gambling with a model of hybridity allows us to recognize the incorporation of multiple traditions into a given poem, object, or ritual as authentic and meaningful, not in spite of but *because* of the dynamic interactions across diverse structures of belief.

Noting the inherent bias in efforts to sift out 'pagan' from 'Christian' or 'magic' from 'religion' in Old English texts, Karen

Jolly has explained that this type of duality results in 'an inadequate model' because it 'gives primacy to a literate mentality that was only just beginning to emerge'.[21] The reality of popular religion involved a 'creative tension with the wider and slower processes of accommodation and assimilation'.[22] In this way, Christian and Germanic, Latin and vernacular, oral and literate modes offered multiple channels of simultaneously competing and overlapping sources of authority and power. Thus, sites of ailment could quite naturally become sites of hybridity, replete with all the potential and danger the process of hybridization implies.

As will be discussed at length in the next chapter, *hybridity* as a cultural metaphor—and even as a biological reality—is far from straightforward, the value of successful hybridization of course being socially constructed and always carrying the risk of usurpation or exploitation of one cultural tradition by another. Yet it is precisely this amorphous, indeterminate, even dangerous nature of Old English remedies that *Hybrid Healing* most directly engages. If we see sites of pain, disease, and ailment as sites of contest, it is largely through its inherent hybridity that Old English medicine disrupts the power structure in the healing texts, as forces of ailment are conquered by forces of healing. As the following chapters seek to show, through complex processes of crossing diverse linguistic, cultural, and medical traditions in the pursuit of health and wholeness, a construct of healing hybridity emerges quite prominently across the Old English corpus.

The texts and the tradition

As noted at the beginning of this chapter, surviving manuscripts leave us with ample texts of remedies, but actual healers can be hard to find. Extant texts offer precious little information regarding who provided healing for the ill and vulnerable, or where and how those suffering could access healing remedies. Aldhelm includes *medicina* in his list of *fisicae artes*, which would seem to suggest that classical medicine was at least to some extent involved in the educational curriculum.[23] Similarly, Bede's *Historia ecclesiastica* includes miracles and stories of healing, especially those associated with John of Beverley, pointing toward the possibility that at least in late seventh-century Northumbria healers were sought in monastic centers.[24] A further detail about these healers is revealed through John of Beverley's criticisms of nuns who sought to perform a phlebotomy outside the authorized lunar period,[25] thus hinting that women also had the authority to perform medical procedures, though their authority at monastic centers here seems to have been subject to men's approval. Additionally, Bede's description of a debate at Lindisfarne regarding whether a tumor over an eyelid would be best treated with a poultice or surgery (Book IV.32) implies not only multiple healers in a given location but also a diversity of medical philosophies and practices.[26]

Though appearances of healers outside the medical corpus are exceedingly rare, we are nonetheless quite fortunate in having extensive collections of the remedies themselves. The two most complete medical compilations of vernacular remedies are found in the late Old English *Leechbooks* (BL, Royal 12 D.xvii)— comprising two books organized roughly in head to foot order (collectively known as *Bald's Leechbook*, from the name found in a Latin colophon at the end of the second book), along with a third book (known as *Leechbook III*)—and a collection conventionally known as the *Lacnunga* (MS Harley 585), which includes almost 200 entries with instruction for healing various ailments.[27] In addition to these vernacular remedies, there are also extant collections translated from Latin into Old English, most notably the Old English *Herbarium*, which is organized by herb rather than by ailment. The Old English *Herbarium* survives in four manuscripts, dating from the tenth to the twelfth centuries: Bodleian Library, MS Hatton 76; British Library, MS Harley 585; British Library, MS Cotton Vitellius C.iii; and British Library, MS Harley 6258B.[28] And beyond these dedicated collections, there are numerous other vernacular charms[29] and remedies scattered throughout various manuscripts, sometimes even inscribed in the margins (such as the metrical charms of Cambridge College Corpus Christi MS 41). Across these eclectic texts, we see tremendous diversity in healing methods, including herbal remedies, songs and incantations, elaborate rituals, and dietary prescriptions. This wide-ranging body of healing lore assists with an equally vast assortment of problems, not

An Old English poetics of health and healing 9

only physical ailments but also challenges ranging from childbirth and dangerous travel to hail storms and even stolen cattle. My goal here, however, is neither a chronological history nor a comprehensive treatment of this vast body of work. On the contrary, this book builds from the central premise that each manuscript, each ailment, even each particular remedy has its own history and deserves—indeed rewards—highly individualized methods of analysis drawing from diverse fields and modes of discourse. Thus, to better analyze the various hybridized medical texts treated here, the book's approach is hybrid as well. Each chapter offers a detailed analysis of a particular text or type of remedy through a methodology that brings together perspectives from two or more conventionally distinct disciplines, always bearing in mind the ever-shifting position of these texts within the dual contexts of oral tradition and literate culture.

A central aspect of this approach involves shifting previously marginalized materials from the periphery to the focal point, and *Hybrid Healing* thus works against entrenched notions of *Beowulf* and heroic narrative verse as the unquestioned center of the Old English poetic universe (and accompanying scholarly discourse). It challenges several long-standing emendations based on expectations for conformity with the epic tradition. Because the book strives to develop a nuanced understanding of the poetics linking healing and verbal arts, *Hybrid Healing* does in some chapters direct its analytical attention specifically towards poetry and oral incantations; however, this project then also seeks to destabilize the privileged position in scholarship of the so-called 'metrical charms' through comparative work across genres of prose and poetry. Viewed as a result of such processes of hybridization, verse portions of healing remedies might be more accurately understood not as free-standing poems to be extracted from the surrounding prose, but as integral components within prosimetric texts, hybrid in form as well as function.

What this volume therefore offers, instead of a comprehensive treatment or representative summary of this corpus, is a case-study approach wherein carefully selected remedies and charm texts are investigated for their insights into how healing was understood and approached in this early medieval period of emerging literacy that continued to derive power from a still-pervasive and ambient oral tradition. This case-study model allows for close readings of individual texts, a strategy that has typically been reserved for more canonical poems of the period, most especially heroic narrative verse and lyric poetry such as the elegies. Such a close focus positions us to appreciate more fully the diverse influences of multiple genres and traditions on any given remedy and thus to resist simple binaries—such as poetry versus prose, Germanic versus Christian, or Latin versus Old English. The book takes as its starting point the endless complexity of the Old English medical tradition and argues throughout that the healing power of individual remedies ultimately derives from the unique convergences of widely disparate traditions and influences, a dynamic and unpredictable process wherein multiple influences are continually joined and rejoined, resulting in forces at once deeply traditional and ever new—a power that is, from this perspective, deeply hybrid.

Overview of chapters

Acutely aware of the benefits as well as the risks of hybridity, both as a biological reality and as a critical metaphor, this book embraces a diverse range of theoretical approaches that collectively build a methodology accounting simultaneously for both the power and the danger of hybridity as a cultural model. The concept of hybridity offers a powerful model for understanding many of the complex and dynamic processes that arise from cultural interactions. However, this model is also one that, if left unexamined, becomes laden with the potential for harmful oversimplification by implying the acceptance—or even glorification—of the exploitation, appropriation, and subjugation that can occur when less powerful groups and traditions are subsumed by force. Thus Chapter 1 endeavors to productively frame the discussion, first situating the concept of hybridity within the historical and agricultural contexts of early medieval England (especially through analysis of the *Æcerbot* land remedy) and then probing the biological basis of the metaphor for parallels that help us appreciate its generative potential as well as its limits. In acknowledging and naming a vast range of ailments and adversities, early medieval medical texts lay bare sites of pain, trauma, and fear, and in so doing they expose sites of vulnerability and contest. Within this space where suffering can be openly contested, the remedies and rituals clearly and forcefully draw from all available power sources, creating healing networks across diverse religious and cultural belief systems. Though the texts produced can sometimes come across to readers accustomed to modern Western medicine as illogical or incongruous, this chapter argues that the process parallels that of biological hybridity, where diverse entities are brought together and crossed in the hopes of—but without the certainty of—positive outcomes. In this construct, sites of pain and adversity in effect become sites of hybridization—embodying all of the hope, risk, danger, and power intrinsic to that process.

Following this foundational exploration of hybridity itself, the core of the book then examines the hybrid nature of healing from the inside out, closely analyzing individual remedies in turn to discover insights concerning healing practices and philosophies more broadly. Chapter 2 starts by bringing oral theory into dialogue with approaches from archaeology in an analysis of the Old English *Herbarium* entry for yarrow, a medicinal herb whose healing properties are deeply connected in traditional lore to the legendary battles of Achilles. The chapter then builds toward analyzing in greater depth an Old English alliterative poem from the margins of Bede's *Ecclesiastical History*, opening 'Ic me on þisse gyrde beluce',[30] a generically hybrid poem in which weapons serve as metaphors for healing and protection. Old English traditional remedies frequently employ weapons (both as metaphors and also as healing implements) to conceptualize disease and to negotiate power over illness and adversity in early medieval England, most obviously through herbs named for weapons (such as *astula regia* ['king's spear'], *garlic* ['spear-leek'], and *sperewyrt* ['spear-plant']) and in instructions requiring knives and even swords as part of healing rituals. Even these onomastic and ritual weapons can provide important glimpses into how 'battles' against ailment might have been understood and imagined by the texts' earliest audiences. And in metaphorically equating items of the most elite warrior's armor—specifically a sword, shield, mailcoat, and helmet—to the four gospel authors, *Ic me on þisse gyrde beluce* essentially elevates figures associated with Christian liturgy to the highest values of loyalty, honor, and protection within the vernacular heroic tradition. Finally, the chapter concludes by discussing several debated matters of editing and translation, most especially a frequent deletion of a repeated half-line *hand ofer head* ['hand over head'] and a commonly accepted emendation of *wega* to *wælgar*, seemingly small choices but ones that have for too long worked against the poetics of weaponry established by the poem and that have important implications for interpretation.

Extending this investigation of weaponry into another poetic charm text, Chapter 3 examines the verse incantation of a metrical incantation in Harley 585 (ff. 175r–176r) 'wið færstice' ['against a sudden pain'],[31] which ascribes pain to spears (*garas*) sent by mighty women from another realm. It is all too easy to dismiss this seemingly incongruous poem as mere superstition or abstract metaphor. But what happens if we look at this incantation in terms of strategies employed within actual Germanic warfare? The speaker—presumably the healer—threatens to return the attack with a flying arrow ('fleogende flane'), and the incantation makes multiple references to smiths forging weapons of iron. This enigmatic incantation is framed on either side by a recipe and instructions involving herbal preparations. So different in tone and content is the incantation from the herbal recipe that some have argued they constitute entirely separate entries in the *Lacnunga*. However, when we bring a more complete awareness of specific weapons and battle strategies to our analysis of the text, we see that this incantation not only operates in tandem with the herbal preparation but emerges from the same underlying logic. Returning to the implications of such matters on choices in editing and translation seen in Chapter 2, an appendix to this chapter then draws from the field of ethnopoetics to offer a newly edited text and translation of the remedy that more fully reflect the complex network of associations at play.

Whereas Chapters 2 and 3 explore plants as weapons in the context of battle, Chapter 4 examines ways that herbs are sometimes invoked as actual sentient beings. Bringing studies in medieval rhetoric to bear on orally performed incantations required by Old English healing recipes, this chapter offers a close analysis of the direct address employed in two medicinal texts within the Harley 585 manuscript in order to communicate with a wide range of plants, specifically *mugwyrt* (mugwort), *wegbrade* (waybroad), *attorlaðe* (identified as cockspur grass or possibly betony), and *mægðe* (mayweed or chamomile) as they appear in the *Lacnunga* within the so-called 'Nine Herbs Charm' and the herbs *ricinum* (castor-oil plant) and *peruica* (periwinkle) as treated in the *Herbarium*. While the charms in the *Herbarium* and the *Lacnunga* both involve direct address in soliciting the respective herbs' assistance, the specific manner in which the herbs are addressed—and, consequently, the relationships implied between healer and herb—differ markedly from each other. Such variation in the two types of address and the attendant methods of persuasion reflect distinct cultural differences between Latinate and Germanic modes of expression and conceptions of herbal healing, yet their juxtaposition within a single manuscript devoted to healing practice nonetheless suggests that these variant strains of thought were not seen as competing or mutually exclusive. As with many aspects of early medieval culture, such variation in the rhetorical devices employed for the persuasion of plants reflects the productive hybridity emerging from Germanic and Latinate influences and helps us better understand healers' complicated conceptions of herbal power.

Chapter 5 turns our attention from matters of composition to questions of transmission and reception, focusing specifically on the mandrake root (*mandragora*) as it appears across manuscript versions of the Old English *Herbarium*. The *Herbarium*, almost exclusively derived from earlier Latin remedies, outlines cures utilizing 138 plants and is preserved in four manuscripts dating from the tenth century to as late as the twelfth. Centering its analysis on the anomalous entry for the anthropomorphized mandrake in a historically neglected manuscript, this chapter challenges the privileging of lavishly produced manuscripts over less visually appealing counterparts. The beautifully illustrated copy of the *Herbarium* in MS Cotton Vitellius C.iii has typically served as an authoritative base text, with the copy in MS Harley 6258B most often being viewed as demonstrating far less care and planning in its production. However, it is precisely the omissions, organizational departures, and other 'flaws' that suggest a close connection of this seemingly lesser text to the actual performance of medical practice. Chapter 5 is thus aimed at helping to rebalance the historical privileging of literate culture over oral tradition in scholarly treatments of the Old English medical corpus, a tendency that risks reading natural variation across versions as 'mistakes' and connections to folklore as irrational. Finally, by drawing especially from Matthew Hall's groundbreaking *Plants as Persons* and Michael Marder's *Plant-Thinking*, this chapter confronts our societal privileging of human over plant. The mandrake—rendered in the illustrated *Herbarium* with face, arms, and legs—may offer an extreme example of anthropomorphism, but a close look at the subtle variations of the plant's characteristics as described across its surviving Old English entries and in the context of the medical texts more broadly also suggests a more inherently collaborative relationship between medicinal plants and healers than the utilitarian models of medicine that typically serve as defaults today. An appendix offers a newly edited and translated text of this entry reflecting the chapter's analysis.

Chapter 6 continues to examine early medieval understandings of medicine, ailments, and bodies, specifically by analyzing ways that remedies in *Bald's Leechbook* challenge modern conceptions of hearing and deafness. Centering discussion around remedies in the third chapter of *Bald's Leechbook*, this analysis brings important work in Deaf studies to bear more directly on our perception of medieval oral/aural culture. Although scholars in Deaf studies have long applied interpretive models from oral theory to analyze the cultural expressivity of signed storytelling, the influence of Deaf studies has yet to be fully felt in the fields of oral theory or Old English studies. In fact, deafness has at times even been used within oral tradition scholarship as a negatively charged metaphor for not appreciating the nuances of oral-connected texts. A hybrid theoretical approach bridging these two fields productively complicates our understanding of early medieval England as a largely oral/aural culture, and evidence from surviving medical texts, law codes, and the archaeological record indicates a range of sensory perception that seems to have been widely recognized. The entries in *Bald's Leechbook* suggest a worldview in which the capacity for hearing, though important in many contexts, was not assumed. Rather, the faculty of hearing itself is described as changing and changeable, in terms of experience rather than identity. Accordingly, the Old English texts describe a wide variety of circumstances that might temporarily or permanently limit one's auditory range at any point in one's life—through such forces as violence, illness, wind, or disease. Thus, examining the Old English complex of remedies involving hearing and deafness in light of Deaf studies and oral theory not only broadens our awareness of health and healing beyond a modern medical model, but even more importantly helps remediate the potential for audism inherent in oral tradition studies and productively complicates our understanding of both hearing and deafness in pre-modern eras.

Chapter 7 then brings us back full circle to the Exeter Book riddle with which we began. This last chapter pans out to cut across genres of Old English poetry, seeking to demonstrate ways that knowledge of Old English healing can inform interpretations of Old English poetry more widely. As ubiquitous as the medieval healer has become in modern film and media, herbal healing and healers are virtually non-existent in Old English heroic verse, and so we can be left with the (false) impression that healing charms and remedies constituted a distinct position in early medieval thought, separate from narrative genres. As we saw earlier, outside of the medical texts, one of the only references left to us in surviving poetry laments a *lack* of healers. Yet this complaint buried within the highly formulaic language of exile and warfare in the Exeter Book's *Anhaga*[32] riddle can nonetheless provide an enormously productive key to interpreting the riddle's warrior persona within a complex network of material objects that have previously been proposed as possible solutions. This chapter explores insights that this seemingly simple riddle can offer into herbal remedies, material culture, and—most of all—into the playful, probing modes of thinking that subtly but powerfully link concepts of deadly warfare and herbal healing in Old English poetry and culture.

Finally, a Conclusion—one that in no way sees itself as ultimately conclusive—first illustrates how approaches from each of the preceding chapters can in turn unlock complex hybridity in a single unassuming remedy (the *Herbarium* entry for *leonfot*). Next, this section brings the chapters more directly into conversation with one another to isolate broader patterns, in a final harvest of sorts. These tendencies include an openness and flexibility that accommodate variation and change, an aliveness that depends upon a deeply collaborative enterprise of healing belief, and a profound empathy that extends beyond the immediate subject of healing to encompass a much larger community.

What we find when we tailor approaches to individual remedies and allow them the space to exist in all their complexity is an underlying empathy for human suffering—not only empathy for the afflicted individual, though that sensitivity is certainly there, but more surprisingly (from a modern perspective at least) empathy for suffering itself. Many first-time readers of *Beowulf* are surprised to feel empathy for Grendel even after he has literally eaten the inhabitants of Heorot. Monstrous though he is, Grendel is shown to suffer physical and emotional pain, even as he brings it. This destabilizing construct is far less jarring, however, when examined through the lens of Old English remedies, where healing plants might also be dangerous and where illness might be brought by entities not necessarily malevolent. What emerges across the book's varied hybrid approaches is that textual and methodological hybridity has the potential now to do the kind of important work hybrids have always done—shifting the power balance, proving time and again that healing power lies in the capacity for change, in newness and growth, in the nature of being animate and alive.

Across these disparate chapters, *Hybrid Healing* seeks to meet the hybridity of tradition with a hybridity of approach, taking the individuality of each medical text and each individual remedy as its starting point. Seldom do Old English remedies provide anything as wholly straightforward as the ailment and cure modern medicine might lead us to expect. Indeed, the inherent ambiguity of these texts asserts itself from the first word that formulaically introduces almost every medical text, *wið*. The dominant meaning of this lexeme when used with the dative, as is reflected in most translations of the remedies, certainly has a sense of confrontation, 'against'. However, then, as now, *wið* had multiple senses depending on context and could also be understood as 'marking association', translated as 'with'.[33] Old English healing remedies and medical texts frequently show us less what we would think of as a cure and more a mindset for living 'with' adversity, in all senses of the word. Awareness of the multivalence that permeates these medical texts therefore opens us to new perspectives on the vast spectrum of human ability and experience in the early medieval period and perhaps even in our own. The chapters that follow seek to more fully and sensitively understand the relationships presented by these texts—relationships with pain, with each other, with healers, and with the very process of healing upon which the medical texts rest. But such explorations can be daunting, carry risks of missteps, and require much care. The next chapter thus begins by unpacking a foundational metaphor that (perhaps like the mandrake discussed in Chapter 5) remains as vibrantly generative as it is deeply fraught: the very concept of hybridity itself.

Notes

1 Lines 10b–12, Riddle 3 in Craig Williamson (ed.), *The Old English Riddles of the 'Exeter Book'* (Chapel Hill, NC: University of North Carolina Press, 1977); numbered as Riddle 5 in George Philip Krapp and Elliott Van Kirk Dobbie (eds), *The Exeter Book*, The Anglo-Saxon Poetic Records [ASPR], vol. 3 (New York: Columbia University Press, 1936. Translations are my own.

2 Throughout this book, I am expressly avoiding the term 'Anglo-Saxon', both because of its ultimately anachronistic implications and because of its now inextricable links to white supremacist agendas. For a thorough, cogent, and intensely personal examination of this deeply fraught term, see Donna Beth Ellard, *Anglo-Saxon(ist) Pasts, postSaxon Futures* (Santa Barbara, CA: Punctum Books, 2019), esp. pp. 16–60. See also Mary Rambaran-Olm's three-part discussion and resource list: 'History Bites: Resources on the Problematic term "Anglo-Saxon"', parts 1–3 (2020), https://mrambaranolm.medium.com/history-bites-resources-on-the-problematic-term-anglo-saxon-part-1-9320b6a09eb7. Accessed 7 July 2021.

3 The word choice is especially striking since the second component of the compound is unnecessary for the line's alliterative requirements.

4 So common has this sense of *hybrid* as a blend of in-person and virtual learning become that by November 2020 usages such as the following in the *New York Times* require no explanation whatsoever: '"I have NEVER been this exhausted", Sarah Gross, a veteran high

school English teacher in New Jersey who is doing hybrid teaching this Fall, said' Natasha Singer, 'Teaching in the Pandemic: "This is Not Sustainable"', *New York Times*, 30 November 2020.
5 The most recent edition of *The American Heritage Dictionary* (*AHD*) defines *syncretism* as the 'reconciliation or fusion of differing systems of belief' (sense 1) and *fusion* (in the metaphorical sense) as 'the merging of different elements' or 'a union resulting from fusing' (senses 3a and b). A *hybrid*, on the other hand, is defined in terms of that which is produced from such unions or mergings, 'the *offspring* of genetically dissimilar parents or stock', '*something* of mixed origin or composition' (s.v. *hybrid*, senses 1 and 2.a.; emphasis added).
6 Elaine Treharne, *Living Through Conquest: The Politics of Early English, 1020–1220*, Oxford Textual Perspectives (Oxford: Oxford University Press, 2012), p. 10.
7 Renée Trilling, *The Aesthetics of Nostalgia: Historical Representation in Old English Verse* (Toronto: University of Toronto Press, 2009), pp. 66–67.
8 Ibid., p. 67.
9 Ibid., p. 69. Homi Bhabha has described 'the hybrid object' as one that 'retains the actual semblance of the authoritative symbol but revalues its presence'. Through this process, culture 'can be transformed by the unpredictable and partial desire of hybridity'. *The Location of Culture* (London: Routledge, 1994), p. 164.
10 Harley 585, folio 160a–163b; Metrical Charm 2 in Dobbie, *Anglo-Saxon Minor Poems*. ASPR. vol. 6 (New York: Columbia University Press, 1942). Woden appears in line 32, and Christ at line 58.
11 See further Chapter 4.
12 Karen Louise Jolly, *Popular Religion in Late Saxon England: Elf Charms in Context* (Chapel Hill, NC: University of North Carolina Press, 1996), p. 12.
13 Nicole Guenther Discenza, *Inhabited Spaces: Anglo-Saxon Constructions of Place* (Toronto: University of Toronto Press, 2017), p. 93. That is, in Discenza's words, 'human and something else, or human less something', p. 93.
14 Hubert Jan de Vriend (ed.), *The Old English Herbarium and Medicina de Quadrupedibus* (Oxford: Oxford University Press, 1984), entry 132, p. 170.
15 Daniel Donoghue, *How the Anglo-Saxons Read Their Poems* (Philadelphia, PA: University of Pennsylvania Press, 2018), p. 82.
16 Dana Oswald, *Monsters, Gender and Sexuality in Medieval English Literature* (Woodbridge: D. S. Brewer, 2010), p. 113.

17 Alf Siewers, *Strange Beauty: Ecocritical Approaches to Early Medieval Landscape* (New York: Palgrave, 2009), p. 142.
18 Maring, *Signs*, p. 156.
19 This remedy appears twice, in the margins of MS 41 CCCC (206) and in Harley 585 (folio 180b–181a). The linguistic hybrid 'reducað' appears only in the Harley manuscript (Metrical Charm 5 in Dobbie, *Anglo-Saxon Minor Poems*). For a full comparison of these two metrical charms in the context of oral tradition, see Lea Olsan, 'The Inscription of Charms in Anglo-Saxon Manuscripts', *Oral Tradition*, 14 (1999), 401–419.
20 Brian Attebery, for instance, parenthetically dismisses the authenticity of a Swedish gravesite containing both Christian crosses and hammers of Thor, quipping that 'someone was hedging his bets', *Stories about Stories: Fantasy and the Remaking of Myth* (Oxford: Oxford University Press, 2014), p. 23. Similarly, in discussing new converts to Christianity who continued to trace their ancestry back to Woden, Toni Mount asserts that 'the new converts must have hedged their bets', *Everyday Life in Medieval London: From the Anglo-Saxons to the Tudors* (Gloucestershire: Amberley Publishing, 2014), p. 32. And in noting the persistence of pre-Christian burial practice into the Christian era, Logan Thompson states that 'pagan warriors, who had only recently converted to Christianity, may have considered it advisable to hedge their bets to guarantee their salvation', *Ancient Weapons in Britain* (Barnsley: Pen and Sword Military, 2005), p. 119.
21 Jolly, *Popular*, p. 18.
22 Ibid. Emily Kesling's excellent work further demonstrates the diversity of the medical corpus, noting that each of the medical texts produced in early medieval England 'reflects the ideas and approaches of different compilers and the different intellectual milieux where they were created', *Medical Texts in Anglo-Saxon Literary Culture* (Woodbridge: D. S. Brewer, 2020), at pp. 6–7. Though her emphasis here is on the tradition's engagement with literary culture, she nonetheless supports an approach that is both/and rather than either/or: 'Rather than *simply* being the domain of history of medicine or folklore, these texts *also* belong to the wider tradition of Anglo-Saxon literary culture', p. 7 (emphasis added).
23 Michael Lapidge and Michael Herren (eds), *Aldhelm: The Prose Works* (Woodbridge: D. S. Brewer, 1979), pp. 42, 96.
24 See further Chapter 6 on John of Beverley's work with a boy unable to speak. Though the outcome of this miracle story should of course not be taken as evidence of typical life, the narrative implies that

the monastery would have been a logical place from which to seek medical help.
25 Book V.3: 'Multum insipienter et indocte fecistis in luna quarta flebotomando' ['You have acted foolishly and ignorantly to bleed her on the fourth day of the moon']. Bertram Colgrave and R. A. B. Mynors (eds), *Bede's* Ecclesiastical History, Oxford Medieval Texts (Oxford: Clarendon Press, 1969), p. 460.
26 Ibid., p. 448.
27 See also Edward Pettit (ed. and trans.), *Anglo-Saxon Remedies, Charms, and Prayers from British Library MS Harley 585: The Lacnunga*, 2 vols (Lewiston: Edwin Mellen Press, 2001).
28 Except where otherwise noted, quotations in the present study follow de Vriend's edition for the Cotton Vitellius C.iii and the Harley 6258B: *Old English Herbarium*.
29 As has been amply noted, the term 'charm' is far from unproblematic. See especially Ciaran Arthur's discussion, *'Charms', Liturgies, and Secret Rites in Early Medieval England* (Woodbridge: Boydell Press, 2018), pp. 8–17. I follow Leslie Arnovick here in applying the term specifically to reference 'a linguistic text representing the illocutionary and/or physical action of a ritual performance', *Written Reliquaries* (Philadelphia, PA: John Benjamins Publishing, 2006), p. 28.
30 MS CCCC 41, 350–353; Metrical Charm 11 in Dobbie, *Anglo-Saxon Minor Poems*. This poem is most frequently referred to as 'The Journey Charm', though it is untitled in the manuscript. In his 1909 edition, Felix Grendon supplied the title 'Siþgaldor' and translated it as 'Journey Spell', drawing from the poem's own reference to a 'sygegealdor', which Grendon translated as 'victory-charm', 'Anglo-Saxon Charms', *Journal of American Folklore*, 22 (1909), 105–237, at 177. In 1948, Godfrid Storms used the title 'Siþ Gealdor', or 'Journey Charm', *Anglo-Saxon Magic* (New York: Gordon Press, 1974. Orig. published 1948), p. 217; however, there is no title or header in the manuscript, and, since any title is an interpretation and this particular title risks undermining the poem's inherent hybridity with the label 'charm', I am opting instead to use the opening line as a working title.
31 Metrical Charm 4 in Dobbie, *Anglo-Saxon Minor Poems*.
32 Because different editors and translators number the riddles differently, I am following Jennifer Neville's new scheme for riddle names. Her titles 'derive from memorable words within the texts themselves, not from proposed solutions', 'A Modest Proposal: Titles for the *Exeter Book* Riddles', *Medium Ævum*, 88.1 (2019), pp. 116–123. This system is effectively employed in Jennifer Neville and Megan Cavell's edited

collection *Riddles at Work in the Early Medieval Tradition: Words, Ideas, Interactions* (Manchester: Manchester University Press, 2020). For ease of reference, I am also noting the numbering of the ASPR edition (Krapp and Dobbie (eds), *The Exeter Book*), which tends to be the default numbering used in current scholarship. *Anhaga*, 'Lone dweller', appears as Riddle 3 in Williamson's edition and as Riddle 5 in ASPR.

33 Cf. Bosworth and Toller, s.v. *wiþ*, Joseph Bosworth, *An Anglo-Saxon Dictionary*, ed. and enlarged T. Northcote Toller (Oxford: Oxford University Press, 1898; suppl. 1921). Online edition available at www.bosworthtoller.com. Accessed 1 July 2021. On the multivalence of *wið* across the body of charm texts (in particular with regard to a remedy for swarming bees, see further Lori Ann Garner and Kayla M. Miller, '"A Swarm in July": Beekeeping Perspectives on the Old English *Wið Ymbe* Charm', *Oral Tradition*, 26.2 (2012), 355–376, at 361–362.

1

With hope and humility: hybridity as theoretical framework

hybrid:

the offspring of two animals or plants of different species....

transferred and *figurative*. anything derived from heterogeneous sources, or composed of different or incongruous elements....

1788 J. LEE *Introd. Bot.* (ed. 4) Gloss. *Hybrida*, a Bastard, a monstrous Production of two Plants of different Species.

1837 T. RIVERS *Rose Amateur's Guide* I. 20 Perhaps no plant presents such a mass of beauty as a finely grown hybrid China rose in full bloom.

1959 E. M. GRABBE et al. *Handbk. Automation, Computation, & Control* II. xxix. 4 The purpose of the hybrid system ... is to combine the advantages noted above for each of the two types of conventional computer....

(*Oxford English Dictionary*)

Two undeniable facts thwart any simple application of hybridity as it relates to early medieval texts. First, *hybridity* in its modern sense existed as neither a term nor a formal practice in early medieval England, making any discussion of Old English hybridity, at least at some level, inherently anachronistic. Second, as long as it has existed in the English language (which was not until the seventeenth century), the term *hybrid* has been a complicated and fraught one, with numerous—sometimes even diametrically opposed—meanings. While these encumbrances necessitate that the concept, as both metaphor and biological reality, be approached and applied with tremendous care, hybridity remains a useful analytical construct, not in spite of, but because of the term's inherent contradictions, its intrinsic tensions, and even its semantic messiness. As I hope to show, in pre-modern medicine and in Old English medical texts in particular, it is in the spaces of conflict and uncertainty that healing power is most often created and invoked. Thus, in this chapter and those that follow, I want to apply pressure to this common metaphor, to push it to its limits and deeply think through how the concept of hybridity—in particular as applied to early medieval healing—can mean much more than simply the bringing together of any two or more unlike parts. Before embracing the potential of hybridity for newness and healthy growth, it is crucial first to recognize and accept the burden of its inherent risks and limitations, most especially the potential of hybridity to subsume or even extinguish, an aspect often overlooked or ignored—in short, to acknowledge the capacity of hybridity to fail.

As part of this effort to interrogate and fine-tune *hybridity* as a theoretical lens, this chapter will first consider the inherent anachronism of medieval 'hybridity' and explore how this modern construct maps onto actual agricultural practices in early medieval England. Next, it will explore the term's complicated history and probe the biological realities of *hybridity*—searching in particular for parallels that keep us cognizant not only of the most frequently referenced *hybrid vigor* but also of such phenomena as *hybrid swamping*, *hybrid sterility*, or even *species extinction*. Far from a simple metaphor, hybridity defies any simplistic expectations and, in so doing, offers a path for understanding illness, disease, and ailment as sites of conquest, as physical and mental spaces where traditions, languages, and modes of thinking merge to effect powerful and compelling change, though not without risk.

Hybridity, crops, and ritual: unknown seed

Though the Latin writings of ancient agronomists include practical guides on soil amendment and plant grafting, surviving records lack confirmation that these were utilized or even available in early medieval England.[1] Indeed, intentional hybridization of plants or animals in any modern sense would have been unknown. That said, farming practice in early medieval England did clearly value diversification of crops and innovation. Debby Banham's extensive work on such practices has shown that early medieval crops 'will have contained a good deal of genetic diversity, possessing as a result more resilience to variations in climate, soils, and cultivation than modern specialized varieties'.[2] As a result, crops included 'a wider range of species and varieties' and 'must have looked a good deal less uniform than the ones we are used to today'.[3] In addition to this genetic diversity, farmers chose to grow crops with mixtures of cereals,[4] and the practice of putting diverse seeds in close proximity in an environment of open pollination increased the likelihood of natural plant hybridity. Thus, even though controlled hybridization is of course a relatively recent phenomenon, naturally occurring hybrids played an important role in the development of new plant species long before the modern era.[5]

This bioarchaeological evidence of crop diversification is corroborated in the text commonly titled *Æcerbot*, a bilingual field remedy found in MS Cotton Caligula A.vii (ff. 176r–178r) and typically dated to the eleventh century. The remedy records verse to be recited in both English and Latin as well as instructions for an all-day ritual requiring multiple participants. Not only is this text the single surviving copy of this particular ritual performance, but it is also the only agricultural remedy of its type, and it is unknown how commonly a ritual such as this might have actually been practiced. The text introduces itself as a *bot* or remedy 'þine æceras betan' ['to better your fields'], but one to be performed as a cure rather than pre-emptively. Though not appearing within one of the compendious medical volumes, it shares with the medical texts instructions to be followed in times of adversity, specifically when land 'nellaþ wel wexan' ['will not grow well']. Crucially, an essential part of the land's healing involves diversification.

The most notable line in this remedy from the perspective of hybridity is a somewhat cryptic line requiring that 'uncuþ sæd' ['unknown seed', l. 46] be plowed into the infertile ground as a supplement to 'namcuþre wyrte' ['plants known by name']. Lisa Moffett notes that 'agricultural traditions are not lightly changed as subsistence farmers cannot afford to take too many risks with unfamiliar crops'; however, experimentation with the unknown, the 'uncuþ', could be seen as the best course of action in times of crisis.[6] As Thomas Hill has noted, 'at least part of the new crop would be from a new strain of seed', thus giving farmers the chance 'of finding the right crop or the right strain of a given crop'.[7] Though in nature hybridization leads far more commonly to sterile hybrids than to new and viable species, the ritual introduction of new seed contributes to an environment where biological hybridity would at least be more likely to occur. And Verne Grant explains that the success of an 'interspecific hybrid' (such as the mixture of cereals required by this ritual) is 'closely correlated with the availability of open habitats', precisely such as that of the ploughed field of the *Æcerbot*.[8] But the possible hybridity of the *Æcerbot* ritual is not limited to the diversification of literal crops and fields, as the ritual also enacts and encourages religious and cultural intercrossings within the healing tradition more broadly. In its instructions, forms of *ælc* ['each' or 'every'] repeatedly reinforce the remedy's impulse toward diversification. The first portion of the ritual requires milk of *each* livestock ['*ælces* feos'], a portion of *each* kind of tree ['*ælces* treowcynnes'], and cuttings from *every* plant known by name ['*ælcre* namcuþre wyrte']. Then the diversity of harvest is ritualized one final time through *ælces* [*each*] near the field remedy's conclusion, when bread is to be baked from '*ælces* cynnes melo' ['from meal of *each* kind'].

Beyond these explicitly agricultural elements of the remedy, hybridity is embedded in other aspects of the text's language as well. Linguistically 'hybrid', the diglossic text is primarily in Old English but provides the most biblically based portion of the incantation in Latin, with inter-lexical glossing (Latin portions in italics):

Crescite, wexe, *et multiplicamini*, and gemænigfealda, *et replete*, and gefylle, *terre*, þas eorðan.

The complexity here is often missed, however. In modern English translations, it is common practice to provide the Latin in its original and translate only the Old English, presumably to better indicate the bilingual nature of the text through implying that the Old English is a fairly direct translation from Latin. Ciaran Arthur's translation follows common practice:

Crescite, grow, *et multiplicamini*, and multiply, *et replete*, and fill, *terram*, the earth.⁹

Most modern English translations similarly treat the Latin and Old English portions as essentially equivalent. But when extracted from the Latin, the Old English 'wexe ... and *gemænigfealda*' actually becomes something ever so slightly new: 'Grow ... and *make manifold*'. On one hand, the verb *manigfealdian* can certainly be rendered as 'to multiply', and *gemænigfealda* is a perfectly reasonable translation for the Latin *multiplicamini*. However, the more subtle connotations of the Old English *gemænigfealda* extend beyond mere multiplication of the same item and imply diversification. The Old English *manigfeald*, in its adjectival form, is defined as 'multifarious, of many kinds, various, consisting of many parts, complex'.¹⁰ The difference in meaning is, from one angle, negligible, but it is precisely such subtle, almost imperceptible changes that lead to new modes of existence, akin to new biological species. What at first glance might look like mere duplication might actually be a wholly new hybrid, created out of diversity. This tendency towards variation—not just multiplication—is a defining feature of the ritual in other aspects as well.¹¹

Additionally, just like most of the so-called 'metrical charms', the *Æcerbot* text is actually prosimetric, alternating prose instructions with verse incantations. In this way, even the manuscript in which the remedy appears evokes elements of hybridity. The Old English *Æcerbot* ritual was copied into the Cotton Caligula A.vii manuscript after the earlier Old Saxon *Heliand*, the two texts together forming a multi-language, multi-genre compilation that Ciaran Arthur has convincingly argued 'emphasize[s] God's power to heal, resurrect and transform the human and spiritual world through formulaic words of power'.¹² This healing takes a distinctly hybrid form in the *Æcerbot*, whose rituals are born from a merging of boundary-marking actions familiar from Christian Rogationtide processions with fertility rituals that predate Christianity.¹³ As Johanna Kramer notes, 'while help is expected to come from God, the earth is nonetheless treated as an entity that can be implored independently'.¹⁴ Most notably, 'eorþan modor' ['earth mother'] occurs just a few lines below references to 'Criste, 7 sancta Marian 7 þære halgan rode' ['Christ, and St. Mary, and the holy spirit']. Here the healing hybridity serves to mediate, as 'divine power is channeled through the practitioners and into the soil itself, whose efficacious role is assumed to lead to the land's healing'.[15] In all these ways and more, this otherwise unprecedented remedy beautifully ritualizes the diversification of crops and demonstrates the power of the poetic tradition to promote agricultural diversification and, ultimately, natural hybridity, and these connections in the unique *Æcerbot* point towards several layers of hybridity inherent in the healing tradition more broadly. The impulse toward hybridization when confronted with adversity runs deep, and, as a cultural metaphor, hybridity is thus an especially powerful one in the context of remedies and medical texts.

Hybridity as metaphor in Old English studies

The use of hybridity as a metaphor for cross-cultural and multigeneric literature is of course not new, and hybridity has long proven a compelling model for understanding Old English poetry and culture in particular, but I want to isolate here a few applications that have been specifically useful in the analysis of performative texts such as early medieval remedies. While most if not all Old English texts produced in early medieval England's era of emerging literacy can be productively examined within what can be understood as the 'oral-literate nexus' of early medieval England,[16] the Old English medical texts, which offer frequent and explicit instructions that incantations, like those of the *Æcerbot*, be spoken (*cweðan*) or sung (*singan*), require us to be especially sensitive to oral/performative contexts.[17] Attesting to the dual roles of orality and literacy within this deeply hybrid mode of signification, a number of remedies require texts to be inscribed on objects, and, whether through writing or through speech, 'the performer, the beneficiary, and the community of hearers or believers affirm the power of words to create a new, hoped for reality among them'.[18] This collective and collaborative aspect of Old English remedies thus reflects a healing practice deriving its power precisely from the nexus of oral/aural, written/visual, and poetic/practical modes of meaning.

The alignment of ritual within the oral poetics of such texts as the *Æcerbot* allows a space for meaningful links between Christian liturgy and the pragmatics of daily life, another important aspect of early medieval medical lore. Heather Maring's study of 'hybrid poetics' offers the fullest exploration to date of the ways by which traditional language can activate liturgical contexts within ritual performance. As but one example, Maring analyzes images of light in Lyric VIII of *Christ*, especially the 'soðfæsta sunna leoma, / torht ofer tunglas' ['truth-fast radiance of the sun, bright beyond the stars']. More than a mere metaphorical representation of the poem's theological understanding of God—though it is certainly this, too—the lines 'could parallel the experience of liturgical participants who intoned or listened to the Advent antiphon after sunset'.[19] Through what Maring terms the tradition's 'ritual poetics', 'the image of souls in the dark awaiting Christ's light chimes with the sensual experience of those in the dark awaiting day'.[20] In a similar way, numerous Old English remedies such as the *Æcerbot* provide a locus where ritual experience and poetic expression draw healing energy from one another.

Consequently, rituals and incantations outlined in such medical texts as *Æcerbot* evoke distinctly ritualized space, a 'performance arena', to use John Foley's term.[21] As will be discussed in the chapters that follow, some remedies extend beyond localized spaces and even imply a full cosmology, in which ailments enter into—or healing power is received from—other-worldly spaces. At other times the medical texts portray the body itself in terms of a physical landscape, a contested space between healer and ailment, a body/battlefield hybrid.[22] And medicinal herbs, of course, form part of the natural landscape even as they are absorbed into the fabric of human life, resulting in another hybrid identity of sorts. As Andrew Scheil has observed, 'space is not exclusively an objective reality; rather what we define as "space" is the result of an overdetermined process, an interaction among bodies and things and the multiple, often contradictory understandings that inform a variety of constitutive elements'.[23] As such, 'place' and 'space' 'are thus hybrid propositions, words that designate that which emerges into human understanding out of an interaction among factors such as human perception, physical environment, representational practices, and historical/ideological forces'.[24] In Old English remedies, power is negotiated not only in literal fields but even on physical bodies. Though not all Old English remedies are intended for human physical ailments—with some prescribed for such adversities as swarming bees, stolen cattle, or hail storms—it would be remiss not to include bodily hybridity in this discussion of hybrid healing. Hybrid bodies and spaces within the wider corpus of Old English writing reveal much about the deeply complex attitudes toward the 'Other' in early medieval England, entities not easily discounted as merely fantastical or monstrous. *Wonders of the East*, for instance, includes numerous illustrations of undeniably hybrid creatures imagined to inhabit such regions as Babylon, Persia, and Egypt, including the *donestre* (a lion-human hybrid) appearing on f. 103v. As Discenza explains, such images visually demonstrate that those producing the manuscript 'found not only distance and danger in faraway peoples but also elements of commonality: monsters fascinate and frighten because they are uncanny, containing elements of both the familiar and the unfamiliar at once'.[25] Descriptions of hybrid creatures, therefore—both in terms of their bodies and the geographies they inhabit—can help forge important cultural connections even as they call attention to departures from the more usual experiences of their intended audiences.

Illness in Old English texts can be interpreted in a similar way, the source of many physical ailments in the underlying medical philosophy understood as beings from other realms, creatures that while distinctly 'other' nonetheless share human commonalities and, in some instances, even participate in human battles. For instance, the remedies known collectively as 'elf charms', which figure prominently in the *Leechbooks* and the *Lacnunga*, operate on the premise that ailments without otherwise known causes result from attacks of 'invisible or hard-to-see creatures who shot their victims with some kind of arrow or spear',[26] a premise exemplified by a remedy in the *Lacnunga* (Harley 585) that offers an herbal recipe and verbal incantation for an ailment affecting the fingernails and eyes and causing the victim to look downward, one that is ascribed to elves as 'wæterælfadle', 'water-elf disease'.[27] Not all remedies are as explicit in that attribution of blame, but the underlying principle across the tradition is important to keep in mind nonetheless: ailments and their remedies operate within a world of heroic battle involving powerful hybrid beings, rendered simultaneously familiar and monstrous, working in potent hybrid spaces.[28]

Limitations and possibilities

Due to the shifting power dynamics inherent in almost any cultural exchange, the concept of hybridity as a literary metaphor is neither unproblematic nor unequivocally positive. In fact, the term itself remains both '[o]ne of the most widely employed and most disputed' in modern critical theory.[29] In a 2008 preface to a special issue devoted to 'Hybrid Forms and Cultural Anxiety', U. C. Knoepflmacher reminds us that our current predisposition to see *hybridity* mainly for its admirable possibilities is a relatively recent phenomenon: 'Since the word "hybrid" so frequently appears in our most positive accounts of new automobiles, new mixed-media forms, and new technological and biological improvements, it seems well worth remembering that earlier cultures were likely to be distrustful, and even fearful, of "mongrel" mixtures they saw as dangerous deformations'.[30] Indeed, the horrendous implications of contaminated purity in earlier mindsets are obvious, but categorically positive attitudes toward hybrid forms are also quite dangerous. Ashcroft, Griffiths, and Tiffin remind us that the term *hybridity* in much scholarship involves 'negating and neglecting the imbalance and inequality of the power relations it references'; as a result, we risk 'replicating assimilationist policies by masking or "whitewashing" cultural differences'.[31]

While it is often tempting to think of hybridity as equivalent to inclusivity, one need look no further than the Old English charms against cattle theft to recognize that such is far from the case. One feature shared among all extant metrical cattle theft charms is a reference to Christ on the cross, a detail that is especially important since in the early medieval tradition 'the cross has the power to reveal what has been illicitly hidden (as God had made known to St. Helen where the cross was buried)'.[32] However, each of these charms then goes on to imply a parallel between the cattle thieves and the Jewish people blamed for Christ's death: 'Jews hanged Christ, did to him the worst of deeds'. Variant spellings in the latter portion of the line within the manuscripts suggest oral transmission—of both the formula and the anti-Semitic thought it conveys—at some point in the process,[33] and Olsan notes that even the phrasing at the beginning of the line ('Iudeas crist ahengon') is actually a vernacularized version of a Latin formula, 'Iudei Christum crucifixerunt', itself a product of an earlier hybridization of Latin language and Christian content.[34] This anti-Semitic vilification is thus introduced into the Old English healing tradition via a hybridization whereby Latinate Christian views are cast in Old English verse.

Such examples also demonstrate that in our exploration of medical texts we would do well to think through the implications of concepts that entered early medieval discourse in already hybridized form.[35] An arguably 'hybrid' combination of elements might be passed from one culture to another whole cloth and could thus be understood as a simple borrowing. The anthropomorphized mandrake root that appears in the Old English *Herbarium*, for instance, had acquired its human/plant hybridity long before the *Herbarium* was translated into Old English. The hybridity in this new context, then, lies less in the dual identity of this creature than in the multiple (far more subtle) ways the mandrake entry itself was transformed through its translation from Latin into Old English and, as Chapter 5 argues, from Old English into early Middle English. In a similar vein, more than two decades ago the *Journal of American Folklore* devoted an entire special issue to the issue of 'Theorizing the Hybrid'. Here Brian Stross described such ongoing transformative processes as part of a 'hybridity cycle', noting that in both culture and biology 'there are no truly "pure" forms, completely homozygous (biologically) or completely homogeneous in composition (culturally), and perhaps never have been. Thus, everything is a "hybrid" of sorts'.[36] It is imperative that we keep this hybridity cycle in mind lest we fall into a dangerous trap of attributing qualities of purity to parent forms and thus privileging that which has come before—for instance, through impossible and deeply problematic quests for 'ur'-texts—or, worse, implicitly accepting overly simplistic evolutionary models that privilege the new 'hybrids' over 'lesser' parent forms.

In many essential ways, hybridity's biological basis—with all its risks and complex implications—makes the metaphor more, rather than less, apt for oral-connected texts produced in the Old English period, perhaps especially for texts connected in such a literal way to living, biological plants. Such a richly complex tradition as the Old English medical corpus deserves a metaphor that offers the multi-layered nuances that the texts themselves provide—and one that at the same time pushes us to treat these texts with caution. In pushing the hybridity metaphor to—and perhaps even beyond—what might sometimes seem reasonable, we can thus not only attain a deeper understanding of the interactions between the literal and associative meanings of the term, but also better appreciate the paradoxes that hybridity as a theoretical construct inevitably creates.

Hybridity as metaphor

Already aware of the rapid proliferation of meanings assigned to the word 'hybridity', Minton Warren published an article attempting to clarify usage as early as 1884. In 'On the Etymology of Hybrid (Lat. Hybrida)', he noted that 'the Romans understood under *hybrida*, strictly speaking, the progeny of a wild boar and a sow'.[37] Once adopted into English, the earliest attested usage in the seventeenth century likewise referred to a 'hog engendered between a wilde Boare and a tame Sow' (*OED*, s.v. *hybrid*). But as even a quick glance at today's *OED* entry shows, the word rapidly acquired negative metaphorical associations that could be applied to people, as in 'She's a wild-Irish borne! Sir, and a Hybride' (1631, B. Jonson *New Inne* ii. vi. 26).[38] In fact, it is not until the nineteenth century that we see the metaphor applied in more neutral contexts as 'anything derived from heterogeneous sources, or composed of different or incongruous elements' (*OED* sense 2.a). By 1860, Charles Darwin himself had used the term metaphorically in praising Asa Gray as 'a hybrid, a complex cross of lawyer, poet, naturalist and theologian'; however, he then immediately followed the comment up with a playful acknowledgment of the term's negative connotations: 'Was there ever such a monster seen before?'[39] Just as genetic hybridity is beginning to be fully understood, its potential 'monstrosity' is already being embraced.

Hybridity as theoretical framework 33

On the other hand, many of the more positive associations with hybridity are based on 'heterosis' or 'hybrid vigor', that is, the 'survival and performance superiority of a hybrid offspring over the average of both its genetically distinct parents'.[40] Hybrid vigor can be understood as the 'conceptual opposite' of inbreeding depression, where there is a 'lack of fitness' resulting from the breeding of closely related individuals,[41] and as a concept has been recognized in scientific investigations since 1876 when Charles Darwin described positive results from the cross-fertilization of plants: 'I raised close together two large beds of self-fertilised and crossed seedlings from the same plant of *Linaria vulgaris*. To my surprise, the crossed plants when fully grown were plainly taller and more vigorous than the self-fertilised ones'.[42] A little over thirty years later, the technique began to be applied more consciously in plant breeding through George Shull's work on corn. James Crow notes that Shull's 1908 paper, 'The Composition of a Field of Maize', 'marked the beginning of the exploitation of heterosis in plant breeding' and sees this new practice as 'surely one of genetics' greatest triumphs'.[43] The term 'heterosis' itself was then introduced a few years later in 1914, and the practice has been employed productively not only for the crossing of two types of plants but also for three-way crosses, four-way, or even more.[44]

As the preceding discussion suggests, hybrid vigor and heterosis are terms often employed interchangeably,[45] the terminology sometimes as difficult to pin down in science as in the study of literature and culture. One distinction sometimes made in biology between hybrid vigor and heterosis involves determination of intent, a challenging if not impossible task, whether in science or in art. Biologist Z. Jeffrey Chen explains that 'in some reports, the term heterosis is restricted to hybrid vigour in crops or crossbred organisms compared with their inbred parents, whereas hybrid vigour applies to natural populations'.[46] This distinction parallels Mikhail Bakhtin's categories of 'intentional' and 'unintentional' hybridization in the discourse of the novel,[47] a differentiation that also productively complicates our understanding of Old English hybrid poetics since very occasionally an Old English text does indeed announce itself as a kind of intentional hybrid. In *Cædmon's Hymn*, for instance, we see the intervention of an angel in Cædmon's dream, whereby he is told to sing of the creation via the traditional poetics of the feast hall. The intentionality here thus renders the hybridity more precisely, an instance comparable more to 'heterosis' than to 'hybrid vigour'. As in biology, however, where the terms are often used synonymously, such distinctions are not always clear. Far more common in the Old English corpus are instances of multiple influences without any context conveying intent or lack thereof. Is the juxtaposition of Christ and Woden in the 'Nine Herbs Charm' intentional or a largely unconscious development in a deeply multicultural world? Does the poem often referred to as 'The Journey Charm' intentionally merge Christian liturgy and Germanic warfare, or do the connections reflect a fundamental underlying mode of thinking? What is perhaps more important to bear in mind is that the biological or cultural hybrid produced—whether through the intervention of heterosis or by the natural process of hybrid vigour—is still an organic, living product in its own right, and the line between intervention and nature is a blurry one at best.

Even murkier than the matter of intent is the question of cause. A 2008 study led by Lanzhi Li reminds us that in the world of biology 'no consensus exists about the genetic basis underlying this very important phenomenon [i.e., hybrid vigor]',[48] even though over a century ago two very different hypotheses, dominance and overdominance, were proposed as explanations. In the dominance model, the benefits of heterosis are attributed to the 'canceling of deleterious or inferior recessive alleles contributed by one parent, by beneficial or superior dominant alleles contributed by the other parent'.[49] The overdominance model, on the other hand, asserts that the 'interactions between different alleles occur in the hybrid, leading to the increase in vigor'.[50] In short, is the perceived superiority the result of suppression of undesirable traits (dominance), or does the interaction itself create a 'synergistic effect on vigor' surpassing both parents (overdominance)?[51] Even in the seemingly objective sciences there is not always a single clear-cut answer. In 'Heterosis: Revisiting the Magic', Zachary Lippman and Dani Zamir state that 'hybrid vigor is determined by non-mutually exclusive mechanisms'; in biological hybrids, certain traits might be diminished due to dominance of others, but at the same time the new hybrid can also become strengthened through interactions of alleles.[52]

Such issues are not new to folklorists. Recognizing that new traditions in folklore frequently result from the dominance of colonization, Timothy Tangherlini stresses that our very notion of 'oral tradition' must be reconsidered within the context of 'colonialism, the postcolonial world, the impact of globalization, and the emergent hybridities that mark the traditions of diasporic populations'; he thus encourages scholars working with technologies of communication to 'explore the manner in which people use oral tradition to reshape their physical and social environments'.[53] Also, both the language used to describe the biological processes and the intriguingly indeterminate conclusions about their cause find striking parallels in the analysis of Old English texts. Returning once again to *Caedmon's Hymn* as a hybrid text, for instance, we see that the text in its extant form can be viewed in terms of both dominance of one tradition over another *and* the interaction of diverse traits. Renée Trilling identifies the tensions here especially succinctly: 'Hybridity thus disrupts Latin's dominance over the vernacular', and the vernacular poetry at the same time 'produces its own authority—so successfully that, in later colonial contexts, English Christianity will come to play the same role in the colonial period that Latin Christianity had in the early Middle Ages'.[54] The hybridity cycle thus continues simultaneously to reify and destabilize current power structures at every stage.

Additionally, in both biology and literature, hybridity operates differently in different contexts. The process of hybridization does not occur in the same ways or at the same rates for all plants. As but one well-studied example, 'the genetic basis or mechanism of heterosis of rice is different from that of maize'.[55] In similar fashion, the hybrid mechanisms at play in the Old English corpus arguably differ significantly depending on whether we are working with elegies or epics, riddles or remedies. Also, for biological hybrids that are 'planted in different environments, the type of gene action may be influenced by environmental effect';[56] some studies go so far as to suggest that adaptedness to environment is actually more important to hybrid success than 'vigor' achieved through genetics.[57] In culture and literature, the questions of environment and influence arguably become even more charged. How can we possibly separate the expertise of the poet in composing from the expertise of the audience in receiving when determining the success of a poetic 'hybrid' drawing power from diverse traditions?

And not only are questions of definition and influence parallel across the fields of biology and literature, but also assignations of value: what constitutes the superior function implied in the term 'vigor'? Any measure of 'vigor' is socially constructed, based on the needs and goals of the participants involved. The mule, for example, is frequently cited in biological discussions of hybridization, valued for traits that make it useful to humans;[58] thus the mule is a successful hybrid by one measure, yet it is typically infertile and so unsuccessful by another.[59] Interestingly, the now inexplicable 'Erce' portion of the *Æcerbot* may be the Old English literary equivalent of the mule. In this remedy, just after seeds are placed on the plough's body, but before the plough cuts into the earth, an incantation opening 'Erce, Erce, Erce, eorðan modor' ['Erce, Erce, Erce, earth's mother'] is required. Among numerous possibilities, it has been proposed that 'Erce' is a corruption of the Latin 'Ecce' ['Hearken'],[60] a verb form related to the Old Welsh *erchim* ['I bid/ask'],[61] the name of a fertility goddess,[62] and, most recently, the second-person subjunctive of the Irish verb *ercaid* ['is abundant, increases, flourishes'].[63] The line remains an enigma because it is unique within the corpus, and I would argue that various ways of reading might have been possible and meaningful even in the text's own time. What all of these interpretations have in common, however, is an understanding of the remedy's reliance upon multiple cultural traditions, a textual entity emerging from hybridity. This particular hybrid, however, seems not to have been reproduced—at least not in any writing that survived to the present day—but, like the mule, its diachronic 'failure' was countered by its success and significance within its own cultural moment as part of a ritual to improve the earth itself.

Of course, when the goal is in fact healthy offspring, the ideal situation for successful hybridization is one in which the parents are different enough to avoid inbreeding depression but similar enough to avoid problems resulting from too extreme a difference, such as hybrid sterility or failure to hybridize altogether. Though usually discussed through different terminology, this line of thinking is also clearly far from new to folklorists. In his still widely used textbook *The Dynamics of Folklore*, Barre Toelken describes the 'twin laws' of the folklore process. Variation, he says 'is not a random or a radical process. Balancing the dynamism of change in performance is the essentially conservative force of tradition itself. The weight of the familiar past continually exerts its subtle pressures on the bearers of these materials'.[64] Tradition bearers 'may institute change, either consciously or inadvertently', paralleling hybrid vigor and heterosis respectively, 'but they will do so chiefly within the framework of the familiar, acceptable, and culturally logical'.[65] Depending on the version, Little Red Riding Hood might take different foods in her basket and ultimately her grandmother might even live or die, but she will always walk through a forest, and she will never wear blue. Similarly, as we shall see throughout the following chapters, the Old English healing tradition retains core elements at the same time that individual remedies respond generatively to new adversities and contexts.

But as we apply the hybridity metaphor to verbal art, it is important to remember that while the benefits of successful hybridization are well-attested,[66] biological hybrid vigor is not always desirable and what is desirable varies depending on context. Attempts at a 'successful' hybrid always carry significant risk. Ever looming, for instance, is the danger of the hybrid's success resulting in the diminishment, even extinction, of the parent forms when new hybrids essentially compete with the native or original populations. In what is known as 'hybrid swarming', 'a population of interbreeding hybrid individuals [...] may affect the genetic integrity of parental populations by genetic introgression'.[67] A related phenomenon is hybrid 'swamping', in which 'population growth rates are reduced due to the wasteful production of maladaptive hybrids', which can in extreme cases 'drive rare taxa to extinction'.[68] Such 'hybrid swamping' has contributed, for example, to the decline of the Icterine warbler, which is being replaced by hybrids of Icterine and Melodious warblers in parts of Western Europe.[69] Additionally, we saw earlier that notions of space and place have figured prominently in discussions of cultural hybridity; in biology the relevant concept is that of 'hybrid zones', wherein 'hybrids occur in a specific area of contact between genetically distinct populations'.[70] In literary analogies, then, the biological issues surrounding *hybrid vigor* as weighed against the dangers of *hybrid swamping* and *hybrid swarms* within specific hybrid zones are easily relatable to the danger of healthy cross-cultural interactions devolving into cultural appropriation or even suppression in a given cultural context or geographical region. It goes without saying, for instance, that the Christian tradition that is hybridized with references to Woden in the 'Nine Herbs Charm' is the same tradition that ultimately rendered the Germanic pantheon extinct.

But there is also the danger of diminishment or extinction resulting from the hybrids themselves being unstable. In the verbal arts, this possibility raises significant questions. How does an originally Germanic remedy retain its integrity as it adapts to new Christian contexts? Or how does a remedy from the classical world survive translation into the vernacular? And how do oral incantations convey their rhetorical force on the manuscript page? Again, we can turn to biologists. One of the most intriguing aspects of biological hybridization involves how a delicate balance is attained so that a hybrid might thrive within challenging circumstances. Barbara McClintock's frequently cited article on genomic shock explains that there are 'shocks that a genome must face repeatedly, and for which it is prepared to respond in a programmed manner'.[71] For these repeated 'shocks', it stands to reason that 'some sensing mechanism must be present in this instance to alert the cell to imminent danger and to set in motion the orderly sequence of events that will mitigate this danger'.[72] The situation becomes more complicated, however, when the genome is confronted with 'challenges that the genome is unprepared to meet in an orderly, programmed manner'.[73] Such is the risk of hybridity.

In these cases, the 'types of response are not predictable' and McClintock's own work stemmed from a goal of 'appreciating how a genome may reorganize itself when faced with a difficulty for which it is unprepared' and how 'major restructuring of chromosome components may arise in a hybrid plant and continue to arise in its progeny sometimes over successive plant generations'.[74] Accordingly, her arguments emphasize the 'importance of stress in instigating genome modifications by mobilizing available cell mechanisms that can restructure genomes, and do so in quite different ways'.[75] And McClintock's ultimate conclusions on the subject are arguably just as relevant to literature and culture as to biology: 'stress, and the genome's reaction to it, may underlie many formations of new species'.[76] Scholars of medieval literature have often employed the concept of hybridity to describe new genres and forms that emerged from responses to subjugation and cultural trauma, a literary equivalent to 'genomic shock'. Tory Pearman's work on women and disability in medieval literature, for instance, explicitly evokes the instability implicit in the concept of 'hybridity', describing Margery Kempe's writing as 'hybrid' while making clear that 'this intermixture did not easily produce a stable "English identity"'.[77] Hybridity involves risk and vulnerability, but also the potential of empowerment. It is this unpredictability of responses to unforeseen challenges that makes hybridization such an apt and compelling metaphor for literature produced in moments of cultural and social change—especially that of the Old English period where increasing literacy engendered fascinating texts produced in the matrix of oral tradition and literate culture. As Stross has noted, the 'difference between the biological hybrid and the cultural hybrid is perhaps not as great as one might at first think. Even biological models are socially constructed after all'.[78]

Hybridity as healing

The chapters that follow show that the very challenges posed by the model of hybridity are precisely those aspects that make the construct a tremendously appropriate one for the study of Old English texts generally and of medical remedies in particular. When not romanticized and when understood as inherently contestatory, hybridity offers a space to 'embrac[e] the subversion and challenge of division and separation'.[79] As with the biological hybrids discussed above, in the Old English medical corpus, power often emerges from unlikely and sometimes seemingly random convergences, and processes of transformation—in this case, the transformations of healing—are often unprecedented and unpredictable. Despite the frequent formulaic promise in the remedies that 'bið he sona hal' ['he will soon be well'], the outcomes and even the paths taken toward healing are far from certain. The approaches and methodologies applied must therefore reflect this sometimes erratic variability.

Accordingly, the metaphor of hybridity can be useful in the context of early medieval healing precisely *because of* rather than in spite of the tensions it produces. Robert Young has noted the dual nature of hybridity, a metaphor 'invoked to imply contrafusion and disjunction (or even separate development) as well as fusion and assimilation'.[80] Building on this notion, Jeffrey Jerome Cohen has argued that 'hybridity in medieval Britain tended to mix both these senses. Never synthetic in the sense of homogenizing, hybridity is a fusion and a disjunction'.[81] This hybrid nature of hybridity itself is integral to the analyses that form the core of *Hybrid Healing*. Hybridity, Cohen argues, 'enticed identities to mutate into forms seemingly beyond the borders of the humanly possible, forms that in fact dwelled alarmingly close to home'.[82] 'Hybridity', he says, 'is so useful because it can never be an absolute category'.[83] As such, hybridity is a fitting construct for the multivocalic and multiform nature of early medieval oral-connected texts, texts that exhibit variation even as they become fixed in manuscripts as representatives of a dynamic, ever-changing tradition within an ongoing cycle of hybridity.

Additionally, as Deborah Kapchan and Pauline Turner Strong have shown while approaching the issue within folklore studies in particular, hybridity's limitations are precisely what invest it with force: 'Because of its ambiguity, the term *hybridity* is bothersome. It threatens to dissolve difference into a pool of homogenization. It is biological, yet resists definition. It is precisely its resistance that forces us to look closely. Under a microscope, the concept transforms before our very eyes'.[84] This ability to transform in living, dynamic ways is what separates hybridity from overlapping concepts.[85] As the following chapters will show, healing in early medieval England was very much understood as a spatial battle, and the site of ailment was in a very real sense a site of conquest. And if, as Kapchan and Strong have suggested, 'the power of hybrid forms can be measured by the threat that their transgressions evoke', in the inherently transgressive act of healing the hybridized remedies and herbs become weapons that are powerful indeed.[86]

Finally, it is important to acknowledge that much of the hybridity apparent in the Old English medical texts—whether through the joining of oral and literate, Christian and Germanic, or Latin and Old English influences—becomes more pronounced within expectations established by modern categories, which of course are not the same as those of early medieval England. But recognizing the interplay is nonetheless a first step to seeing emergent 'hybrid' forms in a holistic way. With these goals in mind, the next chapter thus explores the paradox of healing plants being portrayed as weapons of battle, a situation where the hybrid crossing of Christian theology with vernacular poetics—and also of the liturgical with the literal—leads to a hope for protection and safety that renders the risks of hybridity inherent in these texts ultimately worthwhile.

Notes

1 Jacqueline Fay, 'The Farmacy: Wild and Cultivated Plants in Early Medieval England', *ISLE: Interdisciplinary Studies in Literature and Environment* 28.1 (2021), 186–206, 193.
2 Debby Banham and Rosamond Faith, *Anglo-Saxon Farms and Farming* (Oxford: Oxford University Press, 2014), p. 21. (This particular chapter was authored primarily by Banham, as noted on p. 2.)
3 Ibid., p. 21.
4 Ibid., p. 36. Bioarchaeological evidence further attests to the diversification of cereal crops and related 'dramatic changes' across the ninth through twelfth centuries. Helena Hamerow et al., 'Feeding Anglo-Saxon England: The Bioarchaeology of an Agricultural Revolution', *Antiquity*, 93 (2019), 1–4, at 1.
5 Though the exact statistics are widely debated, somewhere between 'an estimated 30–70% of all flowering plant species have hybridization events in their phylogenetic histories', Jordana Neri et al., 'Natural Hybridization and Genetic and Morphological Variation Between Two Epiphytic Bromeliads', *Annals of Botany (AoB) Plants*, 10.1 (2018), 1c+.
6 Lisa Moffett, 'Food Plants on Archaeological Sites', in Helena Hamerow et al. (eds), *The Oxford Handbook of Anglo-Saxon Archaeology* (Oxford: Oxford University Press, 2011), pp. 346–360, at p. 350.
7 Thomas D. Hill, 'The "Æcerbot" Charm and its Christian User', *Anglo-Saxon England*, 6 (1977), 213–221, at 219.

8 Verne Grant, *Plant Speciation* (New York: Columbia University Press, 2nd edn, 1981), pp. 197, 201. Grant further notes that long before intentional hybridization was practiced through such processes as manual pollination, natural hybrids were a vital aspect of pre-modern agriculture, and that hybrid plants are not uncommon in descriptions of medieval herbals, p. 193.
9 Arthur, *'Charms'*, p. 89.
10 Bosworth and Toller, s.v. *manig-feald* (adj.).
11 See also Bruce A. Rosenberg, who notes the power of bringing together various traditions: 'All the magic one has ever heard of is used to bring the brown fields to life', p. 431, 'The Meaning of *Æcerbot*', *Journal of American Folklore*, 79 (1966), 428–436.
12 Ciaran Arthur, 'Ploughing through Cotton Caligula A. VII: Reading the Sacred Words of the "Heliand" and the "Æcerbot"', *Review of English Studies* 65 (2014), 1–17, at 5.
13 On parallels linking *Æcerbot* with Rogationtide practices, see Johanna Kramer, *Between Earth and Heaven: Liminality and the Ascension of Christ in Anglo-Saxon Literature* (Manchester: Manchester University Press, 2014), pp. 279–283. For further liturgical connections, see Karen Louise Jolly, 'Prayers from the Field: Practical Protection and Demonic Defense in Anglo-Saxon England', *Traditio*, 61 (2006), 95–147.
14 Ibid., p. 183.
15 Ibid.
16 See Mark C. Amodio, *Writing the Oral Tradition: Oral Poetics and Literate Culture in Medieval England* (Notre Dame, IN: University of Notre Dame Press, 2004), esp. pp. 1–32.
17 See Olsan on Old English charms as 'a definable oral genre', 'Inscription', p. 401.
18 Ibid., p. 401.
19 Maring, *Signs*, p. 146.
20 Ibid., p. 147.
21 Foley describes the concept as follows: 'In simplest terms, the *performance arena* designates the locus where the event of performance takes place, where words are invested with their special power'. Foley, *Singer*, p. 47.
22 See further Chapter 3.
23 Andrew P. Scheil, *The Footsteps of Israel: Understanding Jews in Anglo-Saxon England* (Ann Arbor, MI: University of Michigan Press, 2004), p. 198.
24 Ibid.
25 Discenza, *Inhabited*, p. 91.

Hybridity as theoretical framework   43

26 Jolly, *Popular*, p. 134.
27 For an in-depth treatment of the elf charms, see Alaric Hall, *Elves in Anglo-Saxon England: Matters of Belief, Health, Gender, and Identity* (Woodbridge: Boydell Press, 2007).
28 Cf. Asa Mittman's conception of Old English texts as exhibiting 'a theme of cultural permeability, of hybridity', *Maps and Monsters in Medieval England* (New York: Routledge, 2006), p. 13.
29 Bill Ashcroft, Gareth Griffiths, and Helen Tiffin, *Post-Colonial Studies: The Key Concepts* (London: Routledge, 2000), 135. Offering a working definition, Ashcroft et al. state that 'hybridity commonly refers to the creation of new *transcultural* forms within the contact zone produced by colonization' (135; emphasis original). In the case of Old English medical texts, I argue that the body itself becomes the 'contact zone'.
30 U. C. Knoepflmacher, 'Editor's Preface: Hybrid Forms and Cultural Anxiety', *Studies in English Literature: 1500–1900*, 48.4 (2008), 745–754, at 745. Lindy Brady's reservations about the term in her own work on the Welsh borderlands succinctly encapsulates some of the most pressing issues surrounding the concept and term: 'because the word "hybrid" was used to signify monstrosity—either literally or for racist purposes—in medieval (and modern) writings, I will not be using it here'. *Writing the Welsh Borderlands in Anglo-Saxon England* (Manchester: Manchester University Press, 2019), p. 11.
31 Ashcroft et al., *Post-Colonial*, p. 136. They note further, however, that there is nothing inherent 'in the idea of hybridity as such that suggests that mutuality negates the hierarchical nature of the imperial process or that it involves the idea of an equal exchange', p. 137. On past uses of hybridity as a theoretical concept to reinforce notions of racism, see Robert J. C. Young, *Colonial Desire: Hybridity in Theory, Culture and Race* (New York: Routledge, 1995). Young warns of the dangers, and cautions all to use the concept with much care and qualification.
32 Olsan, 'Inscription', p. 406.
33 'gedidon him dæda a wyrstan' (CCCC MS 41); 'dydon dæda a wyrrestan' (Harley 585).
34 Additional examples outside the two metrical charms appear in Latin in CCC 41 and in English in CCC MS 190. For text and translation, see Olsan, 'Inscription', Appendix 3b and Appendix 4, pp. 414–417.
35 Michael Drout has similarly urged scholars to avoid using the term *hybrid* 'to describe any entity that has characteristics taken from more than one source or tradition' and to 'note that *hybrids* come from the combination and intersection of existing entities *after* these have evolved', *Tradition and Influence in Anglo-Saxon Literature: An*

Evolutionary, Cognitivist Approach (London: Palgrave Macmillan, 2013), p. 256.
36 Brian Stross, 'The Hybrid Metaphor: From Biology to Culture', *Journal of American Folklore*, 112 (1999), 254–267, at 258.
37 Minton Warren, 'On the Etymology of Hybrid (Lat. Hybrida)', *The American Journal of Philology*, 5 (1884), 501–502, at 501.
38 The first application to plants, attested in 1788, was equally negative: 'a Bastard, a monstrous Production of two plants of different species' (J. Lee *Introd. Bot* (ed. 4) gloss., *Hybrida*).
39 Charles Darwin, *Life and Letters of Charles Darwin*, vol. 2, ed. Francis Darwin (London: John Murray, 1887), p. 127.
40 Vinay Kumar Baranwal et al., 'Heterosis: Emerging Ideas about Hybrid Vigour', *Journal of Experimental Botany*, 63.18 (2012), 6309–6314, at 6309.
41 R. Rieger, A. Michaelis, and M. M. Green, *A Glossary of Genetics and Cytogenetics: Classical and Molecular* (Springer Science and Business Media, 2013), p. 232.
42 Charles Darwin, *The Effects of Cross and Self Fertilisation in the Vegetable Kingdom* (London: John Murray, 1876), p. 9.
43 James F. Crow, '90 Years Ago: The Beginning of Hybrid Maize', *Genetics*, 148 (1998), 923–928, at 923. Shull also demonstrated that 'selfing' or inbred corn 'led to a reduction of overall growth vigor and yield'. Z. Jeffrey Chen, 'Molecular Mechanisms of Polyploidy and Hybrid Vigor', *Trans Plant Sci.*, 15.2 (2010), 57–71, at 58.
44 See, for instance, Crow, '90 Years Ago', p. 924. Research on maize shows the high potential of triple crosses. G. B. Saleh, D. Abdullah, and A. R. Anuar, 'Performance, Heterosis and Heritability in Selected Tropical Maize Single, Double and Three-Way Cross Hybrids', *Journal of Agricultural Science*, 138 (2002), 21–28, at 21. On naturally occurring three-way cross hybrids, see Zdenek Kaplan and Judith Fehrer, 'Molecular Evidence for a Natural Primary Triple Hybrid in Plants Revealed from Direct Sequencing', *Annals of Botany*, 99 (2007), 1213–1222.
45 See, for example, Rieger, Michaelis, and Green, which in place of a definition for 'hybrid vigor', simply redirects: '→ heterosis', *Glossary*, p. 228. In turn, the entry for 'heterosis' indicates the two terms are indeed synonymous: '= hybrid vigor', p. 219. See also Birchler, Yao, and Chudalayandi's discussion of 'hybrid vigor, or heterosis' as 'the increase in stature, biomass, and fertility that characterizes the progeny of crosses between diverse parents such that the F1 is superior to the better of the two parents', 'Unraveling the Genetic Basis of Hybrid

Vigor', *Proceedings of the National Academy of Sciences in the United States of America [PNAS]*, 103.35 (2006), 12957–12958, at 12957.
46 Chen, 'Molecular', p. 471.
47 Bakhtin defines hybridization as 'a mixture of two social languages within the limits of a single utterance, an encounter, within the arena of an utterance, between two different linguistic consciousnesses, separated from one another by an epoch, by social differentiation or by some other factor'. M. M. Bakhtin, *The Dialogic Imagination: Four Essays*, ed. Michael Holquist, trans. Caryl Emerson and Michael Holquist (Austin, TX: University of Texas Press, 1982), p. 358. For Bakhtin, a defining characteristic of a literary hybrid is its living nature, and his distinction in part lies in the awareness that arguably all living languages are fundamentally hybrid: 'in essence, any *living* utterance in a *living* language is to one or another extent a hybrid', 361 (emphasis original). The intentional hybrid that he posits as integral to the novel's development as a genre implies '*an artistically organized system*', with the specific goal of 'illuminat[ing] one language by means of another', p. 361.
48 Lanzhi Li et al., 'Dominance, Overdominance and Epistasis Condition the Heterosis in Two Heterotic Rice Hybrids', *Genetics*, 180.3 (2008), 1725–1742, at 1725. Similarly, as Chen has noted in connection with maize in particular, 'the molecular bases for this phenomenon remain elusive', Chen, 'Molecular', p. 471.
49 Ibid.
50 James Birchler et al., 'Heterosis', *The Plant Cell*, 22 (2010), 2105–2112, at 2105.
51 Zachary Lippman and Dani Zamir, 'Heterosis: Revisiting the Magic', *Trends in Genetics*, 23.2 (2006), 60–66, at 60.
52 Ibid., p. 60.
53 Timothy R. Tangherlini, '"Oral Tradition" in a Technologically Advanced World', *Oral Tradition*, 18 (2003), 136–138, at 137. In a discussion of more modern technologies, Stross applies the notion to a 'hybrid communicative format, birthed into cyberspace from parent forms of written and spoken communication'. Stross, 'The Hybrid Metaphor', p. 262.
54 Trilling, *Aesthetics*, pp. 67–68.
55 Li et al., 'Dominance', p. 1741.
56 Ibid., 1740.
57 A. Forrest Troyer's discussion of corn and mules, for example, argues that 'adaptedness determines superiority over and above heterosis'. 'Adaptedness and Heterosis in Corn and Mule Hybrids', *Crop Sci.*, 46 (2006), 528–543, at 528.

58 The *Encyclopedia of Environmental Science*, for instance, includes the mule in its entry on 'hybrid', noting that the mule 'is generally stronger and better suited for use as a pack animal or for farmwork than either a horse or a donkey'. John F. Mongillo and Linda Zierdt-Warshaw, *Encyclopedia of Environmental Science* (Rochester, NY: University of Rochester Press, 2000), p. 190.

59 On possible cognitive function in mules, in addition to physical attributes resulting from hybridity, see Leanne Proops, Faith Burden, and Britta Osthaus. 'Mule Cognition: A Case of Hybrid Vigour?', *Animal Cognition*, 12 (2009), 75–84.

60 John D. Niles, 'The Æcerbot Ritual in Context', in John D. Niles (ed.) *Old English Literature in Context* (Cambridge: D. S. Brewer, 1980), 44–56, at p. 55.

61 Audrey Duckert, 'Erce and Other Possibly Keltic Elements in the Old English Charm for Unfruitful Land', *Names*, 20.2 (1972), 83–90, at 86.

62 Dobbie, *The Anglo-Saxon Minor Poems*, p. 208.

63 Caroline Batten and Mark Williams, '*Erce* in the Old English *Æcerbot* Charm: An Irish Solution', *Notes and Queries*, 67.2 (2020), 168–172, at 170.

64 Barre Toelken, *The Dynamics of Folklore* (Logan, UT: Utah State University Press, 1996), p. 34.

65 Ibid., p. 34. For variation within Old English remedies across manuscripts, see Chapter 5. See also John Foley's discussion of 'variation within limits', *How to Read an Oral Poem*, pp. 18, 48 *et passim*.

66 In addition to the many previous studies already cited, see also Matthew J. Hegarty and Simon J. Hiscock, who draw attention to a body of molecular-based studies demonstrating ways 'hybridization can promote adaptive evolution and speciation'. 'Hybrid Speciation in Plants: New Insights from Molecular Studies', *New Phytologist*, 165.2 (2004), 411–423, at 411.

67 P. H. van Tienderen, 'Hybridization in Nature: Lessons for the Introgression of Transgenes into Wild Relatives', in Hans C. M. den Nijs, Detlef Bartsch, and Jeremy Sweet (eds), *Introgression from Genetically Modified Plants into Wild Relatives* (Centre for Agriculture and Bioscience International [CABI] Publishing, 2004), 7–26, at 11.

68 Marco Todesco et al., 'Hybridization and Extinction', *Evolutionary Applications*, 9 (2016), 892–908, at 892.

69 For full details of this phenomenon, see Bruno Faivre et al., 'Morphological Variation and the Recent Evolution of Wing Length in the Icterine Warbler: A Case of Unidirectional Introgression?', *Journal of Avian Biology*, 30.2 (1999), 152–158, esp. p. 153.

70 van Tienderen, 'Hybridization', p. 11.
71 Barbara McClintock, 'The Significance of Responses of the Genome to Challenge', *Science*, 226 (1984), 792–801, at 792.
72 Ibid., p. 792.
73 Ibid.
74 Ibid., p. 799.
75 Ibid., p. 800.
76 Ibid.
77 Tory Pearman, *Women and Disability in Medieval Literature* (New York: Palgrave Macmillan, 2010), p. 173.
78 Stross, 'Hybrid', p. 255.
79 Ashcroft et al., *Post-Colonial*, 138.
80 Young, *Colonial*, p. 16.
81 Jeffrey Jerome Cohen, *Hybridity, Identity, and Monstrosity in Medieval Britain: On Difficult Middles* (New York: Palgrave Macmillan, 2006), p. 2.
82 Ibid., p. 3.
83 Ibid., p. 5.
84 Deborah A. Kapchan and Pauline Turner Strong, 'Theorizing the Hybrid', *Journal of American Folklore*, 112 (1999), 239–253, at 240.
85 Hybridity conveys a dynamism that syncretism cannot: 'hybridity is not simply syncretism renamed but a metaphor that encompasses a broader range of cultural mixtures'. Ibid., p. 248.
86 Ibid., p. 243.

2

Of swords and status: hybridity of metaphor in *Ic me on þisse gyrde beluce*

> Gyf hwylc man hyne begyrdeþ mid þysse wyrte 7 hy on wege mid him bereþ, he bið gescylded....
>
> [If any man encircles himself with this plant, and bears it on the way with him, he is shielded....]
>
> (Old English *Herbarium*, Cotton Vitellius C.iii, f. 46v)

Evincing traits of multiple genres, cultural traditions, and modes of meaning, a 42-line Old English poem inscribed in CCCC MS 41—not in a medical text but in the margins of Bede's Old English *History*—defies categorization in ways that make it a particularly apt focus for our first exploration of hybrid healing. The poem opens with a much-debated ritual whereby the speaker is described as enclosed with a *gyrde*, which can be defined as 'shoot or branch', 'stick or pole', 'rod or staff', and is sometimes even read as *gyrdel*, 'belt, girdle'.[1] Next follows a catalog of adversities against which the ritual presumably protects, ranging from pain ('wið þane sara s(t)ice', ['against the sore pain']) to more general trials ('wið eal þæt lað þe into land fare' ['against all evil that goes across the land']). The text then proceeds to call upon various biblical figures, such as Abraham, Moses, Eve, Sarah, Mary, Peter, and Paul, before metaphorically invoking the four gospel writers as protective military gear, and concluding with a final plea for mercy, friendship, and virtue during travel through this life. Though it is most frequently labeled a 'charm', the connection of this text to the healing charms is, as we shall see, far from straightforward. Even in referencing itself as a *syge gealdor*, the poem is positioned as a sort of heroic/healing hybrid, with *syge* meaning 'victory', especially in battle, and *gealdor* potentially denoting a range of verbal arts from 'poem' and 'song' to 'incantation', 'charm', or 'spell'.² The poem has been variously classified as not only a charm but also a 'prayer',³ a 'lorica', and, perhaps most responsibly, simply a 'formula'.⁴ With all these potentially contradictory possibilities in mind, I therefore reference this enigmatic poem here simply by its first half-line, *Ic me on þisse gyrde beluce*, because any title or previously proposed shorthand risks forcing this emphatically multivalent poem into a generic box and thus denies the very hybridity it so adamantly embraces and depends upon for its meaning.

What I propose here is a new reading of this poem that acknowledges its diverse influences alongside its solid grounding in the Old English medical tradition, a mode in which oral traditional contexts of heroic poetry regularly engaged with Christian contexts of healing practice to produce numerous texts that were generically and culturally hybrid in nature. To this end, the present chapter first sets the stage by examining the period's inherited traditions linking healing and mythic lore through a case-study analysis of a single entry in the Old English *Herbarium*, that of *Achillea millefolium*, or, in Old English, *gearwe*, yarrow. This example will then lead us to explore the signification patterns of heroic imagery—specifically battle gear—across the major Old English medical compilations more broadly, where weapons function diversely as medical tools, as ritual objects, and as descriptive markers in plant names (such as *sperewyrt*). Finally, attention is then turned back to *Ic me on þisse gyrde beluce* as we bring all of these insights from the medical texts, traditional poetry, and the archaeological record to bear simultaneously on this hybrid poem, with important implications not only for its literary interpretation but also for its editing and translation.

Achillea millefolium: Heroic healing

The entry for yarrow (XC; f. 46r-47r) in the Old English *Herbarium* offers an especially compact example of the healing hybridity seen throughout this and subsequent chapters, as epic warfare, traditional narrative, and ritual healing merge powerfully in a single early medieval medical text. Yarrow's Latinate species name

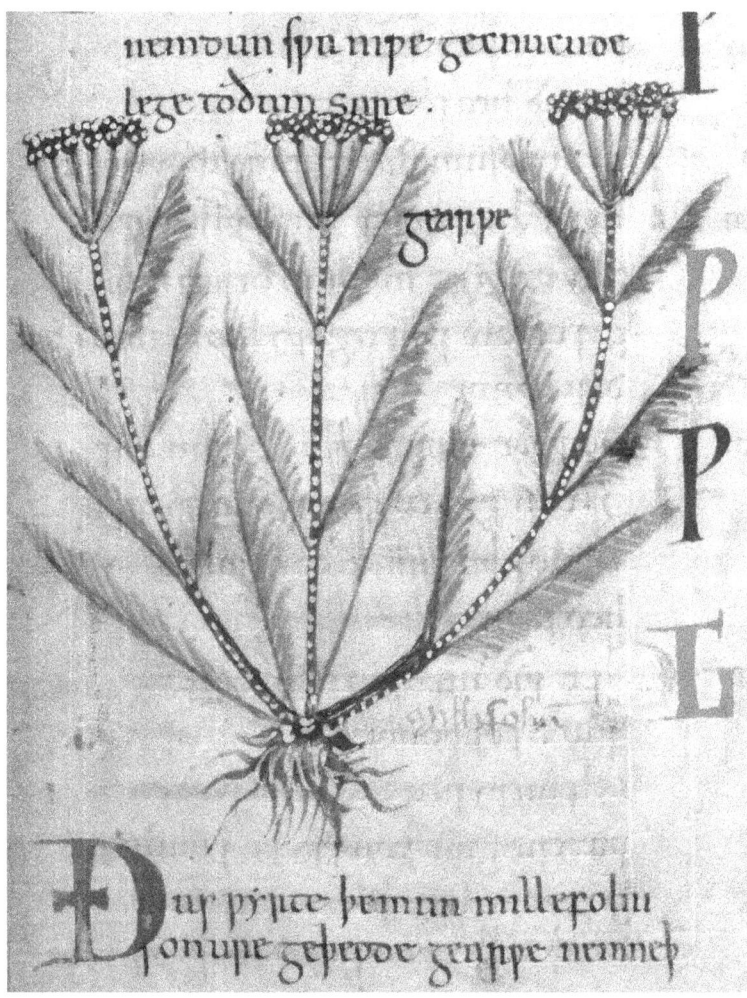

Figure 2.1 *Herbarium* entry for yarrow, *millefolium*, British Library MS Cotton Vitellius C.iii, f. 46r.

millefolium of course serves to help identify the plant by its many feathery leaves, and this feature is illustrated prominently in the MS Cotton Vitellius C.iii.

However, the entry itself in the *Herbarium* opens with an intriguing etiological explanation of the herb's fuller Latin nomenclature,

Achillea millefolium, linking the herb's curative powers explicitly with a narrative involving classical mythology's Achilles:

> Ðas wyrte þe man [millefolium] 7 on ure geþeode gearwe nemneþ, ys sæd þæt Achilles se ealdorman hy findan scolde, 7 he mid þysse sylfan wyrte gehælde þa þe mid iserne geslegene 7 gewundude wæran. Eac heo of sumum mannum for þy genemned ys achylleos, mid þære wyrte ys sæd þæt he eac sumne man gehælan sceolde þam wæs Thelephon nama.
>
> [About these plants that one calls *millefolium* and in our language *yarrow*, it is said that Achilles the ruler had to find it, and with this same plant he healed those who were slain and wounded by iron. Also, because of this, it is called by some *achylleos*; it is said that with this herb he also was able to heal a certain man who was named Telephon.][5]

Achilles clearly functions here as both healer and hero, and this brief but insightful narrative connects with a longstanding tradition, as attested in an entry on the same plant in Pliny's much earlier *Natural History*, from which the Old English medical texts may themselves have been drawing, whether through oral tradition, literate culture, or, most likely, a combination of both:[6]

> Invenit et Achilles discipulus Chironis qua volneribus mederetur. quae ob id achilleos vocatur. hac sanasse Telephum dicitur.
>
> [Achilles too, the pupil of Chiron, discovered a plant to heal wounds, which is therefore called achilleos, and by it he is said to have cured Telephus.] (Book 2 5.xix)[7]

However such connections evolved, even at a quick glance it is quite easy to see how this Old English entry for yarrow operates at the richly generative interface of traditional folklore, classical learning, and herbal medicine. Empowered as it was through a diversity of traditions and modes, this healing hybrid was able to assist with identification of herbs, with transmission of medical knowledge, and—most importantly—with appropriate use and application. In rather subtle ways, the entry's description of the plant's mythic connections would have served quite practical functions: the classical story of Achilles would doubtless have mnemonically facilitated oral transmission, and the narration of Achilles' use of the herb on the battlefield would offer memorable instruction regarding the plant's anti-inflammatory and astringent properties, metonymically associating the herb's name with its specific curative abilities in healing wounds and cuts.[8] Indeed, current ethnobotanic research demonstrates just how powerful the coalescence of oral and written influences has long been—and continues to be—in spreading knowledge about the healing properties of various herbs, including our present example of yarrow. Wendy Applequist and Daniel Moerman, for instance, have shown that yarrow 'is one of the oldest known botanicals used by humans', 'whose use is independently adopted and retained by multiple cultures',[9] and they attribute the spread of the herb's usage to both classical literary texts *and* to oral tradition, noting that the 'oldest surviving texts to record the use of yarrow in the European classical medical tradition are by Pliny the Elder and Dioscorides, both during the first century C.E.', but that 'as for most botanicals, folk use in an oral tradition may have long preceded the plant's appearance in scholarly medicine'.[10] Accordingly, we must accept that it is not an either/or proposition when we seek to understand such texts produced at this intersection of oral tradition and literate culture. Far from an isolated phenomenon, this seemingly insignificant entry in the Old English *Herbarium* reflects much larger patterns, attesting to the healing tradition's essentially hybrid nature as it operates along the intersecting axes of oral/literate, ancient/medieval, and Latinate/vernacular.[11]

Analogues to this entry remind us also that variation is, and has always been, an inherent and accepted aspect of traditional healing—and, more importantly, an incredibly useful one. Just as biological hybrids can be traced back endlessly through past generations, examination of the deeper past of yarrow's medicinal use shows that connections between myth and medicine long predate early medieval healing practice and—no matter how far back we go—cannot be traced to a single monolithic source; variation in practice has always been fundamental to traditional healing. Pliny's discussion of yarrow, for instance, acknowledges and even embraces tremendous variation, never offering a single, definitive recommendation on the herb's use. While such amorphousness is often associated with folktales, it is less typically palatable within modern notions of medicine. However, in contrast to such pharmaceutical ideals, Pliny departs even from the herbal's seemingly core purpose, discussion of the herb itself, as he offers up the possibility that Achilles didn't actually heal with the herb at all, but rather with the rust of his sword:

> alii primum aeruginem invenisse utilissimam emplastris, ideoque pingitur ex cuspide decutiens eam gladio in volnus Telephi, alii utroque usum medicamento volunt.
>
> [Some have it that he was the first to find out that copper-rust is a most useful ingredient of plasters, for which reason he is represented in paintings as scraping it with his sword from his spear on to the wound of Telephus, while others hold both remedies.]

In this way, Pliny's entry goes to great lengths to acknowledge a range of views, and the beliefs of 'others' (*alii*) are mentioned no fewer than six times within an entry of just a few lines.[12] Pliny thus offers his own view of the herb's efficacy as simply one possibility among many. While acknowledgment of such seemingly competing views might appear—from our modern medical perspective—to weaken the authority of Pliny's claims regarding the efficacy of the herb itself, such mentions actually serve to increase the entry's overall utility, providing a medic with herbal means of healing in addition to alternative methods of addressing inflammation from wounds, such as the employment of metal implements.[13] Clearly the healing tradition inherited by early medieval medics in England accepted—and even embraced—variant practices, but across all the variation we see an unequivocal linkage between narrative and medicine.

However, the variation present in the Old English text works in another direction as well: the *Herbarium* does not limit the use of swords to healing battle injuries but, rather, extends the impact of Achilles' discovery from battle wounds to a much wider array of ailments, domestic and military. While the story linking Achilles with yarrow does reinforce the herb's curative properties with regard to battle wounds in particular, the Old English entry also credits yarrow with the ability to heal toothaches, swelling, difficulty with urination, rashes, intestinal and abdominal issues, and even bites of dogs or snakes. These healing properties—effectively transmitted across centuries via stories of Achilles—are widely accepted by medical researchers even today. As part of their argument that *Achillea millefolium* (yarrow) 'should be seen as a very high priority for research funding',[14] Applequist and Moerman cite the herb's 'hemostyptic activity' (that is, its ability to stanch bleeding by contracting blood vessels) as validation for its use to 'benefit conditions such as skin injuries'.[15] But this is not the only established benefit: 'Preclinical studies indicate that it may have anti-inflammatory, anti-ulcer, hepatoprotective, anxiolytic, and perhaps antipathogenic activities'; further, 'studies have also shown that yarrow is generally safe and well tolerated'.[16] Because use on the battlefield is only one of numerous efficacious uses posited in the *Herbarium* entry, it is worth considering that the story also reflects and preserves a deeper, more widespread connection between battle and healing. The potential for shared purposes of sword and plant in healing wounds are explicit in Pliny's *Natural History*, but I would suggest that such connections continue implicitly in the Old English *Herbarium* and that this hero/healer connection aligns strongly with imagery connecting weaponry and healing plants across Old English medical texts more generally rather than only those deriving from classical models, as will be discussed further below.

Collapsing the categories of battle and healing, both classical and medieval medical text entries in effect recast the herb as weapon, the healer as warrior. The debate described by Pliny is not whether or not Achilles had the power to heal, but whether he healed with plants or with weapons. In Old English medical texts, the superficial boundary between plants and weapons blurs further still, and we frequently see herbs themselves described explicitly in terms of spears and arrows. Conversely, we see such implements as swords and knives incorporated into healing rituals and recipes. Accordingly, a more solid understanding of military weaponry can thus transform us into much better readers of the medical texts themselves. Descriptions of material objects—in particular the spears, knives, swords, and armor of the healing remedies—are situated at the intersection of oral tradition and literate culture where complex networks of signification become possible and even small physical details act as effective guides toward deeper levels of interpretation and aesthetic response. Each weapon, each piece of armor, and each battle strategy carry specific social connotations and evoke particular situations of use. Far more than simple metaphors and superstition-inspired abstractions, the physical details of weaponry in these medical texts reveal a deeper and richer understanding of how health and healing were actually understood in early medieval England.

Healing as warfare in Old English medical texts

As we have already seen, the surface-level boundaries separating categories of medicine, folktale, and warfare become far less distinct when we look closely at pre-modern medical traditions. The yarrow entry linking Achilles with medical knowledge would doubtless have been quite appealing in a culture within which battle imagery was ubiquitous across genres and practices, and it is perhaps unsurprising that battle imagery permeated Old English thought in a large number of ways. For instance, traditional wisdom handed down through the Old English maxims teaches that as surely as fish must live in water, kings in their halls, and dragons in their barrows, swords belong in the laps of warriors and spears in their hands:

            Daroð sceal on handa,
gar golde fah.   [...]
            Sweord sceal on bearme,
drihtlic isern.   Draca sceal on hlæwe,
frod, frætwum wlanc.   Fisc sceal on wætere
cynren cennan.   Cyning sceal on healle
beagas dælan.

[A javelin must be in the hand, spear adorned with gold [...]. A sword must be in the lap, lordly iron. A dragon must be in a barrow, wise, proud with treasures. Fish must be in water, to bring forth its kind. A king must be in the hall, to distribute rings.] (*Maxims II* 21–22, 25–29)

This image of the armed warrior was as pervasive as it was powerful, and even the Old English medical texts quite naturally show us a world where plants are named for spears and arrows, where healing rituals employ swords and knives, and where healers can recite poems metaphorically depicting armed warriors or even a full-scale battle. Together, all of these texts challenge conventional, dichotomized categories of modern thought and invite us instead into ambiguous, hybridized spaces—performance arenas populated at once with legendary dragons, natural wildlife, and historical leaders. These mythic, natural, and social worlds are held together in part by a shared material culture that is often conveyed with remarkable specificity, one in which swords, spears, and similar implements are equally at home in medical and military contexts.

Because, as this chapter seeks to show, weaponry functions so importantly within the medical tradition—as ritual objects, practical implements, and rich metaphors—it is imperative that we comprehend weaponry in more than a general, abstract way; as *Maxims II* suggests, it was the precise details of weaponry that worked to firmly ground Old English gnomic wisdom and heroic idealism in real-world battle experience. The ideal spear is one that is adorned with gold (l. 22), and the best sword is made of iron (l. 26). Yet the physical details go beyond the aesthetic, their presence drawing attention not only to beauty and power but also to the bearer's fragility and vulnerability: 'Rand sceal on scylde, / fæst fingra gebeorh' ['A boss must be on a shield, firm protection for fingers'] (ll. 37–38).[17] As Gale R. Owen-Crocker notes, the function and shape of the boss varied widely across the early medieval period, but it consistently served to protect the fingers and hands.[18] Such proverbs readily call to mind images of battle from the epic *Beowulf*, the historical *Battle of Maldon*, or even Old English renderings of biblical narratives such as *Judith* or *Exodus*, which contain numerous expansions of battle scenes in corresponding portions of source texts; weapons and warfare described in these and many other such narrative contexts have been studied extensively.[19] Less fully explored, however, are the equally compelling images of warriors and weaponry that appear in the more practically oriented manuscripts devoted to health and herbal healing. As John Foley observed, overlap across genres—even ones as seemingly far removed as epic poetry and medical manuals—affords 'a built-in opportunity to deepen the resonance' of oral-connected texts.[20] Such resonance as it pertains to the usage of weaponry, warfare, and heroic actions is readily apparent, as even the most cursory glance at the healing texts reveals. The so-called 'Nine Herbs Charm' explicitly praises the herb mugwort for its 'power against the enemy who travels over the earth' ['miht wiþ þa[m] laþan ðe geond lond færð'] (l. 6).[21] A charm against a swarm of bees, which involves a direct address to *sigewif* (that is, 'victory women', l. 9),[22] begins with the same *hwæt* (l. 4) that activates the heroic register in the famous prologue to *Beowulf*.[23] Even those remedies that do not explicitly invoke images of warfare nonetheless present illness and disease as enemies to be conquered, the vast majority of the remedies in surviving manuscripts establishing an agonistic relationship between healer and ailment with the word *wið*, 'against'.[24] The healer thus becomes a hero, and the numerous weapons that appear in the medical texts serve to 'arm' the practitioner in battle against ailments.

Against this backdrop, the practice of naming plants for weapons—a phenomenon we see across all the major Old English medical texts as well as remedies appearing as marginalia—serves the dual function of being both aid to identification and a healer's weapon against disease. For instance, *garclife*, a flowering plant whose nomenclature (literally, 'spear-burr' or 'burdock') 'refers to the towering pointed and spear-like florescence of the plant and its burr-like fruit',[25] appears in the *Lacnunga* (entry cxvi; f. 186r) as part of a lung-salve; in the *Herbarium* (xxxii; f. 186r) with remedies for such ailments as sore eyes, warts, or snakebite; and in *Bald's Leechbook* (II.viii, f.70r and li.2, f. 99v)[26] within recipes for digestive issues and ailing lungs. The still familiar garlic, *garleac*—literally 'spear-leek'—is also referenced in various manuscripts, such as *Bald's Leechbook* (II.xxxii, lvi, and xli) and *Leechbook III* (lxi, f. 122r and lx, f. 122r).[27] Likewise, *sperewyrt*, spear-plant, is included in the *Lacnunga* (cxxxv) within a remedy for pustules and in the *Herbarium* (xcvii) for bladder pain, toothache, and intestinal worms.[28] *Strælwyrt*, 'arrow-wort', appears in *Bald's Leechbook* (I.vi.4, f. 19r) as part of a remedy for tooth pain, so named presumably because 'the forked alignment' of this plant, today known more commonly as club moss, bears 'a great similarity to small arrows sticking in the soil'.[29]

An especially interesting case involves *Herbarium* entry xxxiii for a plant with the native name *woodruff*, the juice of which was to be used in an ointment for leg or foot pain and the roots in a drink for liver problems (Figure 2.2). While the Old English *Herbarium* usually offers fairly close translations of Latin remedies dating back to the fourth and fifth centuries (and there are Latin exemplars for most if not all of the *Herbarium*'s entries), it is important to keep in mind that the translation process was not one of slavish copying but rather of 'merging and adaptation'.[30] For example, the Latin medical text for this particular entry[31] employs *asfodulus* as the primary name for the herbaceous plant, with *astula regia*—which means 'king's spear'—appearing only as a secondary gloss. But all four of the surviving manuscripts of the Old English *Herbarium* opt to retain *astula regia* while dropping *asfodulus* entirely.[32] However, this pattern of emphasizing the plant's connection to a spear makes perfect sense in the entry's new medieval English context, for multiple reasons. First, as we have seen, the use of 'spear' to indicate leaf shape was already familiar in the native plant-naming tradition. Importantly, leaf-shaped spear heads were common in both Roman and Germanic warfare, giving the name a practical function in both the source language and the Old English translation. According to M. J. Swanton's definitive study of spearheads in early medieval England, leaf-shaped blades 'formed a basic component of all spear series throughout Europe', including Roman and English, and among the leaf-shaped variants, those with a slender shape and longer length—not unlike the leaves of the herb known as *astula regia*—were 'by far the commonest leaf-shaped blades found' in early medieval graves.[33] (See Figures 2.2 and 2.3.) Thus, the mnemonic for remembering the plant's shape would seem to have justified the transmission of this particular name from Latin into Old English and across various Old English manuscripts.

The designation 'king's spear' arguably carries social connotations as well. While the shape of *astula regia* might not seem especially connected to kings in particular, in Germanic culture, possession of a spear did connote status. As Swanton explains, for the 'ordinary' individual in early medieval England, 'the spear was possessive of greater significance than either mere poetic fancy or a convenient and singularly destructive weapon; it was the jealously preserved symbol of a free warrior's status in early Germanic

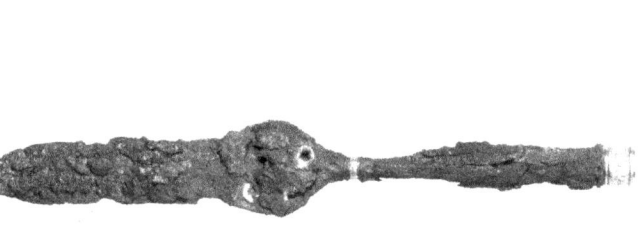

Figure 2.2 *Herbarium* entry for woodruff, *astula regia*, British Library MS Cotton Vitellius C.iii, f. 32r.

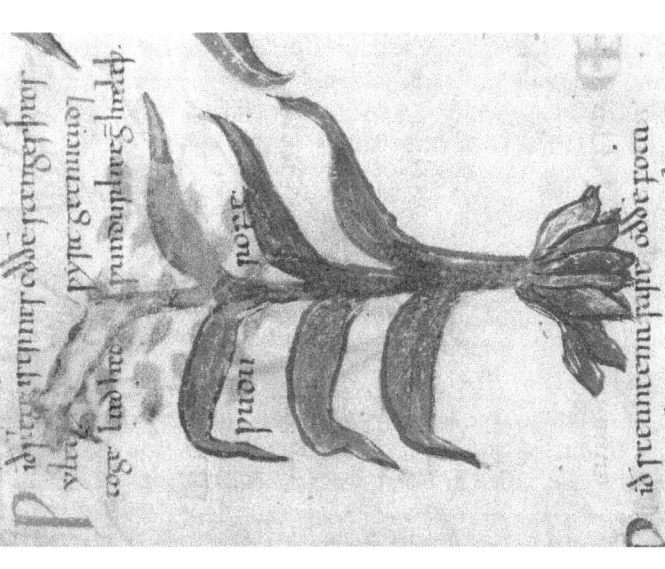

Figure 2.3 Leaf-shaped spear-head, early medieval England. British Museum (Museum number: 1964,0702.491).

society'.³⁴ Tacitus (*Germania* ii.14) reports that even in ancient times only the first-rank soldiers were armed with spears,³⁵ and in Bede's *Historia Ecclesiastica*, a spear is among the accoutrements that the priest Coifi is granted upon his conversion to Christianity (II.13). The spear—and by extension, the plants bearing its name—would thus have long carried positive associations not only with victory over adversity but also with higher social stations, associations conferred by extension onto the healer 'armed' with such resources.

Actual weapons (and household implements that could be used as weapons) also served practical and ritual functions in Old English medical texts. For example, the *seax*, a single-edged knife made from iron, appears frequently in the *Leechbooks* and is used in numerous ways. In *Leechbook III* (entry lxii) it is used to mark the location of the herb *helenium*. In some cases, it is used for surgical cutting, as in entry II.xiii of *Bald's Leechbook* (f. 21r). In other cases still, the seax serves more of a ritual function, as in a remedy for a horse experiencing sudden pain (lxv, f. 106r), where the seax is supposed to have a handle made from an ox's horn, on which there are three brass nails and the following inscription: 'Benedicite omnia opera domini dominum' ['bless all the works of the lord of lords'], a canticle used in Christian liturgy based on a story from the Book of Daniel.³⁶ The inscription called for here elevates a common medieval English household tool to the position of a ritual object linked to both Latin learning and Christian liturgy.

The crossover of weapons and tools into the healing tradition is more natural and logical than it might initially seem when we consider that it was typical in medieval culture for the same bows, arrows, spears, and knives used in battle to have alternative uses in hunting and even everyday household work. Richard Underwood explains that the use of the bow in warfare 'appears to have been limited to a few specialists', though most men would have been trained in archery for hunting purposes.³⁷ John Manley describes the difficulties in isolating arrowheads used for military rather than civilian purposes, offering the view that 'the same arrowhead could be employed for both hunting and warfare in early medieval England'.³⁸ And Nicholas Brooks notes that the spear was 'important as a throwing weapon in hunting and in battle'.[39] But the seax—the most frequently appearing weapon in the *Leechbooks* and *Lacnunga*—is by far the most versatile and ubiquitous such implement in real-world contexts. While there was certainly specialization of use between the long seax and the common seax, as well as differentiation of blade type, there was much overlap as well. As David A. Gale explains, the 'long seaxes have obvious uses as swords'; however, 'the seax must have played a very secondary role as a weapon', and 'in everyday life on the farm and in the ordinary household, the ubiquitous domestic knife was used for eating, skinning, whittling, etc.'.[40] Underwood notes that the majority of individuals, 'both men and women, appear to have carried a knife on a daily basis, presumably used for eating and other domestic tasks. While they were not weapons *per se*, warriors presumably took their knives with them when they went to battle'.[41] The multifunctional seax even makes its way into epic poetry as the weapon with which Beowulf delivers the dragon's final death-blow.[42]

Even the sword, far more specialized for battle use and typically associated with higher rank and nobility, acquires ritual functions in certain remedies. Remedy lxii in *Leechbook III*, for instance, requires crosses to be inscribed specifically 'mid sweorde' ['with a sword'] as part of the preparation before drinking the entry's herbal remedy. The power of the sword's victory in battle is thus transferred to victory over physical ailment, lending ritual force to the final promise of the remedy's power and effectiveness: 'him bið sona sel' ['it will soon be better for him'] (f. 124r). In a culture that made less distinction between weapons and domestic tools across situations of use, it was perhaps more logical and natural for the sword, spear, and seax to figure prominently in the remedies, retaining both domestic and military associations. In this context, the seax could be used both for cutting herbs and for surgical procedures and thus be invested with warlike power against disease; conversely, the sword could bring its military associations into the domestic sphere as part of a ritual preparation of an herbal medicinal drink. The evocation of weapons in poetic incantations for healing can be viewed as an extension of this multifunctionality and multivalence. If we recognize the logic linking healing and battle across these remedies generally, we are in a much better position to understand the weapons appearing in poetic incantations as far more than mere superstition. Herbs in this construct function *as* weapons. We are also now much more fully equipped to examine these remedies individually, and it is with this purpose that we now return to explore the poem *Ic me on þisse gyrde beluce* with which this chapter began.

Arming the traveler: oral poetics and weaponry in *Ic me on þisse gyrde beluce*

The protective poem inscribed in the margins of CCCC 41 calls upon God and various saints and beings for aid and protection while traveling.[43] Quite literally a marginal text, this poem occupies a liminal space within the healing tradition; as Richard Marsden notes, 'the line between prayer and charm' in this text 'may be hard to discern'.[44] Though untitled in the manuscript,[45] the poem is most typically labelled the 'Journey Charm' in modern editions and translations. This convention was begun in 1909 when Felix Grendon added an Old English title, 'Siþgaldor', to the poem.[46] Grendon translated his own title as 'Journey Spell'.[47] Godfrid Storms later picked up the invented title and modified the translation as 'Journey Charm', a convention that has continued to the present day. 'Charm', however, does not fully render the poem's hybrid nature. Karen Jolly, for instance, references the text as a 'prayer',[48] and Thomas Hill argues convincingly for its position within the tradition of Irish *loricae*, that is, 'prayers for safety to be uttered in a time of danger'.[49] As even these few examples of categorization indicate, the text is deeply hybrid in content, form, and genre. Though individual points concerning this hybridity will be the focus in the discussion below, in order to demonstrate the hybrid aspects of this poem more completely, I have also provided at the end of this chapter an appendix presenting a full text and translation of the poem, with choices and notes reflective of the chapter's analysis.

'Ic me on þisse gyrde beluce' in the context of oral traditional healing

Because the poem on pages 350–353 of CCCC 41 beginning 'Ic me on þisse gyrde beluce' has been so frequently anthologized as a 'charm',[50] it is easy to forget that it does not actually appear in a medieval medical collection (and in fact departs in important ways from the recipes that do), nor does it work in quite the same way. Jolly has persuasively argued that the works appearing as marginalia in CCCC 41 as a whole 'were not intended as performative texts, even if they had been copied from manuals that were',[51] and she follows Sarah Larratt Keefer's argument that the texts were instead intended for later copying, as a kind of archive.[52] Jolly's thorough analysis of these collective texts points toward a liturgical function wherein 'the interweaving of these prayers, rituals, and formulas by a single scribe suggests a reassessment of the role of liturgy in everyday life'.[53] While some texts are 'identifiably liturgical', others '*appear* more as remedies because of associations with so-called magical or superstitious charms'.[54]

Of what she terms the 'long formula' or 'prayer' here under consideration (that is, *Ic me on þisse gyrde beluce*), she notes that 'the scribal corrections suggest an effort to emend a text that might have been received orally' and that 'the formula's linguistic anomalies and its metrical qualities suggest oral performance and transmission'.[55] The implicit distinctions Jolly makes here are subtle but important ones: a poem *derived from* but not *intended for* oral performance, a text that *appears* as a remedy but may *function* quite differently. However, it is worth pausing to consider how this text that appears in the margins of Bede's *Ecclesiastical History* might nonetheless still be productively classified as a ritual incantation and, more importantly, how we benefit from considering it alongside medical remedies and charm texts. I do not argue here for any unequivocally oral provenance, but rather that its language and structure resonate powerfully within oral traditional contexts across multiple genres and that we can learn much about this poem and the wider healing tradition by more fully understanding how diverse forces interact within this hybrid text. In particular, I would suggest that the specific weapons associated with the four named gospel authors carry significant connotations within both the larger poetic tradition and the healing tradition, and that these connotations matter significantly for several cruces of interpretation.

In describing what she sees as a 'definable oral genre', Lea Olsan identifies four characteristics shared by most (though far from all) texts often classified as 'charms':[56]

(a) A heading naming the purpose of the charm ... often in the form 'against something' (e.g., *Wiþ færstice* ...)
(b) Directions for performance ('say', 'sing ...'). The directions for the acts associated with a verbal formula may constitute the longest part of the charm and entail ritual as well as practical acts.
(c) The words of an incantation or chant ...
(d) A concluding formula that may vary from a statement such as 'he will soon be well' to more directions for application ...

Though appearing in a different order and in an atypical format, each of these components has still arguably been incorporated into this marginal text implicitly directed towards travelers.

While there is no heading (a) *per se*, the catalog of ailments in lines 2–5 similarly pits remedy (in this case preventive) against ailment through much the same phrasing: 'Wið þane sara s(t)ice, wið þane sara slege, / wið þane grymma gryre, / wið ðane micela egsa þe bið eghwam lað, / 7 wið eal þæt lað þe into land fare' ['Against the sore pain, against the sore bite, against the grim horror, against the great terror that is dreadful to everyone, and against all evil that goes across the land']. The typical charm's directions for performance (b) involve imperatives; however, here the first-person account of the speaker's actions, especially in lines 1 and 6, fulfills much the same function, conveying directions by example rather than command: 'Ic me on þisse gyrde beluce' ['I enclose myself with this branch']; 'Syge gealdor ic begale, sigegyrd ic me wege' ['I sing a victory charm, I carry a victory branch']. Also, the words of the incantation (c) encompass the entirety of the alliterative poem, and the role of the concluding formula 'he will soon be well' (d) is filled in lines 31–40 by the speaker's confident assertions of the happiness and joy that has resulted and/or will result from the prior invocations.

Perhaps even more notably, the speaker in line 6 references his or her own utterance as a *gealdor*, a term that, along with its variant spelling *galdor*, can be glossed as diversely as 'poem', 'song', 'incantation', 'charm', or 'spell' (*DOE*). And while certainly not limited to medical texts, *g(e)aldor* does occur in this corpus with particular frequency.[57] The genre of *galdor* is difficult if not impossible to pin down specifically, but the power attributed to utterances described in such terms is undeniable. Ciaran Arthur's exploration of the term as applied to both authorized rituals and condemned practices indicates that '*galdor* may have been one of the terms that became restricted in usage to signify a dangerous spiritual space'.[58] With reference to the margins of CCCC 41 in particular, Arthur notes that 'the *Old English Bede* contains a condemnatory reference to *galdor* and this appears in the same book of Bede's *History* as the marginal *galdor* ritual [i.e., *Ic me on þisse gyrde beluce*]'.[59] Arthur concludes that '*galdor* was considered an appropriate word to describe a powerful Christian utterance by this scribe in the early eleventh century' despite the condemnation of *galdor* within the main text.

Even more relevant for present purposes, though, the specific reference against *galdor* in the manuscript's main text explicitly links the *galdor* genre with healing practice, *læcedomum*:

Forðon ðe monige ðone geleafan, þe hie hæfdon, mid unrihtum weorcum idledon, ond swylce eac manige in ða tid þæs halgan geleafan, mid þæm hie gelærede wæron, 7 to ðæm dwoligendum **læcedomum** deofulgylda ofsetton 7 scyndon; swa hie þæt sende wite from God scyppende þurh heora **galdor** oþþe lyfesne oððe þurh hwylce hwugu deogolnesse deofolcræftes bewerian mehton.

[For many of them profaned the creed they held by wicked deeds and some of them too, in times of plague, would forget the sacred mysteries of the faith into which they had been initiated and take to the false **remedies** of idolatry, as though they could ward off a blow inflicted by God the Creator by means of **incantations** or amulets or any other mysteries of devilish art.][60]

Whether within Christian contexts (such as the *syge galdor* of the marginal poem) or rejected pagan contexts (such as those within 'læcedomum deofulgylda'), utterances marked as *galdor* were clearly viewed as possessing strong healing and protective powers to be utilized against a range of adversities. However, unlike most incantations identified as *galdor*, the reference in the protective poem in CCCC 41 works against ('wiþ') *anticipated* ailments rather than existing ones; nonetheless, it still clearly taps into the larger healing tradition pitting healer against ailment and was likely to have been read in this context by the poem's earliest audiences.

The poem's placement in the margins of a story about Cuthbert's protection of his spiritual flock evokes a Christian context of pastoral care at the same time that its reference to itself as *gealdor* would seem to go against prohibitions, such as we find in sermons of Ælfric, that 'ne sceal nan man mid galdre wyrte besingan' ['one must not sing/enchant a plant with a charm'].[61] In truth, however, the poem evokes the power of the *galdor* tradition even as it is clearly and deeply embedded in Christian liturgical contexts, a new 'hybrid category of devotional protection'.[62] But this sense of hybridity, as Jolly observes, comes 'necessarily from a modern perspective in which practicality and spirituality are often separate modes, but apparently not at all incongruous to CCCC41's marginal scribe'.[63] 'Although its ostensible purpose may have been protection on an actual physical journey, it can be read allegorically', as a metaphor for 'life as a spiritual journey', 'a familiar trope' in Old English vernacular literature with 'deep roots in British monastic pilgrimage traditions'.[64] In Jolly's astute reading, this marginal poem works in tandem with other texts similarly inscribed in CCCC 41 to suggest a 'reassessment of the role of liturgy in everyday rural life', contributing to a 'larger liturgical agenda' with a strong 'pragmatic concern with everyday life in a rural environment'.[65] The poem appears in the margins alongside Bede's Old English *History*, Book IV.29–30, which narrates Cuthbert's choice to live a solitary life on an island as bishop of Lindisfarne, his subsequent return in response to the monks' needs, and his eventual death,[66] a context that goes far in linking the liturgical implications of the poem with the literal and metaphorical aspects of a journey. But what if we haven't yet explored *all* of the poem's metaphorical possibilities? What if we think about how the poem works as a metaphor, not only for an abstract journey of life but also for the healing practice that so many of its lines clearly evoke? By drawing upon the liturgical context implied by the manuscript in which the poem appears, as well as the medical tradition which the poem's language formulaically suggests, we can discover new fascinating interpretive possibilities that emerge.

To see just how close *Ic me on þisse gyrde beluce* is to the medical text tradition, we can briefly return once again to *Herbarium* entry 90 for yarrow, *millefolium*. After the opening that—as we saw at the beginning of this chapter—links the herb to Achilles himself, there is a series of sixteen remedies for which the plant is recommended. Remedy 14, 'wið næddran slite' ['against snakebite'] includes parallels for several of the key elements in the marginal poem of CCCC 41, specifically the lexemes *wið*, *slite*, *gyrd*, *wege*, and *scyld*:

> **Wið** næddran **slite**, gyf hwylc man hyne be**gyrde**þ mid þysse wyrte 7 hy on **wege** mid him bereþ, he bið ge**scyld**ed fram æghwylcum næddercynne.
>
> [**Against** snake **bite**, if a certain one **surrounds** himself with this plant and bears it with him on the **way**, he is **shield**ed from all snake-kind.]

In the marginal journey poem, these same elements are spread out but are most definitely present and working similarly against— among other adversities—bites, *slege* (glossed by Bosworth and Toller as 'a serpent's sting' [sense 2] and translated as 'bite' by Jolly[67] and others).

Ic me on þisse **gyrde** beluce (1)

[I enclose myself with this **branch**]

wið þane sara stice,   wið þane sara **slege** (2)

[**against** the sore pain, **against** the sore **bite**]

Syge gealdor ic begale,   sige**gyrd** ic me **wege** (6)

[I sing a victory **charm**, I **carry** a victory-branch for myself]

Biddu ... þæt me beo ...   **scyld** Iohannes ... (25, 29)

[I pray ... that for me ... John be a **shield** ...]

From the perspective of someone familiar with medical texts, it would likely be striking that amidst what otherwise appears to be a medicinal remedy there is no mention in this marginal poem of an actual herb—no harvesting instructions, no herbal preparation. Where we would expect to find this information, however, there is instead the enigmatic ritual involving encirclement with the *gyrde*. *Gyrde* in this poem has been translated variously as *stick*, *branch*, *staff*, *belt* (as that of a monk), and *girdle* (as that of military gear). I have translated *gyrde* myself here and in the appendix as *branch* to retain something closer to the herbal healing context evoked immediately afterward through the series of 'wið x' formulae as well as the verb *begalan* ('chant', 'sing') and the poem's own reference to itself as a *gealdor*, though the encircling nature and possibilities for metaphorical harvesting remain the same for most of these translations. Further, 'shoot or branch' is in fact the primary sense of the word, from which the others derive.[68] Likewise, any of the objects proposed as translations could ritually invoke the act of harvesting and thus metaphorically invest the speaker with both protection (from God) and the power to protect (through healing care). But if the *gyrde* of lines 1 and 6 is taken to be an actual plant, a healing herb—following the 'shoot or branch' sense—with which the speaker surrounds herself or himself, the expected elements of a remedy fall more neatly into place, the plant that helps travelers functioning simultaneously at both literal and metaphorical levels, the unnamed herb offering protection against dangers such as snakebites along the route and the metaphorical plant girding the speaker with spiritual protection as well.

    A short remedy against *oman* (most typically understood as the skin disease erysipelas[69]) on f. 186b of the *Lacnunga* offers further intriguing parallels within the dual contexts of healing and ritual as well as additional support for the *branch* translation. In this remedy a *gyrde* that is specifically said to be *grene* (green), thus almost undoubtedly a shoot or branch of some sort, is again used to make a circle around the suffering individual as part of a healing ritual. Like the journey poem in the margins of CCCC 41, this ritual act is also accompanied by a verbal incantation: 'Genim ane grene **gyrde** and læt sittan þone man on ses flore and

bestric hine ymbutan and **cweð**: .... ['Take a green **branch** and let the person sit on the floor and **make a stroke around him** and say: ....']

If we look more closely at the encircling itself in *Ic me on þisse gyrde beluce* (as suggested by *beluce*), the metaphor could go even deeper still. Another arena of ancient and early medieval healing where we see encircling is harvesting rituals. In the *Herbarium* entry for *unfortrædde* or *proserpinaca*, for example, a remedy for eye pain involves a ritual where the plant is encircled by means of a golden ring prior to harvesting: 'bewrit hy abutan mid anum gyldenan hringe' ['write around it with a golden ring']. And again, like the journey poem in the margins of CCCC 41, this ritual has a verbal accompaniment. The incantation is not provided verbatim, but the speaker is told to speak to the plant: '7 cweð þæt þu hy to eagena læcedome niman wylle' ['and say that you wish to take it as a remedy for eyes']. The *Herbarium*'s entry for mandrake (which will be discussed at great length in Chapter 5) also includes a similar ritual of encircling the plant prior to uprooting: 'bewrite þu hy wel hraþe iserne' ['score around[70] it quickly with iron']. The encircling aspect of the action as part of the uprooting is reinforced soon after: 'þu scealt onbutan hy delfan' ['you must dig around it']. Through this lens, the speaker of the journey poem in CCCC 41 is arguably occupying the role of a harvested plant, the encircled subject uprooted and placed directly into the care of God, to be used for healing and at the same time to be protected. This ritual is then followed by litanies evocative of ritual and militaristic power, once again implying the speaker's dual role in this ritual dynamic as both protector and protected, both healing and held—a wild medicinal plant to be harvested and then used as part of God's own healing design.

Rethinking one additional translation choice from the latter portion of the first line in *Ic me on þisse gyrde beluce* lends further plausibility to this reading. Though *helde* is frequently translated as 'grace' or 'protection',[71] its primary sense is simply of being held in keeping, with protective grace as but one possible—albeit hugely important—connotation. This particular text is provided as an example in the *Dictionary of Old English* under sense 2 (s.v. *hyld*), 'safekeeping', which is thus how I have chosen to translate it here and in the appendix. In addition to being the word's dominant meaning, 'safekeeping' also aligns more closely with the sense of something being 'locked',[72] which seems consistent with the bond implied by 'beluce' in the preceding half-line, the speaker encircled—enlocked—for safekeeping. This formulation of 'helde' with a genitive also has additional implications drawn from the wider Old English corpus, with such safekeeping being connected to loyalty and service, as in 'Godes helde 7 on hlafordes' in the Laws of Cnut 23.1 and 'Pharaones helde' in the Old English *Genesis* 42.15. Or in a legal context, 'Godes helde' has been translated by Andrew Rabin as 'rule of God', further emphasizing this sense of obligation.[73] This connotation of fealty is also appropriate to the context of a plant or practitioner being held in safekeeping in part to be of future service, the speaker being not only under the *protection* of God but also—and perhaps even more importantly—in the *service* of God. This poem appears specifically in the margins of Bede's story of Cuthbert in his service as bishop,[74] and it is difficult to imagine a more apt metaphor for pastoral care.

I have offered a number of ways of interpreting this enigmatic line—and many others have been proposed before—so I want to emphasize here that the interpretations need not be mutually exclusive. The unidentified *ic* with which this poem opens invites us to consider all that follows in the paradoxical terms of the riddle tradition. The speaker's identity is perhaps intentionally ambiguous, simultaneously occupying at once the space of the human healer, the healing plant, and the protected traveler. James Paz reminds us that 'in an atmosphere where "orality" and "literacy" coexisted and were interdependent, voice could, quite literally, move across the divide between human subject and non-human object'.[75] In fact, Old English poetry 'invites us to cultivate a lingering fascination' with 'things' that can be interpreted in diverse and thought-provoking ways.[76] This movement is most evident of course in the Exeter Book riddles (see further Chapter 7), but, if we are open to the possibilities, we can see such powerful ambiguity in the medical texts as well. But now let us turn to the nature of the speaker's own power against adversity during journeys (whether physical or metaphorical), a power that is signaled in particular through the traditional idiom shared across medical texts and epic verse in connection with the figure of the noble warrior.

Weapons and status: lines 25–30

The militaristic imagery discussed earlier as present throughout the medical texts emerges forcefully in *Ic me on þisse gyrde beluce* as well, where it helps to foreground the image of the speaker/healer as a high-ranking servant under the direct protection of God. However we might choose to classify this multivalent text—as prayer, charm, liturgy, or lorica—the agonistic relationship with adversity established in its *wiþ* catalog is later reinforced dramatically and powerfully in lines 25–30 through explicit battle imagery. This emphatic connection of herbal healing to weaponry adds multiple significant layers of meaning to the poem, as several costly weapons and items of war gear are invoked metaphorically to correspond to each of the four gospel authors called upon for protection: Matthew as a helmet, Mark a mailcoat, Luke a sword, and John a shield. Weapons here are not just protective in terms of battle, but also invoke protection against illness and adversities faced by travelers far from home.

Biblical parallels for this passage have been extensively noted,[77] especially with the epistle of Paul to the Ephesians (6:14–17):[78]

> Stand therefore having your loins girded in truth, and clothed with the breast-plate of justice, and having your feet shod to the preparation of the Gospel of peace: in all things taking the shield of faith, wherewith you may extinguish all the fiery darts of the most wicked one. And take unto you the helmet of salvation: and the sword of the spirit (which is the word of God).

While this and similar biblical references have been fully probed for metaphorical implications, more literal connections to medieval war gear contemporary with the poem have not been as thoroughly explored, thus limiting our understanding of how this widely acknowledged spiritual metaphor would have been understood by the poem's earliest audiences. From this angle, departures from Ephesians are potentially quite meaningful. As Leslie Arnovick observes, the poem references some of the same weapons as

Ephesians 6 but speaks much 'more concretely of holy defense'.[79] And these concrete details differentiating the Old English poem from the biblical analogue do indeed acquire special significance—particularly in terms of social class—when considered within the context of early medieval military culture.

Taken together, these four battle items—helmet, mailcoat, sword, and shield—are markers of a highly elite status in early medieval England. The best-known assemblage of these items is found in the kingly Sutton Hoo ship burial with one of the richest and most intact collections of grave goods from the period. While weaponed graves cannot serve as an ultimate authority on actual warfare, the selections can certainly enhance our understanding of the symbolic meanings of weapons, meanings that could be—and clearly were—invoked in literary and metaphorical depictions as well.[80] The sword—linked to Luke in the poem—was 'the most prestigious of offensive weapons'.[81] Labor-intensive and costly to make, swords are found in only about 10% of weaponed graves and were often passed down as heirlooms through multiple generations.[82] Likewise, helmets and mail corselets have been found in only a small number of 'very rich' burials, 'indicating that their role as symbols of rank or status may have been much more important than their role in war'.[83] The helmet—the equipment connected to Matthew—occupied a very 'high place in the hierarchy of male military equipment', and only about five have been found to date.[84] Mail—the gear equated with Mark—was also 'a rare luxury' in early medieval England.[85] In fact, 'the rusted remains of only one mailcoat survive' from the period 'and this from the richest deposit ever discovered'.[86] Following this same pattern, the 'wuldre gewlitegod' ('gloriously made') shield metaphorically equated with John would seem to indicate a shield of the type that also denotes high status. Like mail, helmets, and swords, 'decorated shields circulating in society are almost exclusively high-status items'.[87]

Evidence from surviving letters and wills reveals that though weapons are included in over half of all gift-giving cases with named recipients, 'the only weapon types listed as gifts are swords, mail coats, and helmets',[88] precisely those weapons attributed to three of the four gospel authors. The will of Ethelred's son

Hybridity of metaphor 73

Athelstan, which included, among other valuable artifacts, eleven swords, a coat of mail, and two shields, provides further evidence that these particular items circulated together as high-status treasures.[89] A traveler armed with such gear thus would be not only well-protected but also extremely high-ranking. The metaphorical weaponry here manifests a fascinating syncretism of Christian learning and Germanic warrior culture, and the particular weapons chosen effectively fulfill the biblical mandate to arm oneself with Christian ideals while they at the same time convey a very specific social station. But how does the social station of this metaphorical traveler relate to what we know of the world in which the manuscript itself was produced and engaged? And how might the poem's overt image of an idealized warrior operate across socially diverse readerships?

One could of course see the elite weaponry as implying an elite audience, though that audience might be religious rather than lay. Olsan, for instance, argues that the charm's placement in the margins of Book 4, Chapters 29–30, which relate the story of Cuthbert's embarkment on his service as bishop, could suggest an author who 'felt that this protective formula related specifically to the needs of a bishop or someone in a spiritual office'.[90] While the theory of a high-ranking office is indeed quite plausible, neither the scribe nor the intended audience needs to have been high-ranking for the poem to still possess its full rhetorical force, and Jolly has argued for a more modest authorship/readership. The CCCC 41 marginalia, she explains, can be understood as 'the product of a monastic (male or female) scribe, a secular priest in a small collegiate centre, or a manorial priest acting for a lay patron', all figures connected to Christian liturgy but none with credentials likely to be classified as elite.[91] In fact, the diversity of CCCC 41's marginalia leads Jolly to the conclusion that the texts were produced in a rural environment, where 'the scope of orthodoxy' was 'considerably more diverse than that found in major reform centres dominated by prolific authors of texts that have come down to us, such as Ælfric and Wulfstan'.[92]

This more diverse orthodoxy could and did accommodate a wide range of oral traditional materials, and I would suggest that the war gear from traditional heroic oral narrative serves here as a bridge linking the text's (possibly rural) scribe and audience to the culture's highest ideals. The armed warrior is virtually ubiquitous in surviving Old English literature across genres, and, while it might seem on the surface that elite war gear would resonate most powerfully with elite audiences, this imagery from the broader tradition easily serves as an equalizer, a shared set of images metonymically linking Christian liturgy with widely known narratives of bravery, loyalty, victory, and honor—perhaps not unlike how widely known narratives function even today: for instance, while *being* a princess obviously carries class distinctions, stories and films *about* princesses serve as common cultural currency across modern class divisions. What is important is not that the story be directly connected with the past experiences of the audiences but rather that the imagery be familiar and resonant. As such, the elite armament of the gospel authors in the margins of CCCC 41 serves to bridge important cultural gaps. The invocation of weapons following the 'wiþ' catalog of anticipated ailments links Christian liturgy with a distinctly medieval version of preventive care, and the fact that the employed weaponry is decidedly elite elevates the gospel authors and the liturgical connections with many of the highest ideals of the Germanic tradition. With these effects in mind, we can now turn to the importance of preserving such hybridized connections in edited texts and translations.

Battling emendations: lines 26 and 30

The strong associations this passage has with elite military culture argue against two widely accepted emendations to the manuscript text—the frequent alteration of *wega* ['way'] to *wælgar* ['slaughter-spear'] (l. 30) and the common deletion of the half-line *hand ofer heafod* ['hand over head'] (l. 26). Part of the problem is that discussions of metrics and poetics have not always taken into full account the materiality of the objects involved. It is here that that a hybrid methodology merging philological questions with archaeological and historical insights can lead to a greater awareness of the poem's implied protective and healing power. When the poem's weapons are recognized as having grown out of dual contexts—as compelling metaphors within Christian liturgy and at the same time as material objects imbued with ideals of a secular elite warrior culture—longstanding emendations become unnecessary.

The emendation to line 30 was originally made by Holthausen, who altered the manuscript's 'wega Serafhin' ('seraphim of the ways') to instead read as 'wælgar Serafhin' ('the Seraphim a slaughter-spear') in a passage that immediately follows the extended metaphor of the evangelists as protective war gear.[93] However, the emendation's tremendous impact on modern translations, editions, and interpretations comes from its acceptance by Dobbie, whose edition in the Anglo-Saxon Poetic Records (ASPR) has long served as the default standard. In recent years, this version has become even more ubiquitous as it has been copied on numerous websites and thus is often a first stop for many seeking an online text.[94] In editing his ASPR text, Dobbie found the manuscript *wega* 'very unsatisfactory' and explained his decision to follow Holthausen thus: 'Following the identification of the four evangelists with weapons of defence, we expect the *Serafhin* (taken by the poet as singular) to represent a weapon also'.[95] In most cases this emendation has been either quietly accepted or countered only inconspicuously in footnotes or endnotes, and the proliferation of this emendation has led to numerous potential mistranslations and problematic scholarly readings.[96] These emendations have a long history, now entrenched and thus difficult to work against. For interpretations that stop at a basic military analogy, the addition of the seraphim to the military arming metaphor might seem to present no immediate problem. By looking at the poem's weapons in terms of the social connotations indicated from archaeological and historical evidence, however, the addition of the 'spear' actually becomes quite difficult.

While Germanic literature does include examples of warriors armed with a spear or other thrusting weapon along with a sword,[97] the status marker is clearly the sword, and the spear disrupts the social hierarchy established by the poem. Swanton notes the spear's position as a 'symbol of a free warrior's status in Germanic society',[98] and Owen-Crocker also suggests that 'possibly only freemen, of the rank of *ceorl* upwards' would have had the right to carry or be buried with a spear'.[99] Nonetheless, 'the spear is the commonest of weaponry found' in early medieval graves,[100] possessing nowhere near the level of prestige of a helmet or sword. Within the social context established by the poem, it would seem incongruous for one of God's own seraphim to be equipped solely with a significantly lesser weapon—a possession available to any freeman—than the weapons of the highest elite being borne by the human evangelists.

On biblical grounds, too, the emendation has been shown to be unnecessary. Thomas Hill makes the excellent observation that the manuscript reading *wega* not only avoids 'radical emendation' but also retains the poem's treatment of the four evangelists as a unit: 'To the best of my knowledge, the Seraphim are not associated with a spear or spears in any other Insular text of the period, and an emendation that creates an otherwise unattested metaphorical association is problematic'.[101] Heather Stuart objects to the emendation on similar grounds: 'the four Evangelists are mentioned as a structural unit in vv. 27–30, and to introduce *Serafhin* as an extra figurative weapon is to destroy that unit by extending it'.[102] For all of these reasons, then, a return to the manuscript reading *wega* seems the more responsible choice, and indeed the rendering of *wega* is arguably clear as it stands, 'seraphim of the ways',[103] which, as some have suggested, could simply be read as a paratactic construction referring back to John.[104] Such a reading risks disrupting the social hierarchy discussed above by equating John with the seraphim, but the line can also be interpreted as a general wish for the seraphim to be along the traveler's path, a reading that would be fully in line with the spirit of the Old English maxims: 'Wel mon sceal wine healdan on wega gehwylcum' ['It is well for one to have a friend on each of ways'].[105]

The second emendation commonly performed on this section of the poem—the decision to omit *hand ofer heafod* ('hand over head')—is even more widely accepted and less frequently acknowledged.[106] Grendon stated early on that '*hand ofer heafod* appears to me to be an accidental repetition of line 23', the same logic later accepted by Dobbie.[107] However, reading the text in the context of the warrior culture invoked here suggests that the phrase is not necessarily repeated in error. It can instead be understood as a formulaic repetition, common within oral traditional texts, as part of a ritualized request for aid from two distinct groups, first from the 'haligra rof' ['valiant host of holy ones'] (which has often been understood as a reference to saints[108]) and then, in the second instance, from the evangelists. Desire for metrical regularity is one reason that editing the phrase out might initially seem appealing. Editing in a way that retains the half-line alliterative patterns is difficult and has been treated differently among those editors who do retain the manuscript's 'hand ofer heafod'. Storms does not convey half-line breaks, so the issue becomes less relevant, Storms being one of the few to retain both instances of the phrase. Bill Griffiths' edition renders the lines thus, with a half-line break after *hand*: 'þæt me beo hand ofer heafod'. This solution does not seem wholly satisfactory, however, because it breaks the formulaic 'hand ofer heafod', which repeats from 23a.[109] Tupper's much earlier edition treats 'hand ofer heafod' as part of a hypermetric line: 'Biddu ealle bliðu mode þæt me beo hand ofer heafod'. In my own rendering given in this chapter's appendix, I have opted to include 'hand ofer heafod' as an independent half-line:

Biddu ealle bliðu   mode þæt me beo,
hand ofer heafod,

There is ample precedent for single half-lines in this and other charm texts, and, drawing on compelling comparative evidence, John Foley has argued for the integrity of the half-line itself as a viable metrical unit rather than an irregularity, a defining feature of what he terms 'hybrid prosody'.[110] He demonstrates that in instances of 'lexical repetition' creating 'rhythmic modulation'— arguably very much the case here with the repetition of 'hand ofer heafod' from line 23a—this type of 'half-line prosody' is especially common.[111] From this perspective, one might reasonably argue that the 'irregular' half-line is *more* rather than less significant, marked metrically by its very difference.

The retention of *hand ofer heafod* would thus contribute meaningfully to the warrior metaphor and underscore its importance through repetition. Evidence from the broader Old English corpus offers even further evidence for retaining its inclusion. As Anne Klinck has noted in her edition of Old English elegies, line 23a can be connected with two other poetic passages linking head and hands: *The Wanderer*, lines 41–44, in which the speaker describes laying his head and hands, 'honda ond heafod', on his lord's knee; and *Maxims I*, lines 67–68, in which *hond* and *heafod* are associated with the *gifstol* and treasure-giving. 'The gesture of placing head and hands on the knee', Klinck argues, 'certainly seems to have the implication of submission on the one side and protection on the other'.[112] Such a reading builds upon Tupper's earlier but generally overlooked treatment of the phrase, in which he concluded as early as 1912 that '*hand ofer heafod* in the *Journey Spell* carries then the idea of "guardianship" and protection'.[113] If the phrase *hand ofer heafod* does in fact traditionally index a ritualized exchange of loyalty for protection similar to that implied in *The Wanderer* and *Maxims I*, then the repetition is far from redundant, but rather becomes perfectly appropriate in the request for protection from both groups, perhaps even especially so before the explicit connection is made in the succeeding lines between the evangelists and protective armor. A phrase implying an oath of loyalty would serve to validate the speaker's request for protection by framing it within the context of the high-status, heroic warrior culture. This reading does not preclude, but rather can serve to further affirm, interpretations based on religious contexts. Leslie Arnovick (following Godfrid Storms), for instance, offers an equally convincing reading of the image as referring to a hand extended over another's head in a ritual blessing.[114] As with the battle imagery associated with the evangelists, these lines manifest a fascinating hybridity and invite us to think about such images in terms of both Christian typology and Germanic battle. At every stage the text supports—and depends upon—this multivalence.[115]

To add one further possibility to the interpretations already proposed, I would like to suggest that the body itself could provide the 'gyrde' and that the circle implied by 'beluce' could be vertical, rather than horizontal, the 'gyrde' being one's arms, lifting high, 'hand over head'. The combination of the singular 'hand' and the repetition of the phrase could indicate that both hands were intended to be raised individually, one at a time, following the flow of the incantation and ritual. In 1912, Tupper proposed that the 'hand' refers to that of one's lord placed above the 'head' of a subservient subject.[116] However, what if the hands are those of the speaker, and the phrase references a posture of holding one's hands above one's own head, something like the supplicant posture of orans?[117] What if 'beluce' references the motion of the arms rising above the body and head in an encircling, enlocking motion? If we imagine the speaker performing a protective ritual, encircling the body with the hand and arms while incanting the poem's litanies of dangers and corollary protectors, several of the poem's most cryptic elements fall into place, enigmatic repetitions and all. While I am not suggesting that the opening is explicitly in reference to a specifically Roman ritual or posture, it is worth noting that the classical orans might not have been unfamiliar in early medieval England. As but one example, in frescoes from the Lullington Roman Villa in England several figures are portrayed in orans position, hands elevated, if not quite above the head.[118]

And such a posture need not be derived from classical tradition; it could easily have evolved independently as a natural gesture of protection and supplication. Protective rituals linking martial and medicinal arts are far from uncommon. For instance, in an introduction to Qigong exercises, Tianjun Liu explains that the 'purpose of Martial Arts Qigong practice was to protect the self and capture the enemy, focusing outward on the body; the intention of Medical Qigong practice was to cultivate health and prevent illness'.[119] Exercises in tai chi chuan thus often involve bodily movement imagined in martial terms with the specific intent of protecting the body as one would use a 'shield'. One guide suggests moving the hands in circular motions above the head, in front of the chest, and near the body's center, specifically in order to 'create a protective shield'.[120] And a warm-up exercise described in *The Harvard Medical School Guide to Tai Chi* includes instructions to 'circle your hands up the sides of the body and over the head'; the exercise goes on to combine this protective circle with plant imagery: 'imagining you are like a tree with deep roots, guide the energy through your feet into your roots, anchoring you to the earth'.[121] In this context of an embodied ritual, the twice repeated 'hand ofer heafod' could work in tandem with the opening 'ic me on þisse gyrde beluce' to refer to such a vertical circle, or even a horizontal circle performed in prostrate position, with the speaker using his or her hands as a *gyrde* to draw a protective circle 'ofer heafod', a protection that metaphorically functions as a powerful combination of shield, sword, mailcoat, and helmet.

I do not personally see any of these interpretations as mutually exclusive of others. On the contrary, I believe their very force comes from multivalence and the possibility for diverse audiences to experience the same text in manifold ways. As Paul Bradshaw has discussed with regard to modern liturgy, all liturgies 'are essentially multivalent',[122] and this 'essentially multivalent character of worship itself and the multiple meanings' of any given activity can 'co-exist within any group of people celebrating together'.[123] In a diverse early medieval audience I am able to imagine multiple readings of *gyrde*—as 'girdle', 'staff', 'rod', 'shoot', or 'branch', among perhaps others. Similarly, I can imagine the encircling having been diversely interpreted as both literal and liturgical, involving a bishop's staff,[124] a warrior's girdle, or even a gardener's cutting tool.

Throughout this chapter I have proposed numerous ways of reading the various elements of this puzzling poem, and some might find my refusal to take a firm stance frustrating. However, it is crucial to bear in mind that Old English poetry thrives and depends on meaningful ambiguities. Carol Braun Pasternack has long held that the 'ambiguity' or 'doubleness' of traditional utterances 'need not be resolved' into a single 'correct meaning'. Rather, various threads can 'play against each other through their own networks of intertexts' in a 'code of implied tradition'.[125] In this way, reception can be a form of hybridity as well. Following this line of thinking, I believe that the speaker of *Ic me on þisse gyrde beluce* could be read—and was perhaps *intended* to be read—as a traveler, a healer, or a plant. Similarly, I believe that the polysemous *gyrde* could be read—and was perhaps *intended* to be read—as a branch, a staff, a girdle, or a cutting tool. I am also confident that 'hand ofer head' was not a scribal error and could have been read by diverse readers as a ritual act of fealty, as a sign of the cross, or as a protective circle drawn above the head with one's arms—all without contradiction. And what I hope most of all to have added to this conversation in addition to a general openness to this diversity is an awareness of the significance of traditional battle gear within the larger context of medicinal healing. The metaphorical victory of the 'syge gealdor' depends upon metaphorical armor and weapons; thus to understand the metaphor, one that underlies medical texts more broadly, we must also understand how functions of weaponry parallel those of plants.

Far from mere vestiges of superstition, the weaponry employed here and throughout the Old English medical tradition develops from a powerful cultural hybridity, and the emergent poetics of weaponry follows a fairly clear and consistent rationale. The healing logic of the Old English *Herbarium* opts to retain powerful connections linking healers and heroes, swords and herbs, from a shared classical tradition. The leaf-shaped spearhead—a common weapon in Roman and Germanic warfare—quite naturally figures prominently in the Latin-derived *Herbarium* as well as the Old English *Lacnunga* and *Leechbooks* as an accessible aid to identification. Likewise, the *seax*, ubiquitous as a domestic tool and military weapon across early medieval England, displays an equally wide range of uses in the *Leechbooks* as a surgical tool, a harvesting implement, and ritual object. The poem inscribed in the margins of Bede's *Ecclesiastical History*, on the other hand, elevates its subject matter through its metaphorical weapons that would have been associated with only the most elite warriors, equipped with sword, mailcoat, shield, and helmet.

Perhaps it is because poems such as *Ic me on þisse gyrde beluce* do not conform neatly to modern categories of either literature or science and are thus often dismissed as superstition-fraught products of lesser minds that the metrical charms have been subject to such free emendation, with assumptions of error going widely unchallenged. The remedy *Wið færstice* ('Against a Sudden Pain') provides a very different example of how close attention to material artifacts can help counter such tendencies. This complex prosimetric text with its prose instructions for herbal preparation framing a narrative poem also allows us to delve more deeply into the performance/text hybridity manifest in the Old English medical corpus and will therefore serve as the focus of the next chapter.

Appendix

Ic me on þisse gyrde beluce
MS CCCC 41, ff. 350–353

Text and translation

The edition below closely follows Jolly's transcription of the manuscript,[126] adding line breaks and punctuation used by Storms, whose edition is much more faithful to the manuscript than Dobbie's more widely accepted ASPR rendering. Because many of the points in this chapter focused on formulaic language, my translation adheres as closely as possible to the phrasing and sense of the original and reflects consultation of several existing translations. Departures from standard treatment, especially in line 1 and lines 25–30, are explained in the notes and in the preceding chapter.

     Ic me on þisse gyrde beluce   7 on godes helde bebeode.
     Wið þane sara s(t)ice,[127]   wið þane sara slege,
     wið þane grymma gryre,
     wið ðane micela egsa   þe bið eghwam lað,
(5) 7 wið eal þæt lað   þe into land fare.
     Syge gealdor ic begale,   sigegyrd ic me wege,
     wordsige 7 worcsige,   se me dege.
     Ne me mer[128] ne gemyrre,   ne me maga ne geswence,
     ne me næfre minum feore   forht ne gewurþe.
(10) Ac gehæle me ælmihtigi 7 sunu   frofre gast,
     ealles wuldres   wyrdig dryhten,
     swa ic gehyrde   heofna scyppende.
     Abrame 7 Isace   7 swilce men,
     Moyses 7 Iacob,   7 Dauit 7 Iosep,
(15) 7 Evan 7 Annan   7 Elizabet,
     Saharie 7 ec Marie,   modur Cristes,
     7 eac þæ gebroþru   Petrus 7 Paulus,
     7 eac þusend   þira engla
     clipige ic me to are   wið eallum feondum.

(20) Hi me ferion 7 friþion   7 mine fore nerion,
eal me gehealdon,   me[129] gewealdon,
worces stirende.   Si me wuldres hyht,
hand ofer heafod,   haligra rof,
sigerofra sceole,[130]   soðfæstra engla.
(25) Biddu ealle bliðu   mode þæt me beo.
hand ofer heafod,[131]
Matheus helm,   Marcus byrne,
leoht, lifes rof,   Lucos min swurd,
scearp and scir ecg,   scyld Iohannes,
(30) wuldre gewlitegod   wega[132] Serafhin.
Forð ic gefare,   frind ic gemete,
eall engla blæd,   eadiges lare.
Bidde ic nu sigere(s)[133]   godes miltse,
siðfæt godne,   smylte 7 lihte
(35) wind wereþum.   Windas gefran,
circinde wæter.   Simbli gehæle(d)[134]
wið eallum feondum,   freond ic gemete wið,
þæt ic on þis ælmih(t)ian[135] on his frið   wunian mote,
belocun wið þa laþan,   se me lyfes eht,
(40) on engla blæd[136]   gestaþelod,
7 inna halre hand   hofna rices blæd,
þa hwile þe ic on þis life   wunian mote. Amen.

[I encircle myself with this branch[137] and offer myself into the
   keeping[138] of God.
Against the sore pain, against the sore bite,
against the grim horror,
against the great terror that is dreadful to everyone,
(5) and against all evil that goes across the land.
I sing a victory charm, I carry a victory branch;
with victory words and victory deeds, may this avail me.
May no nightmare disturb me, no powerful one trouble me
may nothing dreadful ever come into my life.
(10) But may the almighty one, the son, and the holy ghost save
   me,
the lord worthy of all glory,
such as I heard, the creator of the heavens.

Abraham and Isaac and such men,
Moses and Jacob and David and Joseph,
(15) And Eve and Anne and Elizabeth,
Sarah and also Mary, mother of Christ,
and also the brothers Peter and Paul,
and also a thousand of the angels
I call to myself as a help against all enemies.
(20) They conduct me and protect me and save my life.
They hold me and rule me,
guiding my work. A hope of glory be to me,
hand over head, the valiant holy ones,
the band of victory-saints, righteous angels.
(25) I pray to all, glad in mind
that for me—hand over head—
Matthew may be a helmet, Mark a mailcoat,
light, strong of life; Luke my sword,
sharp and bright edged; John a shield,
(30) wondrously made; Seraphim of the ways.
I go forth; I meet friends,
all the glory of angels, the learning of the blessed ones.
I pray now for mercy of the god of victory,
for a good journey, a calm and light
(35) wind to the shores. I have heard winds,
boiling waters. Always safe
against all foes, I meet with friends,
that I may dwell in peace of the almighty,
guarded against the evil that seeks my life,
(40) established in the glory of angels,
and in the holy hand, the glory of the heavens' kingdom,
as long as I am able to live in this life. Amen.]

Notes

1 *Dictionary of Old English* [DOE], ed. Antonette diPaolo Healey et al., Pontifical Institute of Mediaeval Studies, online edition, http://doe.utoronto.ca. Accessed 15 July 2021. s.v. *gyrd* and *gyrdel*, the latter requiring an emendation of a final 'l'.

2 *DOE*, s.v. *galdor*.
3 See, for instance, Hill's discussion of the poem as it 'corresponds to the liturgy of prayers and blessings offered by the early medieval Church to those who had to undertake dangerous journeys or who went on pilgrimage', or Katrin Rupp's description of the text as 'prayer-like'. Thomas D. Hill, 'The Rod of Protection and the Witches' Ride: Christian and Germanic Syncretism in Two Old English Metrical Charms', *Journal of English and Germanic Philology*, 111 (2012), 145–168, at 155. Katrin Rupp, 'The Anxiety of Writing: A Reading of the Old English Journey Charm', *Oral Tradition*, 23 (2008), 255–266, at 255.
4 On its affinities with the lorica, see, for example, Thomas D. Hill, 'Invocation of the Trinity and the Tradition of the Lorica in Old English Poetry', *Speculum*, 56 (1981), 259–267 and Heather Stuart, '"Ic me on þisse gyrde beluce": The Structure and Meaning of the Old English "Journey Charm"', *Medium Ævum*, 50 (1981), 259–273. Karen Louise Jolly identifies it as 'formula', 'On the Margins of Orthodoxy: Devotional Formulas and Protective Prayers in Cambridge, Corpus Christi College MS 41', in Sarah Larratt Keefer and Rolf H. Bremmer, Jr. (eds), *Signs on the Edge: Space, Text and Margin in Medieval Manuscripts* (Leuven: Peeters, 2007), pp. 135–183, p. 172 *et passim*.
5 As noted above, except where otherwise indicated, quotations from the Old English *Herbarium* follow de Vriend's edition of the British Library MS Cotton Vitellius C.iii. The *Herbarium* is also included in three other manuscripts: Bodleian Library, MS Hatton 76; British Library, MS Harley 585; and British Library, MS Harley 6258B. The brief discussion in this chapter addresses broad patterns shared across all manuscript versions, but for the subtle yet meaningful variation among these manuscripts, see further Chapter 5.
6 M. L. Cameron notes that parallels with Pliny seen in the *Herbarium* 'may imply borrowing, but it may equally be the case that it comes independently from the background common to so much of medieval medicine', *Anglo-Saxon Medicine* (Cambridge: Cambridge University Press, 1993), p. 37. See also a Latin analogue in MS Ca. Montecassino, Archivio della Badia, cited in de Vriend, *Old English Herbarium*, p. 129.
7 Text and translation Pliny, *Natural History* VII, libri XXIV–XXVII, ed. T. E. Page, trans. W. H. S. Jones, Loeb Classical Library (Cambridge, MA: Harvard University Press, 1966), 168–169.
8 See further U. Sellerberg and H. Glasl, whose tests on the efficacy of yarrow extract—especially of flowering material—on blood coagulation yielded positive results. 'Pharmacognostical Examination

Concerning the Hemostyptic Effect of *Achillea millefolium* Aggregat', *Scientia Pharmaceutica*, 68 (2000), 201–206.

9 Wendy L. Applequist and Daniel E. Moerman, 'Yarrow (*Achillea millefolium* L.): A Neglected Panacea? A Review of Ethnobotany, Bioactivity, and Biomedical Research', *Economic Botany*, 65 (2011), 209–225, at 210. Yarrow was among six medicinal plants 'whose pollen was found in a *homo neanderthalensis* grave at Shanidar, dated to 65,000 B.P', p. 210.

10 Ibid., p. 210.

11 Interestingly, *Achillea millefolium* has been shown to hybridize at an especially rapid rate when faced with new ecological environments, the plant itself like the stories it has engendered adapting in new contexts. See Justin Ramsey, Alexander Robertson, and Brian Husband, 'Rapid Adaptive Divergence in New World *Achillea*, an Autopoloyploid Complex of Ecological Races, *Evolution*, 62.3 (2008), pp. 639–653. Many thanks to Rob Laport for this observation.

12 In addition to the two cited above, four more instances of *alii* appear as Pliny continues: 'aliqui et hanc panacem Heracliam, **alii** sideriten et apud nos millefoliam vocant, cubitali scapo, ramosam, minutioribus quam feniculi foliis vestitam ab imo. **alii** fatentur quidem illam vulneribus utilem, sed veram achilleon esse scapo caeruleo pedali, sine ramis, ex omni parte singulis foliis rotundis eleganter vestitam; **alii** quadrato caule, capitulis marrubii, foliis quercus, hac etiam praecisos nervos glutinari. faciunt **alii** et sideritim in maceriis nascentem, cum teratur, foedi odoris, etiamnum aliam similem huic sed candidioribus foliis et pinguioribus, teneriorem cauliculis, in vineis nascentem'. ['This plant is also called by some Heraclean panaces, by **others** siderites, and by us millefolia; the stalk is a cubit high, and the plant branchy, covered from the bottom with leaves smaller than those of fennel. **Others** admit that this plant is good for wounds, but say that the real achilleos has a blue stalk a foot long and without branches, gracefully covered all over with separate, rounded leaves. **Others** describe achilleos as having a square stem, heads like those of horehound, and leaves like those of the oak; they claim that it even unites severed sinews. **Others** give the name sideritis to another plant, which grows on boundary walls and has a foul smell when crushed'. Pliny, *Natural History* VII, pp. 168, 169.

13 This kind of non-judgmental acceptance of variation drawing from traditional stories can also be seen in Book IV, 'De Medicina' ['Of Medicine'], of Isidore of Seville's *Etymologiae*, which acknowledges variant beliefs and stories underlying various remedies through

phrasing such as 'quidam tradunt' ['some say', IV.12.9], and 'credo' ['I believe', IV.9.13]. W. M. Lindsay (ed.), *Isidori Hispalensis Episcopi Etymologiarum Sive Originum*, vol. 1 (Oxford: Oxford University Press, 1911).
14 Applequist and Moerman, 'Yarrow', p. 220.
15 Ibid.
16 Ibid., p. 209.
17 According to Heinrich Härke, shields are among the most commonly buried weapons in the sixth and seventh centuries, found in 45.2% of burials. 'Early Saxon Weapon Burials: Frequencies, Distributions and Weapon Combinations', in Sonia Chadwick Hawkes (ed.), *Weapons and Warfare in Anglo-Saxon England* (Oxford: Oxford University Committee for Archaeology, 1989), pp. 49–61, at 54.
18 Gale R. Owen-Crocker, 'Seldom … does the deadly spear rest for long': Weapons and Armour', in Maren Clegg Hyer and Gale R. Owen-Crocker (eds), *The Material Culture of Daily Living in the Anglo-Saxon World* (Liverpool: Liverpool University Press, 2011), pp. 201–230, at 216. Cf. Richard Underwood's explanation that on a typical shield an 'iron boss, mounted at the centre of the board, covered the grip and protected the knuckles'. *Anglo-Saxon Weapons and Warfare* (Stroud: Tempus, 1999), p. 81.
19 See especially Nicholas Brooks' thorough examination of weapons and armor in *The Battle of Maldon*, Erin Mullally's study of weaponry in *Judith*, and Van Meter's exploration of weapons and warfare in *Beowulf*. In Donald Scragg (ed.), Nicholas Brooks, 'Weapons and Armour', *The Battle of Maldon, A.D. 991* (Oxford: Basil Blackwell, in association with the Manchester Centre for Anglo-Saxon Studies, 1991), pp. 208–219; Erin Mullally, 'The Cross-Gendered Gift: Weaponry in the Old English *Judith*', *Exemplaria*, 17 (2013), 255–284; David C. Van Meter, 'The Ritualized Presentation of Weapons and the Ideology of Nobility in *Beowulf*', *Journal of English and Germanic Philology*, 95 (1996), 175–189.
20 Foley, 'How Genres Leak', p. 79.
21 MS Harley 585, entry 79. Metrical Charm 2 in Dobbie (ed.), *Anglo-Saxon Minor Poems*. ASPR. (See Chapter 4 below for analysis of this poem.) Except where otherwise noted, citations from Harley 585, also known as the *Lacnunga*, are from Edward Pettit's excellent edition, *Anglo-Saxon Remedies*.
22 *Sigewif* could also be understood as singular, possibly referring to the queen. For discussion of this line in relation to beekeeping, see Garner and Miller, 'Swarm', pp. 367–369.

23 On the '*hwæt* paradigm' as a traditional marker, see John Miles Foley, *Immanent Art: From Structure to Meaning in Traditional Oral Epic* (Bloomington, IN: Indiana University Press, 1991), pp. 214–223.
24 The *Lacnunga*, *Herbarium*, and *Leechbooks* all follow this pattern, as the opening remedies of these manuscripts show: 'wið heafodwræce' ('against a headache', *Lacnunga*); 'wið unhyrum nihtgengum' ('against the terrible night-goers', *Herbarium*); 'wið heafodece' ('against a headache', *Leechbook III*).
25 *Dictionary of Old English Plant Names (DOEPN)*, ed. Peter Bierbaumer and Hans Sauer with Helmut W. Klug and Ulrike Krischke. 2007–2009. http://oldenglish-plantnames.org. Accessed 15 July 2021. s.v. *garclife*. Cf. Hans Sauer and Elisabeth Kubaschewski, *Planting the Seeds of Knowledge: An Inventory of Old English Plant Names* (Munich: Herbert Utz Verlag, 2018), p. 220.
26 Except where otherwise noted, citations from the *Leechbook* are from O. Cockayne (ed.), *Leechdoms, Wortcunning, and Starcraft of Early England*, 3 vols (London: Rerum Britannicarum Medii Aevi Scriptores, 1864–66. Reprint 1965).
27 For a complete list of references, see *DOEPN*, s.v. *gar-leac*. The editors clarify that the name refers to the shape of the leaves rather than the garlic root.
28 See *DOEPN*, s.v. *spere-wyrt*. Cf. Sauer and Kubaschewski, *Planting*, p. 220.
29 *DOEPN*, s.v. *strælwyrt*. Cf. Sauer and Kubaschewski, *Planting*, p. 227.
30 Maria Amalia D'Aronco, 'Anglo-Saxon Plant Pharmacy and the Latin Medical Tradition', in C. P. Biggam (ed.), *From Earth to Art: The Many Aspects of the Plant-World in Anglo-Saxon England* (Amsterdam and New York: Rodopi, 2003), pp. 133–151, at p. 144. See also Linda Voigts, who argues that notions of medieval medicine involving 'uncritical copying of antique medical texts must be revised', 'Anglo-Saxon Plant Remedies and the Anglo-Saxons', *Isis*, 70 (1979), 250–268, at 254.
31 The Latin manuscript used for de Vriend's edition and followed here is MS Ca. Montecassino, Archivio della Badia, V. 97. See de Vriend, *Old English Herbarium*, p. 81, MS Ca, entry XXXIII.
32 See de Vriend, *Old English Herbarium*, pp. 80–81 for the manuscript variants as well as a Latin exemplar.
33 M. J. Swanton, *The Spearheads of the Anglo-Saxon Settlements* (London: The Royal Archaeological Institute, 1973), pp. 46, 51.

Notably, the illustration of *astula regia* in the Cotton Vitellius C.iii (Figure 2.2) differs markedly from the corresponding Latin entry in the Monte Cassino, the analogue employed by de Vriend due to the closeness of the texts. Though both illustrations show leaves branching off from the stem, the Monte Cassino shows the leaves in clusters, whereas the leaves of the Old English Cotton Vitellius C.iii far more closely resemble the leaf-shaped spear-heads of Germanic warfare. See Hunger's facsimile of Monte Cassino, Codex casinensis 97, p. 52. Friedrich Wilhelm Hunger (ed.), *The Herbal of Pseudo-Apuleius from the ninth-century manuscript in the abbey of Monte Cassino (Codex Casinensis 97) together with the first printed edition of Joh. Phil. de Lignamine (Editio princeps Romae 1481)* (Leiden: Brill, 1935).
34 Swanton, *Spearheads*, p. 3.
35 Tacitus, *Agricola and Germania*, trans. H. Mattingly, rev. S. A. Handford (New York: Penguin, 1970).
36 See 'The Prayer of Azariah and the Song of the Three Jews' in the non-canonical 'Additions to Daniel', included in the 'Apocrypha' of *The New Oxford Annotated Bible: New Revised Standard Version, with the Apocrypha*, ed. Michael Coogan (Oxford: Oxford University Press, 4th edn, 2010), p. 1543. A version of the verse carved on the knife appears in Daniel 3.35 as part of a litany of praise sung by the three youths in the furnace as they praise God and appeal for help, an especially apt image for an implement that might have been used for rituals connected with healing practice. See also a conjectural drawing of this healer's knife in Stephen Pollington (trans.), *Leechcraft: Early English Charms, Plantlore, and Healing* (Cambridgeshire: Anglo-Saxon Books, 2000), p. 480. The archeological record supports the existence of such handles in actual practice. Kevin Leahy's work on early medieval bone craft tells us that the tangs (the portions of knives that fit into their handles) of some knives 'retain traces left by horn handles with which they were once fitted'. 'Anglo-Saxon Crafts', in Helena Hamerow, David A. Hinton, and Sally Crawford (eds), *The Oxford Handbook of Anglo-Saxon Archaeology* (Oxford: Oxford University Press, 2011), pp. 440–459, at 449.
37 Underwood, *Anglo-Saxon Weapons*, p. 13.
38 J. Manley, 'The Archer and the Army in the Late Saxon Period', *Anglo-Saxon Studies in Archaeology and History*, 4 (1985), 223–235, at p. 223. This is not to say that specialized spears, arrows, and knives created with battle purposes in mind did not exist, but rather that specialized weapons were less widely accessible and that these objects were frequently multi-use. Nicholas Brooks explains that 'as

a standard tool in general use the knife (*seax*) in warfare developed into a single-edged dagger (known by Gregory of Tours as the *scramasax*) or into fine-edged swords, with blades up to 80 cm in length', 'Arms and Armour', in M. Lapidge, J. Blair, and D. Scragg (eds), *The Blackwell Encyclopedia of Anglo-Saxon England* (Oxford: Blackwell Publishers, 1999), pp. 45–47, at p. 46.
39 Brooks, 'Arms', p. 46.
40 David A. Gale, 'The Seax', in Sonia Chadwick Hawkes (ed.), *Weapons and Warfare in Anglo-Saxon England* (Oxford: Oxford University Committee for Archaeology, 1989), pp. 71–84, at p. 80.
41 Underwood, *Anglo-Saxon Weapons*, p. 71.
42 l. 2703. In addition, Grendel's mother uses a *seax* against Beowulf, though he is protected by his mail-shirt (l. 1545). Her choice of weapon is appropriate for both her status as female and her assumed role as avenging warrior.
43 The journey has frequently been understood as metaphorical. See, for instance, Lea Olsan, 'The Marginality of Charms in Medieval England', in James Kapaló, Éva Pócs, and William Ryan (eds), *The Power of Words: Studies on Charms and Charming in Europe* (Budapest: Central European University Press, 2013), pp. 135–164, at p. 149, and Stuart, 'Ic me', p. 268. My reading of its weaponry is compatible with either literal or metaphorical travel, and I firmly believe that it might have been interpreted either way in its early medieval contexts as well.
44 Richard Marsden, 'Biblical Literature: The New Testament', in Malcolm Godden and Michael Lapidge (eds), *The Cambridge Companion to Old English Literature* (Cambridge: Cambridge University Press, 2013), pp. 234–250, at 235.
45 This poem appears in the outer margins of ff. 350–353.
46 Grendon, 'Anglo-Saxon Charms', p. 176.
47 Ibid., p. 177.
48 Jolly, 'Margins', p. 170.
49 Hill, 'Invocation', p. 264. This generic designation was first proposed by Grattan and Singer, though it is Hill's argumentation that demonstrates the larger significance of this Celtic influence on early medieval English literature. J. H. Grattan and Charles Singer, *Anglo-Saxon Magic and Medicine* (Oxford: Oxford University Press, 1952), p. 70. Embedded within the *Lacnunga* (Harley 585, to be discussed further in Chapter 4) is the poem 'Lorica of Lodgen' (ff. 152–157r), suggesting an affinity between medical texts and loricae for early medieval compilers.

50 E.g., Grendon, *Anglo-Saxon Charms*; Dobbie, *Anglo-Saxon Minor Poems*; Grattan and Singer, *Anglo-Saxon Magic and Medicine*; Storms, *Anglo-Saxon Magic*; Louis J. Rodrigues (ed. and trans.), *Anglo-Saxon Verse Charms, Maxims and Heroic Legends* (Middlesex: Anglo-Saxon Books, 1993).
51 Jolly, 'Margins', p. 139.
52 Sarah Larratt Keefer, 'Margin as Archive: The Liturgical Marginalia of a Manuscript of the Old English Bede', *Traditio*, 51 (1996), 147–177.
53 Jolly, 'Margins', p. 146.
54 Ibid., p. 146 (emphasis added).
55 Ibid., p. 170, n. 141.
56 Olsan, 'Inscription', p. 403.
57 Forms of *galdor* or *gealdor* appear no fewer than twenty times in the remedies collectively.
58 Arthur, *'Charms'*, p. 13.
59 Ibid., p. 93.
60 Text: Thomas Miller (ed. and trans.), *The Old English Version of Bede's Ecclesiastical History of the English People* (London: Early English Text Society, 1890), p. 362. Translation: Colgrave and Mynors, *Bede's* Ecclesiastical History, p. 433 (emphasis added).
61 Benjamin Thorpe (ed. and trans.), *The Homilies of the Anglo-Saxon Church*, vol. 1 (London: Richard and John Taylor, 1844), p. 476.
62 Jolly, 'Margins', p. 146.
63 Ibid., p. 146.
64 Ibid., p. 170.
65 Ibid., pp. 146–147.
66 See further Rupp, 'Anxiety of Writing', esp. p. 263.
67 Jolly, 'Margins', p. 171.
68 *DOE*, s.v. *gyrd*.
69 E.g., Bosworth and Toller, s.v. *oman*.
70 This gloss, 'to score around', from Bosworth and Toller (s.v. *bewritan*).
71 e.g., Rodrigues, *Anglo-Saxon Verse Charms*, p. 157; Jolly, 'Margins', p. 171; Arnovick, *Written Reliquaries*, p. 102); Sirr, in Greg Delanty, and Michael Matto (eds), *The Word Exchange: Anglo-Saxon Poems in Translation* (New York: Norton, 2012), p. 495; Rupp, 'Anxiety of Writing', p. 256; Arthur, *'Charms'*, p. 94; Grendon, 'Anglo-Saxon Charms', p. 177; Hill, 'Rod', p. 148.
72 Alongside 'protection', Bosworth and Toller offer 'allegiance' or 'fealty', with the sense of being 'locked' in fealty with reciprocal protection.
73 On this choice, Andrew Rabin writes that he prefers 'the more forceful "rule" or "authority", given the term's etymological link to *healdan*

("govern" or "protect")', 'The Wolf's Testimony to the English: Law and the Witness in the "Sermo Lupi ad Anglos"', *Journal of English and Germanic Philology*, 15.3 (2006), 388–414, at p. 395.
74 Book 4, Ch. 30, Colgrave and Mynors, *Bede's* Ecclesiastical History.
75 James Paz, *Nonhuman Voices in Anglo-Saxon Literature and Material Culture* (Manchester: Manchester University Press, 2017), p. 19.
76 Ibid., p. 27.
77 Marsden, for instance, observes that these 'military metaphors convey the key idea of the spiritual fight which the true wayfaring Christian [...] must wage', and John Hermann refers to these lines as 'an Old English poetic version of the Pauline figure of spiritual armor' (38). Marsden, 'Biblical Literature', p. 235; John P. Hermann, *Allegories of War: Language and Violence in Old English Poetry* (Ann Arbor, MI: University of Michigan Press, 1989), p. 38.
78 Text from Latin vulgate: 'State ergo succincti lumbos vestros in veritate, et induti loricam justitiae, et calceati pedes in praeparatione Evangelii pacis, in omnibus sumentes scutum fidei, in quo possitis omnia tela nequissimi ignea extinguere: et galeam salutis assumite, et gladium spiritus (quod est verbum Dei)'. Translation quoted from Arnovick, *Written Reliquaries*, p. 116.
79 Arnovick, *Written Reliquaries*, p. 116.
80 John Hines, for instance, reminds us that the deceased in these graves 'would appear to be those who did not die on the battlefield, and their weapons, to judge by the criterion of cuts, seem normally to have been unused'. Grave goods, he argues, 'may well represent symbolic rather than practicable weapon assemblages'. 'The Military Context of *Adventus Saxonum*: Some Continental Evidence', in Sonia Chadwick Hawkes (ed.), *Weapons and Warfare in Anglo-Saxon England* (Oxford: Oxford University Committee for Archaeology, 1989), pp. 25–48, at 26, 36.
81 Owen-Crocker, 'Seldom', p. 210.
82 Heinrich Härke, '"Warrior Graves"? The Background of the Anglo-Saxon Weapon Burial Rite', *Past and Present*, 126 (1990), 22–43, at p. 24, 34.
83 Ibid., p. 26.
84 Owen-Crocker, 'Seldom', p. 219.
85 Ibid., p. 226.
86 Ibid.
87 Härke, 'Circulation of Weapons in Anglo-Saxon Society', in Frans Theuws and Janet L. Nelson (eds), *Rituals of Power* (Leiden: Brill, 2000), pp. 377–399, at p. 388.

88 Ibid., pp. 377, 380.
89 Ibid., p. 385.
90 Olsan, 'Marginality', p. 149.
91 Jolly, 'Margins', p. 138. Jolly notes that the 'possibility of a female house cannot be excluded'. (p. 138). On women's writing within monastic communities in early medieval England, see Diane Watt, *Women, Writing and Religion in England and Beyond, 650–1100* (London: Bloomsbury, 2020), esp. pp. 21–39.
92 Jolly, 'Margins', p. 139.
93 F. Holthausen, 'Zu Altenglischen Dichtungen', *Beiblatt zur Anglia XXXI*, 31 (1920), 25–32, p. 31; cited in Dobbie (ed.), *Anglo-Saxon Minor Poems*, p. 218.
94 E.g., www.oepoetry.ca/ (accessed 12 January 2021) and www.sacred-texts.com/neu/ascp/a43_11.htm (accessed 2 February 2021).
95 Dobbie, *Anglo-Saxon Minor Poems*, p. 218.
96 Marsden accepts Dobbie's emendation, translating as 'deadly spear', 'Biblical Literature', p. 235. Stuart provides the emended ASPR reading in the text of her article, but in an endnote expresses reservations about Dobbie's reading, which 'although quoted here is not accepted as suitable', p. 273. Judith Vaughan-Sterling gives the text as *wælgar* and includes this line as part of larger point about the poem's 'penchant for heroic imagery', 'The Anglo-Saxon *Metrical Charms*: Poetry as Ritual', *Journal of English and Germanic Philology*, 82 (1983), 186–200, at 190; Lois Bragg likewise translates as 'Seraphim my spear', noting in her analysis 'the depiction of the four evangelists and the seraphim as armor and weapons', 'The Modes of the Old English Metrical Charms', *Comparatist*, 16 (1992), 3–23, at 16–17; S. A. J. Bradley's is one of numerous translations following the emendation, 'my spear', *Anglo-Saxon Poetry* (London: J. M. Dent, 1982), p. 549. The potential for confusion and misreading is especially apparent in Peter Sirr's dual-language edition in the widely available anthology edited by Delanty and Matto, *The Word Exchange: Anglo-Saxon Poems in Translation*. The Old English text here gives the emended form '**wælgar**' in bold, consistent with a common online manner of indicating that an emendation of some sort has occurred; the facing-page translation, however, gives 'path', which would seem to follow the manuscript *wega* instead, pp. 496–497. Clearly, more consistency and greater understanding are needed with regard to these lines.
97 *Egil's Saga*, for instance, describes both Egil and his opponent Berg-Onund as carrying a spear or hauberk in one hand while also girded with a sword. For a modern English translation of this passage, see

Egil's Saga, Bernard Scudder (trans.), (New York: Penguin, 1997), pp. 116–117.
98 Swanton, *Spearheads*, p. 3.
99 Owen-Crocker, 'Seldom', p. 205.
100 Ibid., p. 205.
101 Hill, 'Rod', p. 149.
102 Stuart, 'Ic me', p. 273.
103 Or, as Storms translates, 'Seraphim of the roads', *Anglo-Saxon Magic*, pp. 218–219.
104 Though a full treatment of this reading is somewhat outside the scope of the present analysis, see Grendon and Storms for examples of translators presenting the seraphim in apposition with John. Grendon, who retains manuscript *wega*, saw the military language employed with respect to the gospel authors as sufficient for the context, claiming that the Germanic 'notion of God's kingdom as a military power can easily be recognized in these suggestive metaphors', Grendon, 'Anglo-Saxon Charms', pp. 179, 149; Storms, *Anglo-Saxon Magic*, p. 219.
105 *Maxims I*, l. 144.
106 The emendation is frequently accepted in scholarship on the this poem (e.g., Stuart, 'Ic me', p. 262; Hill, 'Rod', p. 147; Rupp, 'Anxiety of Writing', p. 259; Vaughan-Sterling, 'Anglo-Saxon', p. 190), as well as editions (e.g., Rodrigues, *Anglo-Saxon Verse Charms*, pp. 156–157). Unlike words or characters that are added or modified, an omission cannot be italicized or put in bold and thus frequently leaves no trace. The 'hand ofer heafod' perceived as extra is left untranslated without comment, for instance, in R. K. Gordon, *Anglo-Saxon Poetry* (London: Everyman, 1954), p. 91, and also Sirr's dual-language version in Delanty and Matto, *Word Exchange*, pp. 496–497.
107 Grendon, 'Anglo-Saxon Charms', p. 221. Krapp and Dobbie, *Exeter Book*, p. 217.
108 See, for instance, Hill, 'Rod', p. 148.
109 Bill Griffiths, *Aspects of Anglo-Saxon Magic* (Norfolk: Anglo-Saxon Books, 1996), p. 202.
110 Foley, 'Hybrid Prosody', p. 284.
111 Ibid., 287.
112 Anne Klinck, *The Old English Elegies: A Critical Edition and Genre Study* (Montreal: McGill-Queen's University Press, 1992), p. 114. See further the treatments of this half-line by Leslie and Tupper: R. F. Leslie (ed.), *The Wanderer* (Manchester: Manchester University Press, 1966), p. 74; Frederick Tupper, 'Notes on Old English Poems', *Journal of English and Germanic Philology*, 11 (1912), 82–103, at pp. 97–100.

In *Egil's Saga* as well, we see a ritual greeting that involves Egil approaching a king in a gesture of humility. He lowers his head and embraces the king's feet, an act which would presumably require one or both hands to be placed above his head (chapter 60).

113 Tupper, 'Notes', p. 100. Tupper translates the relevant lines as follows: 'In sanguine mood I solicit, that mine be sovereign protection: Matthew my helmet [...]'.

114 Arnovick, *Written Reliquaries*, pp. 115–116.

115 Jolly has noted that the CCCC 41 participates in 'a larger pattern of liturgical/medicinal behavior', shared by the *Lacnunga* and *Leechbooks*, which similarly 'borrow Latin prayers from liturgical and devotional books to use for specific ills', 'Margins', p. 167.

116 Tupper, 'Notes', p. 98.

117 Grendon speculates about this possibility but does not fully pursue it: 'The passage is obscure. Can it refer to a lifting of the hand over the head, an attitude that might have traditionally accompanied certain prayers? Elevation of the hands while praying was common enough' ('Anglo-Saxon Charms', p. 221).

118 On the *orans* pose, see Megan Henvey, 'Crossing Borders: Re-Assessing the "Need to Group" the High Crosses in Ireland', in Cynthia Thickpenny, Katherine Forsyth, J Geddes, and Kate Mathis (eds), *Peopling Insular Art: Practice, Performance, Perception: Proceedings of the Eighth International Conference on Insular Art, Glasgow 2017* (Oxford: Oxbow Books, 2020), pp. 179–187, at 181.

119 Tianjun Liu (ed. and trans.), *Chinese Medical Qigong* (London: Singing Dragon, 2010), p. 42.

120 Shoshanna Katzman, *Qigong for Staying Young* (New York: Penguin, 2003), p. 63.

121 Peter M. Wayne, with Mark L. Fuerst, *The Harvard Medical School Guide to Tai Chi* (Boston: Shambhala Publications, Inc., 2013), p. 81. Many thanks to Marjean Liggett for help with these connections.

122 Paul Bradshaw, 'Difficulties in Doing Liturgical Theology', *Pacifica*, 11 (1998), 181–194, at 181.

123 Ibid., p. 194.

124 Klaeber, for instance, suggested the interpretation Kreuzes-stab, '*Belucan* in dem altenglischen Reisesegen', *Beiblatt zur Anglia*, 40 (1929), 283–284.

125 Carol Braun Pasternack, 'Post-Structuralist Theories: The Subject and the Text', in Katherine O'Brien O'Keeffe (ed.), *Reading Old English Texts* (Cambridge: Cambridge University Press, 1997), pp. 170–191, at 177.

126 Jolly, 'Margins', pp. 170–171.
127 Manuscript *sice*.
128 Frequently emended to *mere*.
129 Manuscript *men*.
130 Manuscript *sceote*.
131 This rendering retains the manuscript reading of this much debated line, which is discussed at length in the present chapter.
132 As is discussed in the chapter above, ms *wega* here is frequently emended without comment to *wælgar*.
133 Jolly explains that 'sigere', emended by Dobbie and Storms to *sigeres*, is 'the same colour as the margin text, perhaps added later. The "d" of "godes" is dark, as if overwritten or corrected later'. 'Margins' 171, n. 146.
134 Manuscript *gehælepe*.
135 Storms emends to *ælmihtian*. See Jolly, 'Margins', 171, n. 149.
136 Manuscript *bla blæd*.
137 The *DOE* offers the following as its first definition (1.a.) for *gyrd*: 'long straight slender shoot or branch growing upon or cut from a tree, bush, etc.; twig, stick'. Though most translations of this text have rendered *gyrde* as something closer to 1.b ('stick or pole') or 1.b.i ('rod or staff'), I am opting for the primary sense here, which aligns with the contexts of herbal healing suggested later in the text. A smaller number have read *gyrde* here as 'girdle'. As an object encircling the speaker, this meaning would not be inconsistent with the interpretation put forth in this chapter, and it is quite possible that the poem's earliest readers might have read this multivalent word in all of these ways.
138 This particular text is provided as an example (referred to as 'Metrical Charm 11', following the numbering in Dobbie's ASPR edition) in the *DOE* under sense 2 (s.v. *hyld*), safekeeping. See further the discussion on this choice found earlier in this chapter.

3

When healers are heroes: hybridity of battle in *Wið færstice*

Sæt smið, sloh seax.

[A smith sat, forged a knife.]

(*Wið færstice*, l. 11)

Bogan wæron bysige. Bord ord onfeng.

[Bows were busy. Shield caught point.]

(*Battle of Maldon*, l. 110)

The remedy commonly known as *Wið færstice* ['Against a Sudden Pain'], which appears in Harley 585 (*Lacnunga*, entry cxxvii), evidences the fundamental hybridity of form and function also found in *Ic me on þisse gyrde beluce*. Like the protective formula of CCCC 41's marginalia, *Wið færstice* employs powerful war imagery; however, this more explicitly medical text depicts not the individual, idealized warrior on a solitary journey, but rather an all-out battle fought with a full artillery of the most common weaponry found in early medieval England. Nevertheless, the remedy's prose instructions and verse incantation venture beyond the mere fear of adversity and provide a path to confront the reality of severe and sudden pain. Through its combination of herbs, rituals, and poetry, this deeply hybrid remedy offers and enacts empowerment in the face of suffering.

Wið færstice opens simply enough with a prose assertion of the remedy's purpose against sudden pain and a list of three herbs to boil in butter. Next comes a 26-line poem in alliterative verse, presumably an incantation, narrating a fierce attack of approaching female riders and the speaker's own attempts at retaliation;

following the poem there is then a final brief command to dip a knife in liquid. On its surface this entry might seem rather uncomplicated, but its precise interpretation has actually been far from straightforward. Stephen Glosecki once observed that 'quibbles creep in over almost every line of this lyrical charm',[1] with much of the debate connected to the poem's treatment of weaponry. Similarly, Thomas Hill explains that 'there are many phrases and even whole lines of the charm which are wholly opaque',[2] and Alaric Hall notes that the text has 'challenged scholars since the nineteenth century'.[3] A significant portion of this text's mystery revolves around the relationship of the incantation to the herbal preparation; the poetic incantation of *Wið færstice*, fraught with images of war, is so seemingly disconnected from the rest of this otherwise unremarkable preparation of an herbal salve that some have argued for it to be analyzed in complete separation from the remedy as a whole,[4] and the incantation's value has too often been reduced to vestiges of 'primitive' magic.[5] Where the previous chapter argued that warfare and healing are integrally connected through the hybridity of the Old English healing tradition, this chapter extends the implications of such linkages, arguing that the incantation and herbal preparation of *Wið færstice* actually work closely in tandem, effectually enacting a full-fledged battle between healer and ailment. In short, neither the ritual nor the incantation is complete in isolation. Rather, the two modes converge in an essentially hybrid remedy. The whole being more than the sum of its parts, the two enigmatic components complement and reinforce one another, establishing a unified front against the sudden affliction.

The goals of the following exploration are twofold: 1) to more precisely discern what the poem's medical battle means in terms of actual Germanic weaponry and warfare, and 2) to create a text and translation of the Harley 585 entry that renders visible the significant patterns linking healing, ritual, and warfare. As I hope to show, considering the poem's weapons quite literally, with an interpretation grounded in archaeological evidence, not only helps resolve seeming ambiguities in the poem, but also reveals a coherent logic underlying the remedy's healing power, one that powerfully links the cryptic incantation to the surrounding instructions for herbal preparation. Accordingly, the text and translation in the appendix reflect this chapter's reading and create a framework for future analysis, underscoring the parallels between the ritual and the incantation as well as parallel structures within the incantation itself. The methodologies here thus rely heavily upon not only archaeological approaches to early medieval England—such as were important in the previous chapter—but also scholarship in ethnopoetics, in particular that which has stemmed from Del Hymes' belief that part of our responsibility as scholars of verbal art deriving from oral tradition is to produce rhetorical analyses, texts, and translations that reflect the cultural expectations and traditions in play.[6]

In his own experimental ethnopoetic transcription of the opening of *Beowulf*, John Foley freely acknowledged that we will of course never be able to recover the exact relationship of any text on the manuscript page and its active performance in early medieval England; nonetheless, he argued that we 'can't afford to ignore the expressive dimensions' emerging from its connection to oral tradition.[7] In the case of Old English medical texts, characterized by frequent commands to speak and sing during the preparation and performance of healing and protective practices, the importance of recovering such links seems even more urgent. As can be seen in the pages that follow, the patterns in *Wið færstice* that emerge are deeply meaningful, revealing a concept of healing far more logical and consistent than has sometimes been assumed. The implications for the editing, translation, and interpretation of not only *Wið færstice* but also other equally enigmatic texts are thus potentially quite significant and wide-reaching. To this end, the analysis here begins by confronting a series of thorny questions raised by the poem through a combined awareness of the remedy's underlying poetics and the realities of medieval battle from which it draws.

The chaos of early battle and poetic ambiguity: lines 1–10

The first stage of the battle in this poetic incantation is, quite naturally, an attack from approaching enemies, in this case 'mihtigan wif' ['mighty women'] (l. 6): 'Hlude wæran hy, la, hlude, ða hy ofer þone hlæw ridan' ['Loud were they, lo, loud, when they rode over the mound'] (l. 1). The folk epidemiology underlying this and many other Old English remedies assumes that ailments without otherwise known causes result from attacks of 'invisible or hard-to-see creatures who shot their victims with some kind of arrow or spear',[8] so the riders can easily be interpreted as the implied source of pain. Not to be defeated in this medical battle, the healer in turn orders the sufferer to 'Scyld ðu ðe nu' ['Shield yourself now'] (l. 3). However, the specifics of the battle that ensues have been much debated.

Stod under linde: who is under the shield?

The next half-line, 'stod under linde' ['stood under a (linden) shield'[9]] (l. 5), has raised many questions about the narrative context, since 'stod' can designate third or first person and can thus be variously translated as 'I stood' or 'he/she/it stood'.[10] Parallels in historical and literary battles, however, suggest that this ambiguity would not have been as problematic for early medieval audiences as for modern scholarship, and that such confusion arguably contributes to the battle's realism. For instance, this opening battle of the healer against the mighty women is paralleled by the *Battle of Maldon*'s description of the historic 991 battle against a Viking invasion, a battle that also begins in earnest with a fierce exchange of flying arrows and spears, and protection from wooden shields: 'Bogan wæron bysige. Bord ord onfeng' ['Bows were busy. Shield caught point'] (l. 110). Just as the metrical incantation does not specify who is under the shield, *Maldon* does not specify whose shield caught whose point, the seeming implication being that in this early stage of fighting arrows and spears are flying everywhere and each side is shielding itself from the other. The subject could be the speaker, any warrior (male or female), or even a supernatural being (in the case that the subject is understood as 'it').

While such specifics remain uncertain, what is most important is the fierceness of this initial onslaught: 'Biter wæs se beaduræs' ['Bitter was the attack'] (l. 111). Nicholas Brooks' discussion of weaponry in *Maldon* notes that 'preliminary bombardments' occurred 'before the two armies closed for hand-to-hand fighting' and that 'the practice was to reuse the enemy's projectiles;'[11] this strategy is also paralleled in the speaker's oath that 'him oðerne eft wille sændan' ['I will send them another back'] (l. 8). In a context of actual warfare, the ambiguity of the subjectless *stod*—retained in the appendix's translation—grammatically contributes to the chaos in a fierce and fast-paced battle where individuals are difficult to distinguish from one another and everyone on both sides is presumably seeking protection from shields.

Gar, flan, speru: who is fighting with what, and does it matter?

Another source of confusion in the poem lies in the relative interchangeability of terms such as 'darts', 'javelins', and 'arrows' to refer to its missile weapons, a feature also shared with *Maldon*. The speaker, for instance, returns *garas* ['spears'] (l. 7) with a *flane* ['arrow'] (l. 9); *Maldon*, too, intensifies the chaos of early battle through the inclusion of flying *speru* (l. 108) and *garas* (l. 109), as well as the 'flanes flyht' ['flight of arrow'] (l. 71) and Æscferð's shooting of a *flan* (l. 269). The Old English poem *Judith*, which notably also includes both male and female fighters, similarly exhibits this kind of alternation, as the battle between the Bethulians and Assyrians begins with archery, the missiles flying from hornbows variously referred to as a *flan, gar*, and *stræl* (ll. 220–224):

>   Hie ða fromlice
> leton forð fleogan   flana scuras,
> hildenædran   of hornbogan,
> strælas stedehearde;   styrmdon hlude
> grame guðfrecan,   garas sendon [...].
>
> [Then they quickly
> let showers of arrows [*flana*] fly forth,
> battle-adders, from the hornbows,
> hard arrows [*strælas*]; grim warriors
> loudly raged, sent spears [*garas*]...].

This interchangeability not only gives poets of these and other texts flexibility with regard to alliterative requirements; the variation on kinds of arrows and throwing spears also adds to the sense of chaos that each of these texts conveys during missile warfare, a chaos that beautifully parallels the mixing and boiling of the diverse herbs being prepared in *Wið færstice*,[12] as reflected in the parallel columns through which the text is presented in the appendix at the end of this chapter. When these parallels are viewed in terms of physical/verbal hybridity, the emergent ritual acquires a coherence heretofore seen as lacking and, far more importantly, manifests a powerful and holistic sense of healing purpose.

Hy gyllende garas sændan: who/what is yelling?

The chaotic tension of missile warfare in the poem is furthered by the syntactical ambiguity in its description of the attack in which 'hy gyllende garas sændan' (literally, 'they yelling spears sent', l. 7), where *gyllende* could easily modify either the mighty women or the spears they sent, both being possible renderings in the context of battle in early medieval England.[13] The lines above in *Judith*, for instance, offer one of many examples of fierce warriors approaching loudly, *hlude* (l. 223). Thus, the women could indeed be yelling, but perhaps even more plausible in the context of early medieval battle patterns is that the flying spears and arrows are themselves *gyllende*. John Manley notes that while some Germanic cultures did employ archery at close-range, in early medieval England bows and arrows were used more regularly for long-range fighting,[14] and, of course, the longer an arrow remains in the air, the stronger, faster, and louder it becomes, making this image quite apt for the arrows flying from approaching—but still somewhat distant—attackers. Alaric Hall supports his own translation 'shrieking spears' with evidence from *Widsið*, which offers the half-line 'giellende gar' (l. 128).[15] In the context of the battle chaos being depicted, either reading is appropriate, and, as Edward Pettit has stated, 'an oral performance might well exploit the potential ambiguity of the syntax and render both senses available at the same time'.[16]

But the more important aspect to keep in mind here is that literary and historical evidence suggests the missile weapons so prominent in the early lines of *Wið færstice* are being used specifically to mark an enemy's approach and the beginning of battle. Richard Underwood explains that 'before battle lines joined and warriors risked all', warriors in early medieval England 'would attempt to thin the enemy ranks with missiles. This would begin with archery'.

Hybridity of battle in Wið færstice 103

This strategy then eventually led 'to the hand-to-hand combat'.[17] If we think of archery and the use of projectile weapons as preliminary to close combat (if the spears are yelling) and bear in mind that yelling would also be appropriate for warriors approaching from a distance (if the women are yelling), the poem's next section, involving weapons best employed at close range, becomes less an abstract metaphor of fighting illness and more a precise tactical choice in seeking close contact with sources of pain only after careful preparation.

Close fighting, close reading: lines 11–24

In its second half, the incantation of *Wið færstice* shifts the focus from flying and hurled weapons used at a distance to those that require close proximity, most particularly knives and spears. This portion of the poem is then paralleled by instructions to dip a knife in liquid, presumably the previously described herbal salve intended for application to the site of pain. But, just as in the earlier half of the remedy, this later section also presents interpretative ambiguities.

*Sæt smith / syx smiðas sætan:
whose side(s) are these smiths on?*

In lines 11–14, the poem introduces first a single smith and later six smiths forging weapons appropriate for close fighting. This section of the poem has caused much debate as to which side these smiths are assisting. Glosecki, for instance, argues that all of the smiths are 'forgers of pain',[18] whereas Storms asserts that the individual smith and the group of smiths are all forging weapons on behalf of the healer.[19] Minna Doskow makes a strong case for seeing a division of the smiths 'into two groups, the single good one followed by the six evil ones'.[20] In fact, all of these readings are quite plausible. If we continue to see the battle as relatively balanced between two sides, however, then it can perhaps become easier to accept the persistent ambiguity presented in the text. In a battle with opposing forces applying a shared set of tactical strategies, it would be expected for both sides to then follow the initial exchange of missile weapons with similarly balanced preparations for the next stage of battle, hand-to-hand combat. With each successive stage of battle, the very indeterminacy that precludes clear distinctions between opposing sides brings into sharper focus a reciprocal relationship binding the healer's remedy to the pain it seeks to lessen.

Lytel iserna: iron knife or small sword?

Another much-discussed question regarding this section of the text involves precisely what weapon the first smith is forging. The manuscript reads, 'sæt smið sloh seax lytel iserna' [lit., 'a smith sat, forged a *seax*, small, of iron(s)']. As with the protective poem in the margins of CCCC 41, assumptions of scribal error have led to editing and translation choices that are arguably unnecessary and that sometimes work against the specific type of battle set up by the poem's elaborate imagery.[21] As Figure 3.1 below shows, there is no indication of omitted material between *lytel* and *iserna*.

Nonetheless, in an attempt to correct perceived irregularities in the meter, Grendon set a powerful precedent by editing the lines with inserted ellipses as follows:

    sæt smið   sloh seax lytel
    ... iserna   wund swiðe

Dobbie later retained the same ellipses, and subsequent editors have even inserted 'wæpen' as an alliterating element with 'wund'.[22]

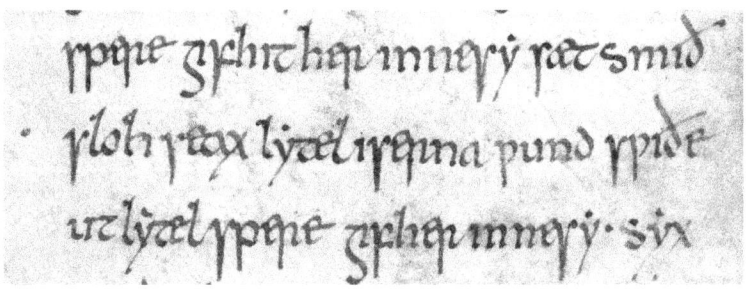

Figure 3.1 *Lacnunga* entry, lines 11–12. British Library MS Harley 585, f. 175v.

As an alternative to these rather heavy-handed emendations, the reading of this portion as 'little knife of iron parts',[23] an interpretation followed by Doane[24] and later Pettit—who states that '*lytel iserna* seems to be in apposition to *seax*'[25]—is most in line with the poetics of weaponry and is the form thus presented in the edited text of the appendix here. In this rendering, '*lytel iserna*' qualifies what type of *seax* is being forged, since, as noted in the previous chapter, size could vary significantly. This reading also meshes with the perspective of Pettit, who on the grounds of metrics and performance argues that the tendency of some scholars to see *lytel* as instead directly modifying, and thus placed on the line with, *seax*, 'spoils the line's massed and balanced *s-* alliteration' and 'the exact syllabic balance' of the two half-lines.[26]

As Glosecki has aptly noted, the incantation is 'obviously a performance poem' characterized by 'rhythmic utterance' and 'balance'.[27] However, if we accept A. J. Bliss's argument for the integrity of the half-line as a viable—albeit uncommon—metrical unit rather than an abnormality driven by error, the manuscript reading is still quite viable without overly disrupting the performative balance.[28] But perhaps more importantly, the manuscript reading is also completely in keeping with the underlying battle ethos of the poem. If we see *lytel iserna* in apposition with *seax*, we can understand the line thus: 'a smith sat, forged a knife, a small one, [made] of iron pieces'. Since the *seax* 'occurred in long and short varieties (54–76 cm and 8–36 cm respectively)',[29] the designation of the iron as '*lytel*' could potentially be quite important in clarifying the nature of the *seax* being forged and indicating precisely what type of combat was forthcoming. And certainly little pieces of iron being forged together in a *seax* could also serve as a helpful reminder to continue mixing the herbs, which in turn will be 'forged' into weapons of healing.

A more literal, archeology-based reading of this poetic battle can also help resolve another source of confusion in the line—the precise meaning of *iserna*, which has been translated by some as the material iron and by others as a metonymic reference to swords.[30] But the specific battle context here—which employs common rather than elite weaponry—would argue strongly for a small knife made of iron, thus also remaining true to the grammatical case of the genitive *iserna*, rather than for a 'sword'. While it is possible that the poem is invoking a sword as a symbol of elite power (or that some audiences may have understood the multivalent text in this way), all other evidence in the poetic battle would seem to suggest a much more common mode of warfare, one fought with the spears, bows, arrows, and knives that would have been widely available to a far greater number.

In this way, the weaponry serves as an equalizing element across opposing groups, reaffirming the reciprocal and balanced nature in the poetic battle between the 'mihtigan wif' ['mighty women'] and the healer, who, in the first stage of battle, exchange equally powerful missile weapons. If the next stage of battle also remains balanced, with smiths forging on both sides, a *sword* is less likely than an iron *seax*, a tool/weapon more widely available to all social classes and frequently carried by women as well as men.[31] Noting parallels of female agency linking the metrical charms with the epic *Beowulf*, Sara Frances Burdorff observes that the *seax* of *Wið færstice* is 'the same weapon Grendel's mother wields against Beowulf'.[32] Spears, too, seem to have been at least somewhat less gendered than swords, and there is evidence for small spears being worn and carried by women as trinkets,[33] making the *wælspera* (the 'slaughter spears' that are depicted as being forged a few lines later in the poem) and knives an especially likely combination of weapons in this battle with approaching female riders as it escalates from missile warfare to direct combat.[34]

The power of repetition and the promise of healing

Interspersed sporadically throughout the poetic incantation, various forms of the phrase 'ut lytel spere' ['out, little spear'] appear (ll. 4, 10, 13, 15). This spacing of a refrain may seem to lack regularity, inconsistently repeated as it appears to be. In fact, the seemingly random appearance of lines invoking the 'lytel spere' at lines 4, 10, 13, and 15 has led to perceptions of a structural 'irregularity' that 'leaves much to be desired'.[35] However, when we keep in mind the poem's systematic progression toward hand-to-hand fighting with spears and knives, the refrain's spacing acquires a clear and compelling logic. These imperatives, directed toward the singular, specific source of the pain (the little spear), punctuate the incantation with increasing frequency, first with five lines between refrains, then two, and, finally, just one. The refrains thus serve as increasingly urgent reminders of the battle's most important goal, to send the source of pain away and thus restore balance and healing to the suffering victim. The refrain is indented in the text of the appendix to highlight this important pattern.

Also, on a practical level, as Cameron explains, incantations that 'appear superficial' could often serve time-keeping functions in the absence of modern watches and clocks, ensuring that herbs or liquids were boiled or mixed for the proper amount of time.[36] Martha Bayless's experimental work with medieval methods of bread-making, for instance, demonstrates the practicality of timing in units of *Pater Nosters*.[37] In the case of Wið færstice, the timing of the incantation is far from random and operates meaningfully at both the figurative and literal levels: in the context of the narrated battle, the increasing anticipation of the final, decisive stage of close fighting corresponds to the diminishing poetic space between refrains. And while this figurative battle is being narrated through the incantation, the actual herbs are presumably still boiling in the butter, coming closer and closer to fruition as an herbal salve; the compression of the refrains as the incantation continues could thus serve as an audible reminder to the practitioner of when to end the preparation and apply the salve. Such a method of reminding is still quite powerful even today, similar in some ways to the increasing frequency of alerts on some car models when gas is running low, or on alarm clocks that increase in volume and frequency the longer one continues to snooze.

In the context of these increasingly frequent reminders that the battle's climax is now approaching, the assurance of aid following the final recitation of the refrain thus becomes recognizable as a powerful *beot*, a formalized oath commonly uttered in Old English heroic poetry prior to battle.[38] Such a pledge as those made by Beowulf prior to fighting each of the epic's monstrous antagonists 'summoned to any given narrative present in which it occurred a whole network of interlaced and interdependent meaning(s)', most notably characterizing admirable resolve before battle.[39] After completing preparations for his final battle against the dragon, for instance, Beowulf 'spræc beotwordum' ['spoke pledge-words'] (l. 2511): 'ic wylle ... fæhðe secan, mærðum fremman' ['I will ... seek battle, perform with glory'] (ll. 2513–2515). Immediately after this *beot*, Beowulf shares some last words with his retainers, the Geats he is protecting, and begins the final confrontation.

Wið færstice follows a surprisingly similar pattern to that found in *Beowulf*, as a pledge of victory precedes the final confrontation with the source of pain. By the point of the final refrain, preparations for the final stage of the narrated poetic battle and also the herbal mixture are now complete, and the healer is at last in a reasonable position to promise aid: against pain in flesh, blood, or limbs caused by shots from a wide array of supernatural beings, 'nu ic wille ðin helpan' ['now I will help you'] (l. 22), a pledge repeated two lines later in slightly different form: 'ic ðin wille helpan' ['I will help you'].[40] Just as Beowulf follows his *beot* with acknowledgment of a higher power's role in determining the outcomes—'swa unc wyrd geteoð, metod mann gehwæs' ['as fate allots us, the measurer of each of men'] (ll. 2527–2528)—the healer, too, follows her or his promise to help with the invocation of a higher being: 'helpe ðin drihten' ['May your lord help you'.][41] But the battle is still not quite yet won.

Aftermath: healing and hope, lines 25–26

Nim þonne þæt seax, ado on wætan: what happens next?

Following the incantation, the remedy calls for a knife to be plunged into liquid: 'Nim þonne þæt seax, ado on wætan' ['Then take that knife, put in liquid']. As noted above, we do not see the actual hand-to-hand combat in the poem. But in these final lines we instead witness the surrounding physical actions of the remedy working most directly and explicitly in conjunction with the poetic incantation to complete the battle. The incantation's lengthy explication of the early, preparatory stage of battle has been recited precisely during the period needed for preparation of the herbs. Most likely, the herbs would have then been applied as part of a salve directly to the skin, with a knife.[42]

Cameron has offered a detailed discussion of the uses of the herbs mentioned in this remedy, concluding that 'all three herbs have been recommended for muscular and joint pains, hence useful against "sudden stitch", when applied as a salve to the aching parts'.[43] If the sterilized knife (having been dipped in the boiling liquid) was used to apply the herbal salve, this application could easily be seen as the medical equivalent of direct and close-up combat with the ailment itself.[44] In the logic provided by the remedy, the herbs *themselves* become weapons, consistent with the naming of plants after weapons, as seen in all of the major medical texts and discussed in Chapter 2.[45] The metaphorical thus becomes quite literal as the knife, through its application of the salve, becomes the primary instrument of healing, effectually concluding the battle. The medical preparation and application then quite neatly parallel the events of battle described in the poetic incantation. In summary, Table 3.1—which complements and demonstrates the relevance of the edited text and translation at the end of this chapter—makes salient the structural segments of the remedy and shows how the text's seemingly enigmatic poetic portions correspond to both actual battle practices and also the instructions for herbal preparation framing the incantation.

The mixing of herbs parallels the frenzied flight of arrows and javelins in both directions, as enemies begin to draw close, to blend. The direct application of the resultant salve in turn parallels the ensuing one-on-one-battle, close enough to be fought with a knife or dagger. In recognizing the patterns outlined in Table 3.1, we can more readily see that battles against illness—like battles against military opponents—have distinct stages. The poetry in *Wið færstice* beautifully and powerfully reminds us of the importance of careful preparation without ever losing sight of the ultimate goal. And the link, of course, is the simple *seax*, which functions as a powerful weapon forged by smiths within the inset heroic poem and as a healer's curative implement in the outer preparation of the medicine.

Once we are able to see the compelling logic linking healing and battle in this individual text, we are in a better position to recognize less obvious connections between the worlds of epic poetry and traditional healing lore, connections that complicate meanings in both

Table 3.1 Rhetorical structure of *Wið færstice*

Action	Incantation

Statement of remedy's purpose against pain	I. First stage of battle: fighting at a distance (ll. 1–10)
	  A. Preparation
	    i. Approach of female riders (1–2)
	    ii. Command to shield oneself (3)
	        Refrain (4)
	  B. Fighting
	    i. Taking cover under shield (5)
	    ii. Exchange of spears and arrows (6–9)
	        Refrain (10)

Preparation of remedy: Chaotic exchange of weapons // mixing and boiling of herbs	II. Second stage of battle: close combat (11–24)
	  A. Preparation
	    i. Forging of *seax* (11–12)
	        Refrain (13)
	    ii. Forging of spears (14)
	        Refrain (15)
	    iii. Litany of desired outcomes—*gif* catalog (16–22a)
	    iv. Promise to help—comparable to heroic *beot* (22b)
	  B. Fighting
	    i. Engagement –*þis þe* catalog (23–24a)
	        [*þis* = application of herbal preparation]
	    ii. Reiteration of promise or *beot* (24b)

Application of remedy: Close combat // application of salve with knife	III. Aftermath (25–26)
	    i. Anticipation of desired outcome, enemy's flight (25)
	    ii. Command to be whole (26a)
	    iii. Call for Lord's help (26b)

arenas. The next and final section of this chapter will explore these wider implications for our understanding of Old English literature and culture. As this and the previous chapter have demonstrated, battle operated as an important metaphor for healing across Old English medical texts, suggesting a powerful influence of heroic epic poetry upon the genre of verbal healing. What might be less obvious to modern readers is how the healing tradition reciprocally could have worked to sustain the genre of heroic epic. Though healers as such do not appear explicitly in heroic poetry, formulaic patterns evocative of the medical texts most certainly do, creating a powerful network of signification across genres, and a reader attuned to the logistics of healing as warfare might see subtle but meaningful connections, as this chapter's final section demonstrates.

Broader contexts

Healing, heroism, and sustainability

In modern medical models where poetic literature is typically far removed from visits to doctors, it can be easy to lose sight of how poetic narrative and medicine nourish each other. Within some living oral traditions today, however, a sustaining interconnectedness linking healing and heroism is not uncommon in traditional narrative.[46] For instance, King Gesar, famous within the Mongolian epic tradition, acquires precious medicine as he accumulates power, thus embodying the delicate balance between healing and heroism.[47] Medicine and armor are also explicitly juxtaposed in the Mande epic of *Sunjata*. For instance, an important arming scene of Sunjata—a hero who possesses tremendous powers of healing—is directly preceded by interactions with vessels of his medicinal water:

> In the morning he bathed in the water of his seven medicine pots.
> He took his battle axe and hung it on his shoulder.[48]

Such connections are, in important ways, similar to those we saw in the yarrow entry of the Old English *Herbarium* in Chapter 2, where the healing properties of this herb, also known as *Achillea millefolium*, are shared in part via a story of the epic Achilles. So realistic are the *Iliad*'s depictions of battle wounds and trauma that the idea of Homer as a medic was captured in Ezra Pound's *Cantos*: 'It is said also that Homer was a medic / who followed the Greek armies to Troas' (Canto 80).[49]

In such instances as these, however, the inherent value of the epic tradition is reinforced by the incorporation of heroic elements into practical daily life. In turn, elements in the remedies that are shared by the epic tradition lend credibility and authority to the healing remedies themselves. But these connections between healing and heroism can exist in even more complex associative networks. One comparative example[50] that is particularly enlightening for understanding a wider range of healing practice is a modern Serbian charm against skin infection (likely erysipelas) that has been well analyzed by John Foley. Drawing examples from his own fieldwork with South Slavic oral traditions, Foley has discussed overlap across genres in terms of a natural ecosystem:[51]

> To appropriate a biological metaphor, oral poems inhabit an ecology of verbal art. Neither poems nor performances nor genres can be isolated without doing violence to that ecology, without changing them into something they aren't.

In myriad oral traditions, 'various genres annex diction and narrative patterns that seem to attach principally to no single genre, but are shared at the level of the larger poetic tradition'.[52] Thus, Foley cautions against isolating epic from other verbal arts, noting that the epic tradition often works in concert with other genres such as charms, laments, proverbs, and even genealogies. And it is in this Serbian charm that Foley finds an especially compelling example of the linkage between charm and epic.

The charm, as performed by Desanka Matijašević, opens with the following lines:[53]

Otud ide crveni konj,
Crveni čovek, crvena usta,
Crvene ruke, crvene noge,
Crvena griva, crvene kopite.
Kako dodje, tako stiže,
Ovu boljku odmah diže;
I odnose i prenose,
Preko mora bez odmora.

[Out of there comes the red horse,
the red man, the red mouth,
the red arms, the red legs,

the red mane, the red hooves.
As he comes so he approaches,
he lifts out the disease immediately.
He carries it off and carries it away
across the sea without delay.]

Out of context, these lines are rather cryptic and potentially quite confusing to readers unfamiliar with the traditional idiom. As Foley has explained, however, the Serbian healer, or *bajalice*, is here 'enlisting a heroic ally, a man on horseback to help rid the world of the intrusive red disease and take it back to where it originated and where it properly belongs—in the "red" world'.[54] This logic of disease being introduced into the human realm from an other-worldly opponent is actually quite similar to what we see in much Old English medicine,[55] but where the Old English remedy casts its fight against pain in terms of a Germanic battle, the Serbian charm invokes a distinctly South Slavic image of the horse and rider, a common motif in South Slavic epic tradition.[56] This small connection is only one of many places where overlap across diverse genres can be explained in terms of a culture-encompassing ecosystem of mutually nourishing and enriching poetic forms. Such evidence from living oral traditions as well as from long-textualized but clearly oral-derived ancient poetry suggests that a crucial aspect of sustainability as related to oral poetry involves a deep interconnectedness across diverse genres. The result is an understanding of generic diversity as a vibrant, dynamic system of exchange and mutual reciprocity. In the Serbian charm, the folk epidemiology does not require 'killing' the source of disease, but rather *returning* it. The goal, Foley explains, is 'to rid the world of the intrusive red disease and take it back to where it originated and where it properly belongs'.[57] This particular healing logic reminds us that battle metaphors within medical texts do not automatically imply extermination as the goal, and a closer look at the precise language surrounding the poetic battle in *Wið færstice* alongside a parallel in *Beowulf* also suggests that a less inherently binary model of healing and battle is appropriate within the Old English tradition as well.

Hlude wæron, la, hlude: heroes and healers

Keeping this idea of mutually sustaining genres in mind helps us read connections between the opening lines of *Wið færstice* and an unlikely comparand in *Beowulf* as more than mere coincidence. Reciprocal relationships across genres would logically be quite natural given the homogeneity in verse form shared by Old English poetry,[58] yet the absence of healers in heroic verse makes such connections much less transparent. Nevertheless, lines 322–329 of the epic resonate powerfully with the opening of *Wið færstice* as they describe the approach of Beowulf and his men to the hall Heorot, where they arrive armed and ready for battle against the monstrous Grendel:[59]

... **hringiren scir**
song in searwum, þa hie to sele furðum
in hyra **gryregeatwum** gangan **cwomon**.
Setton sæmeþe side **scyldas**,
... Byrnan **hringdon**,
guðsearo gumena. Garas stodon
sæmanna searo, **samod ætgædere**....

[... **Bright iron rings**
sang out on their gear **when they first came**
marching into the hall in their **terrible armor**.
Sea weary ones put down their broad **shields**.
... The byrnies **rang out**,
battle-gear of the warriors. Spears stood,
gear of sea-men, **all together**....]

Thematically, both passages narrate the approach of troops and anticipate battle between heroic warriors and hostile alien beings; the monstrous Grendel in the epic parallels the anthropomorphized bearers of pain in the medical text.[60] More subtly, both texts note the audible force of the troops. The loudness of the approaching enemy in *Wið færstice* ('Loud were they, lo, loud') is matched by the sounds of the clanging armor in *Beowulf* ('their bright iron rings sang out', ll. 322–323; 'byrnies rang out', l. 327). Both poems also reference the presence of shields: *Wið færstice* includes directions to 'shield yourself now', and the epic not only describes the 'hand-linked mail-coats' and 'terrible armor' of Beowulf and his men (ll. 321–322, 324), but, more relevantly, includes the statement that the men set aside their shields, 'setton sæmeþe side scyldas' (l. 325).

Even structurally, the descriptions of the approaching forces exhibit strong similarities. The phrasing of the approach of enemies in Wið færstice, 'when they rode', is syntactically parallel to the approach of Beowulf's men in the epic, 'when they first came' (l. 323), both sharing the formulaic construction 'þa hie/hy ...' [third person, past tense, plural verb of motion] (ll. 323–324). Most importantly, both passages highlight the unified front of the troops, so common in depictions of the Germanic *comitatus*, riding together in Wið færstice and marching together in Beowulf.[61] The resoluteness of purpose is made especially explicit in Wið færstice, where the warriors are described as 'anmode' ['of one mind'], parallel to the spears in the Beowulf passage, which are 'samod ætgædere' ['all together'] (l. 329).

Intriguingly, these parallels align Beowulf and his men not with the healer of Wið færstice, but with the rapidly approaching riders whom the healer works against. The parallels impact meaning in both directions, complicating binaries that align healers against disease, heroes against monsters. Within the heroic narrative of Beowulf, awareness of the parallels intensifies our awareness of the threat that Beowulf and his men initially pose, possible carriers of metaphorical disease, dangerous threats to the very social fabric of the Danes. However, the depiction of Beowulf's troops as potentially threatening is not followed by any military altercation; rather, Beowulf quite quickly proves himself to be the Dane's most forceful ally. Less obviously, Wið færstice also complicates the status of its own approaching riders as unequivocal enemies. Notably, no sword in this incantation is ever thrust directly into an enemy, no foe ever explicitly said to have been harmed—in spite of the poem's extensive references to weaponry and battle. Rather, the approaching threat simply retreats, in a healing restoration of balance: 'Fleo þær on fyrgenhæfde. Hal westu, helpe ðin drihten'. ['May it fly there to the mountaintop. Be whole. May your lord help you'.] In Beowulf, the approaching hero is both the approaching threat *and* the force that restores balance by sending Grendel away from Heorot. If we apply a similar logic to the metrical charm, the approaching female riders actually resolve the pain themselves, by flying to the mountains, the victim's suffering ended not through sheer violence but through an arguably cooperative endeavor that follows the *threat* of violence.

Of course, these blurred boundaries between ally and enemy or healer and harm are just one further manifestation of the ambiguity that pervades *Wið færstice*, a feature shared even on the linguistic level by the single most common word in Old English healing: *wið*. Like almost every remedy in Old English medical texts, entry cxxvii of the *Lacnunga* opens with 'Wið', historically most common with the sense of 'against' yet eventually connoting cooperative effort in the modern English sense of 'with'.[62] But such grammatical ambiguity (or at least what appears as ambiguity for modern readers) in the Old English *wið* is quickly resolved when we look at the approach of Beowulf's men as parallel to the approaching riders of *Wið færstice*. Beowulf's presence, initially perceived by the coastguard as potentially threatening, becomes Heorot's eventual salvation. Similarly, a site of pain, such as that of *Wið færstice*, can quickly turn into a site of healing, if—and only if—the healer/warrior works *wið*, in both senses of the word, the source of ailment. By viewing epic and medical texts alongside one another, we thus see early medieval literature actively working against what have today become common stereotypes of polarizing violence.[63] In isolation, the opposite 'sides' of battle in *Wið færstice* might seem unambiguous, but examined in the context of the larger generic ecosystem, within which a potential foe works towards a shared solution, the binaries quickly break down. Just as Beowulf returns Grendel to the mere, the healer of *Wið færstice* calls upon potential threats to return to the mountaintop from which they rode. The ultimate goal is not violence in itself—though violence might nonetheless ensue—but bodily balance and order, where what might be a disease in one realm can be restored to a healthy position in another.

Far from mere vestiges of superstition, the employment of weaponry in *Wið færstice* and throughout Old English medical tradition follows a fairly clear and consistent logic. As we saw in the previous chapter, the protective poem inscribed in the margins of Bede's *Ecclesiastical History* appropriately references metaphorical weapons that would have been associated with only the most elite warriors; *Wið færstice*, on the other hand, appears in a commonplace medical text and employs correspondingly commonplace weapons—primarily arrows, flying spears, and a knife. But this everyday hunting equipment could also be easily transferred to the more specialized context of the battlefield, whether in real life or within epic poetry, and thus these many different types of power drawn from multiple cultural contexts are all channeled via this imagery into herbal remedies and ritual practices for healing. This particular healing logic is in alignment with medieval thought more widely. Viewing medieval medicine within larger cultural and poetic contexts, Peter Dendle has convincingly shown that 'for the early Middle Ages, Nature was largely an enemy, an obstacle to be surmounted' and that 'plants, animals, and the very elements war against each other ... nature against nature'.[64] At the same time, however, there is an interconnectedness that 'counteracts the inherent hostility of Nature: at any time, any created thing . . . can suddenly erupt into an overflowing of power or energy for the benefit of human kind'.[65] Yet it is equally important to bear in mind that the ultimate goal of battle preparations needn't be eradication or brute violence; they could—with strategic care—result in peaceable restoration of balance. Accordingly, by combining our knowledge of material culture, military tactics, and historical context with the seemingly far-removed fields of oral poetry and traditional medicine, we come to a much richer understanding of how traditional healers negotiated power over illness and adversity in early medieval England. The next chapter pushes this logic further still: if the site of ailment is a metaphorical battleground and herbs are equated with weaponry, what does it mean for a healer to direct ritualized speech toward the healing herbs themselves?

Appendix

Wið færstice
MS Harley 585, ff. 175r–176r

Text and translation

Wið færstice is a complex text that defies conventional categories of interpretation, and the edited text and accompanying translation on the next page reflect its intricacies. Seeking to render the remedy on its own terms and recover its underlying logic of healing, the formatting of both the edited text and the translation depart in important ways from long-standing conventional treatment of Old English verse. Most significantly, the presentation provided here attempts to convey not only poetic structure and lexical meaning, but also rhetorical patterns and syntactical repetitions that can serve as powerful interpretive guides.

The standard method of editing Old English verse in half-lines goes far in revealing poetic form and acoustic features such as alliteration and stress patterns. But some texts—and I argue that *Wið færstice* is among these—remain more enigmatic than necessary, in large part because rhetorical structures that would likely be somewhat obvious in performance are more easily missed on the printed page. In editing *Wið færstice*, my most important goal has been to convey the close connection between herbal preparation and poetic incantation. I have thus created two columns, one for the herbal remedy's presentation (on the left side of the page) and a second for the poetic incantation (on the right).[66] As explained in this chapter, my working assumption (one based both on evidence from surviving medieval medical texts and on common practice in modern traditional healing) is that the incantation would have been recited not after but *during* the preparation of herbs, as is not infrequently prescribed for incantations in other medieval remedies. This editing format thus frees the remedy from textual restrictions of linearity and indicates a relationship between prose and poetry that is parallel rather than sequential.

A second editing goal has been to convey meaningful patterns within the poetic incantation itself. Ethnopoetic transcription often seeks to 'show the nature of the architecture of verse patterns',[67] and it is in this spirit that the text as presented here seeks to visually reinforce rhythms and patterns more easily heard than seen. Because different patterns become more apparent in Old English than in modern, the text and translation each convey different levels of patterning. The edited text conveys the prosody, following the typical format of full and half-line breaks for the poetic portions based on patterns of alliteration and stress. The translation meanwhile applies different formatting techniques designed to expose repeated phrasing and sentence structures.[68] This dual approach models many aspects of transcription and translation used by Toby Langen for Lushootseed oral narrative. Langen transcribes a Lushootseed story narrated by Mariah Moses in a manner that 'emphasizes the innate rhythms and internal echoes of the phrases being spoken',[69] a format that parallels the typical rendering of Old English verse to emphasize patterns of stress and alliteration. In contrast, however, Langen's translation was also designed 'to emphasize structural, not acoustic, features'.[70] Accordingly, in my modern English translation, I also follow Langen's practices where 'indentation calls attention to circular or concentric figuration and variations on episodic patterns', italics mark 'rhythmically heightened delivery' (specifically the incantation's refrain), and spacing indicates 'episode boundaries and bridge passages between episodes', such as phases of battle depicted as the poem advances.[71]

Finally, my edited text and corresponding translation reflect several departures from conventional treatment, most notably the following:

> ll. 4, 10, 13, 15: The treatment of the 'ut, spere' lines as offset from the main text is meant to underscore the refrain's important role in punctuating the stages of battle, as discussed earlier in this chapter.
> l. 5: Although the syntax is undeniably awkward in modern English, the word order in the translation retains the semantic ambiguity of *stod*'s grammatical ambiguity in the original Old English.
> l. 5: The translation 'I' is the most commonly proposed subject (e.g., Michael Collier, 'Against a Sudden Stitch', in Delanto and Matto, *The Word Exchange*; Pollington, *Leechcraft*; Rodrigues, *Anglo-Saxon Verse Charms*; Glosecki, *Shamanism*); 'it' is preferred by Hall, *Elves*, and Jolly leaves the subject unstated, noting that '*stod*

Hybrid healing

Action	Incantation
[f. 175r, ll. 5–7] Wið færstice, feferfuige and seo reade netele ðe þurh ærn inwyxð, and wegbrade, wyll in buteran.	[f. 175r l.6–f. 176r l. 6] Hlude wæran hy, la, hlude, ða hy ofer þone hlæw ridan, wæran anmode, ða hy ofer land ridan. Scyld ðu ðe nu, þu ðysne nið genesan mote. Ut, lytel spere, gif her inne sie.

(5) Stod under linde,   under leohtum scylde,
þær ða mihtigan wif   hyra mægen beræddon
and hy gyllende   garas sændan.
Ic him oðerne   eft wille sændan,
fleogende flane   forane togeanes

(10)   Ut, lytel spere,   gif hit her inne sy.

Sæt smið,   sloh seax,
lytel iserna,   wund swiðe.

Ut, lytel spere,   gif her inne sy.

Syx smiðas sætan,   wælspera worhtan

(15)   Ut, spere,   næs in, spere

Gif her inne sy   isenes dæl,
hægtessan geweorc,   hit sceal gemyltan.
Gif ðu wære on fell scoten   oððe wære on flæsc scoten
oððe wære on blod scoten

(20) oððe wære on lið scoten,   næfre ne sy ðin lif atæsed;
gif hit wære esa gescot   oððe hit wære ylfa gescot
oððe hit wære hægtessan gescot,   nu ic wille ðin helpan.

[f. 176r l. 6–7]
Nim þonne þæt
seaxado on
wæton.

þis ðe to bote esa gescotes,   ðis ðe to bote ylfa gescotes,
ðis ðe to bote hægtessan gescotes;   ic ðin wille helpan.

(25) Fleo þær   on fyrgenhæfde.
Hal westu,   helpe ðin drihten.

Action	Incantation
Against a sudden pain:	Loud were they, lo, loud, when they rode over the mound,
	were single-minded, when they rode over land.
feverfew and the red nettle, which grows in through a building, and waybroad.	Shield yourself now, you are able to survive this evil.
	Out, little spear, if it be in here.
	[He/she/it/I] stood under linden, under a light shield, where the mighty women readied their strength
Boil in butter.	and they yelling spears sent.
	I will send them another back, a flying arrow back in the other direction.
	Out, little spear, if it be in here.
	A smith sat, forged a knife, a small piece of iron, severe wound.
	Out, little spear, if it be in here.
	Six smiths sat, made slaughter-spears.
	Out, spear, not in, spear.
	If herein be a piece of iron, work of a hag, it must melt.
	If you were shot in the skin or were shot in the flesh,
	or were shot in the blood
	or were shot in a limb, may your life never be harmed.
	If it were gods' shot, or it were elves' shot
	or it were a hag's shot,
	now I will help you.
Take then the knife, dip in liquid.	This to you as a remedy for gods' shot,
	this for you as a remedy for elves' shot,
	this for you as a remedy for hag's shot;
	I wish to help you.
	May it fly there to the mountaintop.
	Be whole.
	May your lord help you.

is unclear'.[72] I have included 'she' as a possibility in my own translation, not only grammatically viable but also contextually appropriate, given the approaching female riders.

l. 12: ASPR edits with 'lytel' on previous line. Taking the meaning metonymically, some have translated *isern* as sword.[73] See further this chapter's discussion above on the rationale for reading *iserna* literally, in apposition with *seax*.

l. 25: Manuscript *fled*. *Fleon* and *fleogan* both being strong verbs, *fled* requires emendation. On various proposed emendations, see Dobbie (ed.), *Anglo-Saxon Minor Poems*, p. 213. I am here adopting the emendation to *fleo* (proposed by Grimm and Sweet in the nineteenth century), taking the form as the present subjunctive singular of *fleon*. *Fleo* requires less intervention than other common proposals, such as *fleoh* or *fleah*, and follows the rhetorical logic of the poem's larger structure. See *DOE*, s.v. *fleon*.[74]

Notes

1 Stephen Glosecki, *Shamanism and Old English Poetry* (Shrewsbury, MA: Garland, 1989), p. 109. For a list of translations and editions along with a detailed overview of scholarship on this text prior to 2001, see Pettit, *Anglo-Saxon Remedies*, pp. 212–261.
2 Hill, 'Rod', p. 160.
3 Hall, *Elves*, p. 1.
4 Howell Chickering's reductive yet still highly influential analysis, for instance, recommends separating the incantation, which he considers 'a masterpiece', from the lesser remainder of the remedy on the grounds that 'as modern readers we bring only an aesthetic appreciation to the charm, not a real belief' and thus 'can only perceive the literary force of its verbal magic'. 'The Literary Magic of *Wið Færstice*', *Viator*, 2 (1971), 83–104, at 95, 104.
5 Storms, *Anglo-Saxon Magic*, p. 143.
6 Del Hymes, *'In vain I tried to tell you': Essays in Native American Ethnopoetics*, with new preface by the author (Lincoln, NE: University of Nebraska Press, 2004. Orig. publ. 1981), p. 6 *et passim*. Hymes' experimental approach was initially developed for editing narratives belonging to first peoples along the North Pacific coast. Many of these texts that had originally been transcribed in run-on prose in the early twentieth century could be seen as inherently poetic when transcribed in

ways that underscored recurring patterns, taking advantage of indentations, spacing, and other typographical features to expose what Hymes saw as a narrative's 'architecture', p. 7.
7 Foley, *How to Read an Oral Poem*, pp. 102–107, 103.
8 Jolly, *Popular*, p. 134.
9 While a minority translate *linde* as linden tree, the majority assume a metonymic reference to a shield made from linden or a similar wood.
10 On choices in handling *stod*'s subject in modern English translations, see Appendix, note to l. 5.
11 Brooks, 'Weapons', p. 208.
12 In the case of *gar*, the ambiguity is inherent in the word itself. While *flan* refers consistently to projectile weapons, 'arrow, dart' (*DOE*, s.v. *flan*), and *stræl* likewise indicates 'arrow, shaft, dart' specifically (Bosworth and Toller s.v. *stræl*), the primary sense of *gar* offered in the *DOE* is simply 'weapon with a pointed head'. Sense 1.a is 'spear, javelin', and 1.a.i is 'a weapon that is hurled or thrust'. Perhaps 1.c best encapsulates what I myself see as the sense here: 'used metonymically in phrases referring to battle or warfare in general' (*DOE* s.v. *gar*).
13 The variation in translation reflects this ambiguity as well: Hall (*Elves*), Hill ('Rod'), Bjork (*Old English Shorter Poems*), and Rodrigues (*Anglo-Saxon Verse Charms*) translate as *gyllende* modifying *garas*; Pollington (*Leechcraft*) and Collier ('Against a Sudden Stitch', in Delanty and Matto, *Word Exchange*) are among those who have *gyllende* modifying women; Jolly (*Popular*) retains the ambiguity, 'they screaming spears sent', p. 139.
14 Manley, 'Archer', pp. 229–230.
15 Hall, *Elves*, p. 2.
16 Pettit, *Anglo-Saxon Remedies*, p. 240.
17 Underwood, *Anglo-Saxon Weapons*, p. 23.
18 Glosecki, *Shamanism*, p. 108.
19 Storms, *Anglo-Saxon Magic*, p. 146.
20 Minna Doskow, 'Poetic Structure and the Problem of the Smiths in Wið Færstice', *Papers on Language and Literature*, 12 (1979), 321–326, at 325.
21 McGillivray's *Old English Reader*, another likely place for first-time readers to encounter the poem, supplies *wæpen* in the presumed gap, which restores the perceived irregularity in meter, *Old English Reader* (Toronto: Broadview Press, 2011). Perhaps it is because these poems conform neatly to modern categories of neither literature nor science, and thus are often dismissed as superstition or products of lesser minds,

that the metrical charms have been subject to such free emendation and that assumptions of error go so widely unchallenged.
22 E.g., McGillivray, *Old English Reader*, p. 143.
23 Dobbie, *Anglo-Saxon Minor Poems*, p. 143.
24 Doane, A. N, 'Editing Old English Oral/Written Texts: Problems of Method (With an Illustrated Edition of Charm 4, *Wiþ Færstice*)', in Donald G. Scragg and Paul E. Szarmach (eds), *The Editing of Old English: Papers from the 1990 Manchester Conference* (Woodbridge: D. S. Brewer, 1994), pp. 125–145, at 143.
25 Pettit, *Anglo-Saxon Remedies*, p. 244.
26 Ibid., pp. 245, 246.
27 Glosecki, *Shamanism*, p. 106.
28 A. J. Bliss, 'Single-Half-Lines in Old English Poetry', *Notes and Queries*, 18.12 (1971), pp. 442–449, at p. 448. On the integrity of single half-lines in Old English charms specifically, see further Foley, 'Hybrid Prosody'.
29 Owen-Crocker, 'Seldom', p. 203.
30 See, for instance Hall, *Elves*, p. 2, and Collier, 'Against a Sudden Stitch', p. 483 (in Delanty and Matto, *Word Exchange*), which show the smith forging a small sword. Jolly (*Popular*, p. 139) and Hill ('Rod', p. 159) are among those who translate *iserna* as the material iron.
31 Gayle Owen-Crocker notes that in burial practice, swords were typically limited to graves accorded to men, 'Seldom', p. 201. In contrast, knives are among those described as 'standard' goods in female furnished graves', Andrew Reynolds, *Anglo-Saxon Deviant Burial Customs* (Oxford: Oxford University Press, 2009), p. 72. Any such general patterns must be approached with great caution, however, as new possibilities in genomic testing have called into question gender assumptions based on weapons found in furnished graves. An especially egregious example of such misidentification involves a biologically female occupant of a tenth-century grave in Birka, Sweden, furnished with a sword, two shields, and other items indicative of a high-status warrior, who was assumed to be male from the initial excavation in 1878 until 2017. See Neil Price et al., 'Viking Warrior Women? Reassessing Birka chamber grave Bj.581', *Antiquity*, 93 (2019), 181–198.
32 Sara Frances Burdorff, 'Re-Reading Grendel's Mother: *Beowulf* and the Anglo-Saxon Metrical Charms', *Comitatus: A Journal of Medieval and Renaissance Studies*, 45 (2014), 91–103, at p. 98.
33 Gale R. Owen-Crocker, 'Dress and Identity', *The Oxford Handbook of Anglo-Saxon Archaeology*, David A. Hinton, Sally Crawford, and Helena Hamerow (eds) (Oxford: Oxford University Press, 2012), pp. 91–118, at 106.

34 For discussion of gender and the slaughter-spears, see, for example, Pettit, *Anglo-Saxon Remedies*, pp. 242–246.
35 Storms, *Anglo-Saxon Magic*, p. 143.
36 Cameron, *Anglo-Saxon Medicine*, pp. 38–39.
37 Her recipe for thin hearth-cakes (Old English *cycel*) notes that 'six or seven Lord's Prayers' worth of time should do it. (Remember, this was how they measured duration.) Don't hurry over the prayers'. Martha Bayless, 'How to Make Anglo-Saxon Bread: Version 2', Early English Bread Project, post from 13 May 2017, https://earlybread.word press.com/2017/05/13/how-to-make-everyday-anglo-saxon-bread-version-2-hearthcakes-or-kichells/. Accessed 7 July 2021. In a more grim example of elements of liturgy used for time-keeping, the *Textus Roffensis* calls for the hot iron of an ordeal to be laid upon coals for the duration of a mass, not removed 'oð ðæt þa æftemestan collectan' ['until the final collect']. F. L. Attenborough (ed. and trans.), *The Laws of the Earliest English Kings* (New York: Russell and Russell, Inc., 1963), p. 172. See further Sarah Larratt Keefer, 'Ðonne se cirlisca man ordales weddigeð: The Anglo-Saxon Lay Ordeal', in Stephen Baxter, Catherine Karkov, Janet L. Nelson, and David Pelteret (eds), *Early Medieval Studies in Memory of Patrick Wormald* (London: Ashgate, 2009), pp. 353–367, at 357.
38 Cf. Beowulf's promise to Hrothgar that he will defeat the monstrous Grendel (ll. 679–685). For an early articulation of the *beot*'s role in Old English poetry, see Stefán Einarsson, 'Old English *Beot* and Old Icelandic *Heitstrenging*', *PMLA*, 49 (1934), 975–993. On the traditional force of the *beot*, see further Amodio, *Writing*, pp. 146–156.
39 Ibid., p. 156.
40 For fascinating discussions of the supernatural beings that appear in these lines, see especially Glosecki, *Shamanism*, pp. 106–131; Hall, 'Rod', pp. 1–3; and Pettit, *Anglo-Saxon Remedies*, pp. 247–255.
41 Storms claims that this line must be 'a later, Christian, addition' that 'differs in atmosphere' from the previous promise of aid, *Anglo-Saxon Magic*, p. 149. However, the parallels with Beowulf's *beot* and subsequent deference to *wyrd* prior to his final battle suggest a shared traditional pattern.
42 Some early work on this remedy assumed that the *seax* was to 'be used on some dummy representing the evil spirits'. Grendon, *Anglo-Saxon Charms*, p. 215, n. 29; but as early 1911, A. R. Skemp saw an inherent logic in the view that *wætan* references the herbal salve, a liquid that could have been applied to the site of pain with the knife, as butter is

spread on bread. Skemp, A. R., 'The Old English Charms', *Modern Language Review*, 6 (1911), 289–301.
43 Cameron, *Anglo-Saxon Medicine*, pp. 143–144.
44 While Cameron's explanation is certainly convincing, the logic is still consistent if the knife is used for other purposes, such as surgical incision or a ritual of sympathetic magic, as suggested by Storms, *Anglo-Saxon Magic* p. 149. However the *seax* might be used, it unquestionably ends the battle through close-range fighting. For discussion of various theories regarding this final instruction, see Pettit, *Anglo-Saxon Remedies*, pp. 259–260.
45 Even some of our most basic vocabulary speaks to a long-standing overlap connecting the worlds of plants and weapons, and evidence from historical linguistics indicates that many of our earliest metaphors go from plants to weapons rather than the other way round. As just one example, our word *blade*—used for blades of grass and blades of swords alike—ultimately derives from Proto-Indo-European *bhel-, 'thrive, bloom', *American Heritage Dictionary [AHD]*, 'Indo-European Roots', s.v. *bhel-[3].
46 Such paradigms of sustainability and oral epic were the focus of the Chinese Academy of Social Sciences Forum, International Summit on Epic Studies: Toward Diversity, Creativity, and Sustainability (November 17–18, 2012, Beijing). I am grateful to the Chinese Academy of Social Sciences, the Institute of Ethnic Literature, and the Center for Oral Traditions Research for the opportunity to participate in the forum's productive and enlightening discussions, which inform much of the analysis here.
47 In Douglas Penick's rendering (based to a great extent on the works of Chögyam Trungpa Rinpoche), for example, Gesar is told by Padma Sambhava that he must seize medicine treasuries as he conquers lands if his kingdom is to thrive. *The Warrior Song of King Gesar* (Minneapolis, MN: Mill City Press, 2009), p. 17.
48 There are many versions of this epic. This translation is based on the performance of Djanka Tassey Condé (ll. 4368–4369), David C. Conrad (trans.), *Sunjata: A West African Epic of the Mande Peoples*, narrated by Djanka Tassey Condé (Indianapolis: Hackett Publishing Company, 2014).
49 Ezra Pound, *The Cantos of Ezra Pound* (New York: New Directions Books, 1934), p. 523. Koutserimpas, Alpantaki, and Samonis note that the *Iliad* retains a 'plethora of medical information' with description of 147 injuries, and that such detail characterizes Greek mythology more widely as well. Christos Koutserimpas, Kalliopi Alpantaki, and George

Samonis, 'Trauma Management in Homer's *Iliad*', *International Wound Journal*, 14.4 (2017), 682–684, at 682).
50 For a thoughtful and probing study on questions of ethics, with regard to comparative work and medical texts in particular, see Erin Sweany's contribution to the special issue *Indigenous Futures and Medieval Pasts* (edited by Tarren Andrews and Tiffany Beechy): 'Unsettling Comparisons: Ethical Considerations of Comparative Approaches to the Old English Medical Corpus', *English Language Notes*, 58.2 (2020), 83–100.
51 Foley, *How to Read an Oral Poem*, p. 188.
52 Foley, 'How Genres Leak', p. 101.
53 Text and trans., John Miles Foley. Desanka Matijašević was the pseudonym used by the woman who performed this charm. She was 55 at the time and lived in Orašac. Also present at the performance were anthropologist Barbara Kerewsky Halpern and Desanka's 7-year-old grandson Marko. For full text and translation of this charm in two variants, and context on the larger tradition, as well as details on this deeply collaborative fieldwork, see John Miles Foley, *Singer*, pp. 117–120. See also Barbara Kerewsky Halpern and John Miles Foley, 'The Power of the Word: Healing Charms as an Oral Genre', *Journal of American Folklore*, 92 (1978), 903–924.
54 Foley, *How to Read an Oral Poem*, p. 193.
55 On more prosodic connections between South Slavic and Old English charms, see Foley, 'Læcedom and Bajanje: A Comparative Study of Old English and Serbo-Croatian Charms', *Centerpoint*, 4 (1981), 33–41.
56 On the typical scene of 'Readying the Hero's Horse' in South Slavic epic, see John Miles Foley (ed. and trans.) *The Wedding of Mustajbey's Son Bećirbey as performed by Halil Bajgorić* (Helsinki: Academia Scientiarum Fennica, 2004), p. 197, and *Immanent Art*, pp. 124–133.
57 Foley, *How to Read an Oral Poem*, p. 193.
58 On the uniformity of verse within Old English oral poetics, see Amodio, *Writing*, pp. 34–39.
59 Quotations from *Beowulf* are from R. D. Fulk, Robert E. Bjork, and John D. Niles, *Klaeber's* Beowulf (Toronto: University of Toronto Press, 4th edn, 2008). Bolded sections highlight parallel motifs from *Wiþ færstice*.
60 See also Vaughan-Sterling, who notes that 'the part of Grendel … is taken over in the *Charms* by omnipresent evil spirits, who plague man', 'Anglo-Saxon', p. 188. Glosecki draws further connections between Grendel and disease spirits, arguing that in Old English narrative verse 'forces of evil—and simultaneously disease—' are 'embodied in march monsters like Grendel', *Shamanism*, p. 178.

61 On the ideal of *comitatus* in Old English verse, see Amodio, *Writing*, pp. 47–51.
62 In both Old and modern English, the preposition could accommodate a range of conflicting senses, but the more common sense in Old English was 'against', 'in the way of', or 'opposite' (Bosworth and Toller, sense 1.e and 1.f). In contrast, the *American Heritage Dictionary* gives 'in the company of' as the primary meaning and 'against' only as sense 18, as in 'wrestling *with* an opponent'.
63 In 'No More Militaristic and Violent Language in Medicine', Jing-Bao Nie et al. argue convincingly that metaphors of cancer as a 'war' and disease as a 'killer' can actually cause harm. Jing-Bao Nie et al., 'No More Militaristic and Violent Language in Medicine', *The American Journal of Bioethics*, 16 (2016), 3–11.
64 Peter Dendle, 'Plants in the Early Medieval Cosmos: Herbs, Divine Potency, and the *Scala natura*', in Peter Dendle and Alain Touwaide (eds), *Health and Healing from the Medieval Garden* (Woodbridge: Boydell Press, 2008), 47–59, at 48, 49.
65 Ibid., p. 50.
66 The more typical format, used by Dobbie, numbers the lines sequentially, with the ritual instructions constituting lines 1–2 and the incantation beginning on line 3. McGillivray's edition treats the poem as a discrete unit, beginning the numbering with the first line of the poem and including the more standard ASPR numbering in parentheses. For an interactive version of this edition, see http://people.ucalgary.ca/~mmcgilli/ASPR/MCharm4fram.htm. Accessed 1 June 2021.
67 Hymes, '*In vain*', p. 11.
68 Because line breaks do not always correspond to these syntactic units, line numbers are not provided in the translation.
69 Marya Moses and Toby C. S. Langen, 'Reading Martha Lamont's Crow Story Today', *Oral Tradition*, 13.1 (1998), 92–129, at 94.
70 Ibid., p. 95.
71 Ibid.
72 Jolly, *Popular*, p. 205.
73 E.g., Hall, *Elves*, 3; Collier, 'Against a Sudden Stitch', in Delanty and Matto, *Word Exchange*, p. 483.
74 J. Grimm, *Deutsche Mythologie* (Berlin: F. Dümmler, 1875), p. 1192. Henry Sweet, *An Anglo-Saxon Reader* (Oxford: Clarendon Press, 4th edn, 1884), p. 123.

4

To persuade a plant: hybridity of rhetoric in Harley 585

Gemyne ðu, Mucgwyrt, hwæt þu ameldodest....

[Remember, Mugwort, what you declared....]
(*Lacnunga*, MS Harley 585, folio 160r)

Wyrt ricinum, ic bidde þæt þu ætsy minum sangum....

[Ricinum plant, I ask that you be present at my song....]
(Old English *Herbarium*, MS Harley 585, folio 93v)

In the Old English *Herbarium*, entry 93 (for the herb named in the header variously as *wælwyrt*, *ellenwyrt*, or *ebulus*)[1] includes a remedy 'wið næddran slite' ['against snakebite'] that requires the following Latin incantation to be spoken (*cweð*) three times over the plant as it is harvested: 'Omnes malas bestias canto' ['I sing/enchant all evil beasts']. An English paraphrase is promised immediately after, 'þæt ys þonne on ure geþeode ...' ['that is then in our language ...']. However, though the Latin verb is in the first person[2] with the practitioner assuming healing agency, the Old English translation intriguingly recasts the verb into the imperative: 'Besing 7 ofercum eale yfel wilddeor' ['Sing and overcome all evil wildbeasts'], implicitly transferring both volition and agency directly to the plant itself. The addition of *ofercum* then further intensifies the plant's active role in the battle to come. Both of the herb's native names as provided in the remedy, *wælwyrt* and *ellenwyrt*, also reinforce the implications of agency in warfare, *wael* translated as 'battle' or even 'slaughter' and *ellen* literally meaning 'strong' but also connoting personal courage and bravery, as well as heightened emotion.[3] In an alternative reading, the difference in the mood distinguishing the Latin and Old English verbs could be connected to the charm's performativity. In this reading, the Old English imperative 'sing' and 'overcome' could be seen as the scribe/manuscript directing the practitioner, who would in turn chant the Latin incantation, in first person: 'I sing', 'I overcome'.[4] Diverse audiences could have read the remedy in different ways. Yet, though either of these readings might have been viable for the manuscript's earliest audiences and neither requires grammatical emendation, so entrenched is the scholarly default to Latin that modern translations of the Old English paraphrase often render both *besing* and *ofercum* as first-person singular verbs to match the Latin, not withstanding the fact that they lack the Old English first-person indicative personal endings.[5] As we shall see, there are important implications for such seemingly small differences in the translation, editing, and interpretation of this and other human/plant exchanges, differences that in turn highlight the need for deeper exploration into the precise nature of Latin and vernacular speech in the remedies, specifically speech directed towards plants.

To that end, this chapter applies a hybrid methodology drawing from the fields of rhetoric and oral tradition to better understand what such speech acts might teach us about herbal healing in medieval England across both Latinate and Old English traditions. Building from previous scholarship that has addressed productive connections between healing charms and rhetoric at a general level and numerous studies devoted to identification of rhetorical devices within vernacular verse in particular,[6] the present exploration isolates the particular mode of verbal discourse within the broadly conceived genre of medical lore involving persuasive speech directed toward plants. After a brief examination of such rhetoric within medieval healing practice more widely, this chapter then explores the Harley 585 manuscript as a hybrid compilation of medical knowledge, including both the Latin-derived Old English *Herbarium* and the distinctly vernacular compilation known as the *Lacnunga*; in particular, the central analysis will focus on particular rhetorical devices employed in speech directed towards plants, specifically apostrophe, personification, prosopopoeia, anaphora, chiasmus, and metonymy in the *Herbarium* entries for *ricinum* and *peruica* and the so-called 'Nine Herbs Charm' of the *Lacnunga*.

Verbal healing in early medieval England

To be clear, the vast majority of Old English remedies provide little more than a formulaic indication of adversity ('wið X') followed by straightforward instructions for remedy, and accordingly there are actually very few instances of incantations explicitly directed towards plants. Yet the spoken word is nonetheless woven intermittently throughout every major surviving medical text. Although far from the norm, scattered speech acts such as the incantation to be recited over *wælwyrt* metonymically signal an underlying—and distinctly pre-modern—healing logic, one characterized by a powerful healing hybridity. Collectively, if not individually, Old English medical texts manifest at once as verbal art, ritual expression, and medical practice and guide us toward a deeper understanding of the complex relationships binding practitioner, sufferer, ailment, and healing materials, all of which are characterized at different points as having sentience and agency. Speech towards plants reveals healing in Old English as a deeply collaborative endeavor, one that extends significantly beyond human agency alone.

But to more fully understand the subtleties of the language directed toward plants, a sufficiently nuanced understanding of medieval rhetoric is needed as well, one that extends beyond its more usual home in Latin learning and that allows for meaningful overlap between oral and written modes of communication. Martin Camargo has noted many ways that medieval rhetoric 'encompassed both oral and written discourse and permeated a broader range of social practices than those enumerated in the treatises devoted specifically to the discipline itself'.[7] Also recognizing the deep interconnectedness of rhetoric and orality, John Foley viewed the 'rhetorical transformation of traditional oral forms' as essential to any genuine understanding of oral-connected texts, such as those surviving in Old English manuscripts; 'continuity of reception of a work that stems from oral tradition but which survives as a text', he argued, 'will depend on the reader's ability to recognize the rhetorical signals that are the bequest of performance and tradition, and then to credit these signals with the institutionalized meaning they carry as a dedicated register of verbal communication'.[8]

The tremendous diversity of cultural influences that shaped speech acts in Old English healing practice thus requires not only acknowledging but even embracing a certain degree of inherent variability within the category of 'medieval rhetoric', especially for early medieval England where the relationship 'between Latin rhetoric and the vernacular tradition' remains 'elusive' at best.[9] As Louise Bishop has aptly noted, in medieval and early modern medicine, 'healing, bodies, and words are linked materially, rhetorically, historically, and philosophically'.[10]

Previous chapters have sought to show how the amorphous body of medical literature from early medieval England defies much of our modern categorical thinking, and rhetorical speech acts must be understood as far more important than mere ornamental flourishes to healing practices; for many medieval and early modern cultures, words held 'the power to expose, cause, and even cure infection'.[11] As Lisi Oliver and Maria Mahoney astutely observe in their discussion of rhetoric and anatomy in the early Middle Ages, 'a single rhetoric is not sufficient for the portrayal of the ultimate reality',[12] which is why I have limited analysis here to this very specific phenomenon of speech to plants as manifest within the single Harley 585 manuscript. But by focusing so precisely on the variations of verbal rhetoric employed in the persuasion of plants, we can come to a more nuanced understanding of how early medieval medical practitioners viewed themselves more generally in relation to the world of medicine and the healing plants that they employed in their remedies.

Hybrid healing and the Harley 585

Offering a unique opportunity for comparison of remedies drawn from Germanic tradition alongside those translated fairly literally into Old English from known Latin sources, the MS Harley 585 is a particularly apt focal point for studying the rhetorical aspects of an early medieval healing practice that had long been viewed as a collaborative enterprise with the herbs themselves. This manuscript contains both the Old English *Herbarium* (folios 1r–101v), which renders translations of remedies collected almost entirely from Latin compilations, and also the medical text widely known as the *Lacnunga* (folios 130r–193r), which comprises a miscellany of charms and remedies, including a number of poetic incantations in alliterative Old English verse.[13] And where the *Lacnunga* is organized (albeit loosely) around ailments, the *Herbarium* arranged remedies pharmaceutically by herb. Yet as different as these two medical texts are from one another at a surface level, the compiler's choice in including both collections together suggests that the two works were nonetheless seen as offering parallel and complementary modes of herbal healing for early medieval practitioners.

Among the significant performative features shared by both texts within this manuscript are directives for speech to herbs: specifically *mugwort*,[14] *wegbrade* (literally 'way-broad'[15]), *attorlaðe* (literally 'venom-hater'[16]), and *mægðe* (chamomile[17]), as treated in the *Lacnunga* within the so-called 'Nine Herbs Charm'; and *ricinum* (*ricinus communis L.*, or castor-oil plant) and *peruica* (*vinca maior L.*, or periwinkle plant), as treated in the *Herbarium*.[18] While both texts incorporate speech to plants, however, the specific ways that the healers are called upon to persuade these respective herbs manifest distinctly Germanic and Latinate rhetorical tendencies. Together, these two modes of persuasive speech reflect the cultural hybridity inherent in the healing tradition.

Representing the more distinctly Germanic healing practice, the 'Nine Herbs Charm' of the *Lacnunga* invokes the power of nine herbs to be employed against nine poisons. This metrical charm opens by itemizing and praising the individual herbs (ll. 1–29). Next, the poem moves into a more collective treatment of the nine together, providing mythopoetic contexts ultimately attributing the herbs' powers to Woden (ll. 30–40) and then elaborating on the many poisons and ailments against which the herbs are said to hold power (ll. 41–57). Then, in a telling illustration of this healing tradition's deep hybridity, the poem concludes with an invocation of Christ. Following these poetic portions of the text are instructions for preparation of the herbs into a paste and salve along with directions to sing the charm over the plants themselves and also into the mouth, ears, and sores of the person to be healed. The portions of this metrical charm that involve direct addresses to herbs all occur within its first thirty lines.

The context for directly addressing herbs is markedly different in the *Herbarium*, as this text adheres closely to the organization of its Latin models in providing more discrete entries ordered individually by herb. Periwinkle's entry in the *Herbarium* attributes the plant with power over numerous afflictions, ranging from mental conditions such as *deofolseocnyssa* ['devil sickness'] to venoms from snakes and even to abstract troubles such as envy or fear. After this list of possible uses, the entry then provides an incantation to recite prior to picking the herb, concluding with a brief admonition to be 'clean' when picking the plant. The entry for *ricinum*, which follows the same general structure, more directly targets threats from the natural world—specifically hail, lightning, and other rough weather. As with *peruica*, *ricinum*'s potential applications are followed by an incantation spoken to the herb, invoking the power of God in bringing the herb's powers to full effect. In both of these Old English entries, the incantation is provided first in Latin, followed by an Old English rendering.[19]

The macaronic nature of this entry with its mixed languages helps us to see that while the *Herbarium* remedies do indeed have identifiable Latin antecedents, such texts should not be viewed as any less integral or 'authentic' than their vernacular counterparts in medieval English medicine; the scribal choice to translate these Latin-derived entries into Old English across various manuscripts suggests their full incorporation into the broader healing tradition, encompassing both vernacular and Latinate modes of meaning.[20] And if we shift our focus from origins to performativity, the two linguistically and culturally distinct texts emerge in ritual performance as complementary, at times even overlapping, modes of healing. From this perspective, the Latinate origins of the incantations are inherent to the charms' power.

So apparently significant to the remedy was the incantation that the *h* at the beginning of the Latin version's address to *herba ricinum* is separated with a dot from what precedes, begins a new line, and is enlarged relative to the surrounding text (shown in Figure 4.1). It is also marked with red rubrication. The beginning of the incantation directed toward periwinkle is likewise marked with an enlarged capital, rubrication, and the beginning of a new page (shown in Figure 4.2).

Hybridity of rhetoric in Harley 585 135

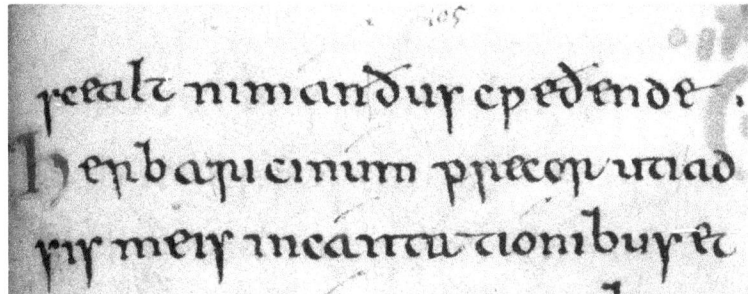

Figure 4.1 Entry for *ricinum*, British Library MS Harley 585, f. 94r.

This textual signaling of the beginning of an oral performance is consistent across all manuscripts produced during the Old English period. In Cotton Vitellius C.iii, the *h* in 'Herba ricinum' is kept on the same line, but it follows a dot and is capitalized and larger than the surrounding text. The *T* beginning the incantation 'Te precor' is marked even more clearly in this manuscript, not only rubricated and in a larger script but also beginning a new line (though there is still ample empty space in the line above) and set off in the left margin, a mode of marking typically reserved in this manuscript for new remedies (f. 72v). (See Figure 4.3.)

In the twelfth-century Harley 6258B, a manuscript that will be discussed at length in the next chapter, even though the *h* in *herba ricinum* is not rubricated or placed at the beginning of a new line, it is still slightly larger than the surrounding text and distinguished from the preceding text (f. 34r). Similarly, the initial *T* in 'Te precor' follows a period and is capitalized in a very slightly larger script than that of the surrounding text, though again it does not begin a

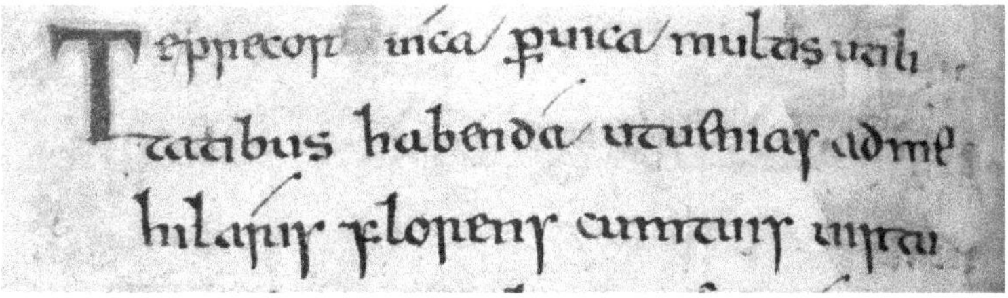

Figure 4.2 Entry for periwinkle, British Library MS Harley 585, f. 96v.

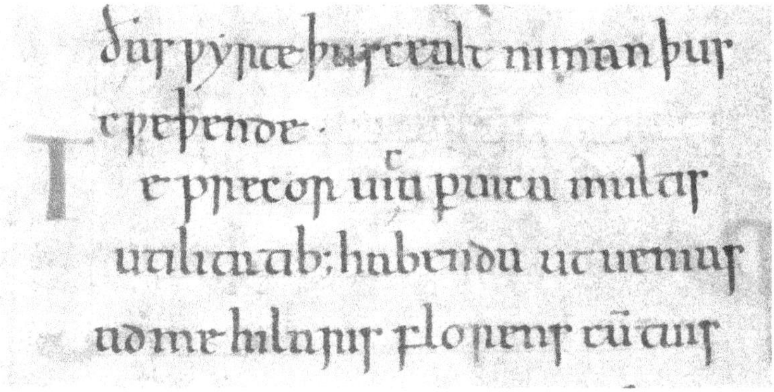

ðas wyrte þu sceealt niman þus
cweþende ·
Te precor uinca puinca multas
utilitatib; habendu ut uenias
ad me hilaris florens cũ tuis

Figure 4.3 Entry for periwinkle, British Library MS Cotton Vitellius C.iii, f. 72v.

new line and is not rubricated (f. 32r). On the other hand, the Old English version of the incantation is not set apart or distinguished in such ways within any of the manuscripts. Even in the most lavish Cotton Vitellius C.iii, *ricinum* was written without any special care, with missing characters, the *ci* inserted above the main line.

Indeed, the fact that the incantation is provided first in Latin and then only afterwards translated into Old English—in a text that otherwise silently converts Latin remedies into the Old English vernacular—suggests that the rhetorical power of the spoken address must have been seen as deriving at least in part from its language, with the Latin and the vernacular playing complementary, but not interchangeable, roles within the healing economy. The reduplication of the incantation in Latin and Old English thus provides important information as to how these remedies might have been understood by early readers of the text. The fact that the translation was thought necessary at all implies an audience of healers reading and performing the charm who were not assumed to have reading knowledge of Latin. Just as importantly, however, this presentation in the manuscript indicates that even though the implied speakers of the incantation were not assumed to know Latin, they were still expected to speak to the two plants *in* Latin. In short, it was important for the speaker to know what the words meant, but the meaning alone was insufficient for the charms' rhetorical power; the words had to be understood in English but voiced (at least the first time) in Latin itself. This linguistic code-switching within Old English charm texts reflects a productive hybridity in ritual performance that depends not only upon the voicing of diglossic texts but also upon dual rhetorical strategies in the persuasion of the herbs. It is this crossing of linguistic and rhetorical traditions that enables the potential for empowering hybridity within the healing register.

The very phenomenon of speaking to herbs activates a fairly specialized register. Most herbal remedies in the Harley 585 manuscript (and also in the wider healing tradition) that include verbal components at all dictate that the incantations be recited *over* herbs or, even more generally, provide words that can be spoken *about* herbs. But the six herbs involved in these particular herbal remedies from the *Herbarium* and the *Lacnunga*'s 'Nine Herbs Charm' are not only spoken to directly, but are also called upon explicitly to perform tasks to aid the speaker. This shared framework across the two texts allows us to identify and explore subtle differences between strategies of persuasion *towards* herbs with regard to their Latinate and Germanic registers respectively.

The richness and complexity of this hybrid healing has at times been overlooked since those moments calling for speech towards plants have often been dismissed as mere superstition.[21] But the concept of a healer as a rhetorician is less anachronistic than it might otherwise seem when we take into account that during the medieval period, especially in parts of Europe, 'medical prediction, as an art dependent on personal skills such as memory and conjecture, was taught with the aid of the liberal arts of rhetoric and logic'.[22] Drawing evidence in part from the large number of orations given by physicians, Siraisi has demonstrated that premodern medicine participated actively in what was a 'still largely rhetorical culture'.[23] Though short in length compared with more conventional persuasive arguments in public speeches or other such fora, the incantations of Old English medical texts nonetheless employ a range of strategies in their solicitation of herbal healing power, strategies related especially closely to the rhetorical figures of *apostrophe*, *personification*, *prosopopoeia*, *chiasmus*, *anaphora*, and *metonymy*.

I want to stress that in using these classical rhetorical terms I am not positing a conscious or intentional employment of classical rhetoric by medieval scribes or medics.[24] As Janie Steen explains, historical evidence is 'too weak' to show that Old English poets were trained in the arts of rhetoric; however, 'it is clear that Latin rhetorical devices did find their way into vernacular verse', or at the very least that the Latin demonstrates more widely-employed rhetorical devices.[25] Whether or not the employment of rhetorical figures was in conscious emulation of classical authors, vernacular poets' 'close reading and absorption of works by Christian Latin authors could have exercised a much deeper influence on their own compositions than any diligent burrowing in Latin rhetorical manuals'.[26] This line of thinking is entirely consistent with the linguistic and cultural hybridity typical of oral and oral-connected texts. While it might be tempting to align vernacular/Latin categories with oral/literate learning, the reality of the situation is more complex. Focusing specifically on the Old English *Herbarium* but with regard to the larger 'early medieval world', Van Arsdall argues for 'a system of apprenticeship'—one notably encompassing both vernacular *and* Latin healing traditions—in which the written texts that survive today were only 'a secondary resource' to the 'unwritten text[s]' in 'the voice of the teacher and the memory of the apprentice healer'.[27] While in terms of origin the *Herbarium* arguably comes from a more 'literary' tradition, and the vernacular *Lacnunga* a more 'oral' one, in social practice neither had meaning outside of oral and aural performance. From a synchronic perspective, then, the two texts offer contemporaneous models for verbal healing.

Thus, the nature of the connections between these two medical texts in the Harley 585 is indeed complicated. On one hand, the *Lacnunga* clearly reflects a more Germanic mode of healing than the Old English *Herbarium*, for which almost every remedy can be traced to a known Latin source. On the other hand, the compiler of the Old English *Herbarium* was selective, and it stands to reason that the choices reflect a tendency to incorporate charms bearing features already familiar and meaningful to early medieval audiences. Although the incantations of both of the manuscript's compilations share certain rhetorical strategies, then, the *ways* these features are employed reflect distinct, but nonetheless complementary, ideologies and concepts of healing derived from a productive syncretism of the Latinate and Germanic medical traditions.

Apostrophe, personification, and prosopopoeia

The very speech act of addressing the herbs in the two medical texts within MS Harley 585 invites comparative exploration of the interrelated rhetorical devices of apostrophe, personification, and prosopopoeia.[28] However, while the incantations in both the *Herbarium* and the *Lacnunga* use seemingly similar types of direct address in soliciting the respective herbs' assistance, the methods by which the herbs are addressed—and, consequently, the relationships implied between healer and herb—differ markedly. Within the *Herbarium*, herbs are assumed to enter the human realm from elsewhere during each charm's performance. *Ricinum*, for instance, is asked to 'be present': '[I]c bidde þæt þu ætsy minum sangum' ['I ask that you be present at my songs'] (CLXXVI 22–23);[29] Periwinkle is similarly invited: '[I]c bidde ... þæt ðu glæd to me cume' ['I ask ... that you gladly come to me'] (CLXXIX 20–21),[30] even though in both cases the speaker is presumably already in possession of the physical herbs. The effect in these Latin-derived remedies is thus a separation of the spirits of the herbs from the physical plants themselves, a very different state of affairs from that implied in the 'Nine Herbs Charm' incantations, where the formulaic language employed not only assumes that the herbs' spirits are already present but that the herbs have been sentient all along.

Two of the four direct addresses to plants in the 'Nine Herbs Charm', for instance, imply such long-term awareness for the herbs by opening with an invocation for them to remember: 'Remember, Mugwort' (1), and 'Remember, Maythe' (23).[31] The address to Way-broad does not explicitly invoke a verb of memory, but it does likewise operate from the assumption that the herb is already innately strong—animate, listening, and ready to be persuaded: 'Ond þu Wegbrade, wyrta modor, eastan op[e]ne, innan mihtigu ...' ['And you, Way-broad, mother of herbs, open from the east, mighty within ...'] (7–8). The address to Attorlaðe also presumes that the herb's healing power is already with the speaker in the present moment, 'now'; the supplicant asks not that the herb come to join the speaker from another location, as in the *Herbarium*, but rather to act in the present location, at once: 'Fleoh þu nu Attorlaðe seo læsse ða maran' ['Put to flight now, Attorlaðe, the lesser [and] the greater'] (21–22). More than an artificial rhetorical device, this employment of direct address suggests a powerful collaboration between practitioner and plant.

Defined broadly, apostrophe[32] and personification are unquestionably prominent features in each of these particular incantations; in both the Latin-derived and vernacular incantations, the herbs are addressed directly, their capacity to hear and discern human speech anthropomorphically implied. When one considers the wider corpus of Old English literature, it stands to reason that vernacular remedies would incorporate such devices and that Latin remedies sharing similar tropes would be selected for inclusion. Apostrophe, for instance, is a natural corollary to prosopopoeia, long recognized as 'a recurrent favorite' in Old English poetics and a device that is especially pronounced in the Old English riddles as a way for the inanimate characters to speak.[33] Its inverse, speech to characters through apostrophe, would likely also have been a natural and compelling mode of persuasion in early medieval England.[34] To the extent that the incantations assume sentient auditors capable of comprehending human speech, all of these addresses toward herbs employ some degree of personification as well, with the marked difference that the personified addressee is presumed present in the *Lacnunga* but not already so in the *Herbarium*.

Exploring these ideas of presence and absence a bit further, we find that the seemingly illogical request for Ricinum from the Latinate *Herbarium* to 'be present', or for Periwinkle to 'come' when presumably the practitioner is already in presence of the herbs, can actually be explained through varied conceptions that existed for personification and apostrophe within medieval rhetoric. As defined in the classical *Rhetorica ad Herennium*,[35] personification (*conformatio*) as a figure of speech had more than one sense:

> Personification consists in representing an absent person as present, or in making a mute thing or one lacking form articulate, and

attributing to it a definite form and a language or a certain behaviour appropriate to its character.[36]

The *Herbarium*'s direct address, then, implies the first, more specialized of these senses, representing an absent person as present, whereas the Old English 'Nine Herbs Charm' already assumes the hearer's presence and employs only a broader form of personification. Here the Latin charm, as might be expected, adheres more closely to the more particularized rhetorical practices of classical texts.

A similar pattern holds with apostrophe. While the incantation of the 'Nine Herbs Charm' employs apostrophe in the more general sense of direct address, the *Herbarium* reflects its more restricted sense as reflected in such texts as the *Rhetorica ad Herennium*: 'Apostrophe [Exclamatio] is the figure which expresses grief or indignation by means of an address to some man or city or place or object'.[37] By focusing more directly on the speaker's needs, the speaker of the *Herbarium*'s incantations comes much closer to this state of grief or indignation than the implied speaker of the 'Nine Herbs Charm'; where the 'Nine Herbs Charm' appeals to shared positive memories between the speaker and herbs regarding distinctly earthly events, the *Herbarium*'s remedies focus instead on bringing the herb's spirits from another realm to that of the troubled speaker. Thus, in a manner more consistent with classical apostrophe and personification, the direct addresses in the *Herbarium* place the speaker explicitly in the role of plaintiff or supplicant, with the current need and desired outcome to be granted by the herb (in its abstract and distant form) given primary importance.

In fact, the implication of this more supernatural audience has led some scholars (e.g., Dendle) to refer to these incantations as 'prayers',[38] and this sense of supplication to a higher power is especially reinforced in the final line of the incantation to Periwinkle, which invokes the 'naman ælmihtiges Godes se þe het beon acenned' ['name of God almighty, who bade you to be born'].[39] The plant is thereby reminded of its indebtedness to God and thus in turn to the speaker, who is invoking God's name. The reminders in the 'Nine Herbs Charm', however, operate on very different assumptions. Rather than invoking God's past deeds, the speaker appeals to the herb's *own* past deeds, relating—or in some cases merely alluding to—stories of past power in the hopes of rekindling it for the future. More than a supplication, the incantations of the 'Nine Herbs Charm' invoke a shared sense of honor and duty, appealing to the herbs as heroic comrades.

To this end, in typical Germanic heroic fashion,[40] Mugwort and Maythe are both reminded of specific accomplishments (and also their own rhetorical skills that helped make them known), events alluded to but not described. Mugwort is reminded of a public declamation from its past as follows (1–2):

> Gemyne ðu, Mucgwyrt, hwæt þu ameldodest,
> hwæt þu renadest æt Regenmelde.
>
> [Remember, Mugwort, what you declared,
> what you brought about at Regenmelde.]

This phraseology is paralleled by the reminder to Maythe of a similar declamation (23–24):

> Gemyne þu, Mægðe, hwæt þu ameldodest,
> hwæt ðu geændadest æt Alorforda.
>
> [Remember, Maythe, what you declared,
> what you finished at Alorforda.]

Way-broad, however, is reminded not of a specific event but of more general past accomplishments (7–9):

> ofer ðy cræte curran, ofer ðy cwene reodan,
> ofer ðy bryde bryo- / dedon,[41] ofer þe fearras fnærdon;
> eallum þu þon wiðstode 7 wiðstunedest.
>
> [over you carts creaked, over you queens rode,
> over you brides trampled, over you bulls snorted;
> you withstood and crashed against all then.]

Significantly, the reader or user of the 'Nine Herbs Charm' is reminded of the origins of the plants as a creation of Woden,[42] and Christ is also, near the end of the poem, posited as an opposing force to sickness.[43] Thus, presumably the incantation *could* have appealed to these higher powers in a fashion parallel to that seen in the *Herbarium* but did not. The contrasting approaches, though, are not due solely to differing belief systems; instead, the more significant difference lies in what rhetorical strategy is believed most convincing to the *plants*. The Latin-derived *Herbarium* appeals to the herb's shared sense of indebtedness to God, while the Old English text appeals to the herbs' sense of duty and heroism based on their *own* inherent strengths. There is an implicit hierarchy in the Latin text as well; by addressing the plant 'in God's name', the speaker asserts dominance over the plant. The speaker of the 'Nine Herbs Charm', on the other hand, shares a similar goal of enlisting the plant's healing power but does so by appealing to it as a comrade.[44]

The two types of address and subsequent methods of persuasion reflect cultural differences between Latinate and Germanic modes of expression and conceptions of herbal healing.[45] Yet, as different as the two types of direct address are in these respective texts, their juxtaposition within a single manuscript devoted to healing practice nonetheless suggests that these variant strains of thought were not seen as competing or mutually exclusive. As with many aspects of early medieval culture, such variation in the rhetorical devices employed in the persuasion of plants reflects the productive syncretism of Germanic and Latinate influences, a pattern that becomes even more pronounced when we look at patterns of repetition.

Anaphora and chiasmus

As with apostrophe and personification, the shared uses of anaphora and, to a lesser extent, chiasmus in the *Lacnunga* and *Herbarium* also reveal distinct patterns of difference. Though present in both texts, anaphora is much more pronounced in the 'Nine Herbs Charm' of the *Lacnunga*, a pattern consistent with the great appeal that such patterns of structural repetition seem to have had for vernacular-connected texts during this period more generally. Bede, for example, as an individual influenced heavily by both the Germanic and Latinate traditions, not only privileges anaphora with its own entry in his *De schematibus et tropis* (defining it as 'when the same utterance is repeated two or more times at the beginnings of verses'[46]), but also employs it as one of the most frequent rhetorical devices in his own homilies.[47] The 'Nine Herbs Charm' also relies heavily on anaphora at several points, but especially so during the incantations directed toward the herbs themselves.

A significant effect of anaphora is to reinforce through repetition and rhythm the concepts being paralleled. Through this structuring device, the incantations of the 'Nine Herbs Charm' underscore the inherent power of the herbs themselves. The 'þu miht wið' ['you have power against'] sequence (ll. 4–6) directed toward Mugwort, for instance, highlights the power the herb has over various foes (emphasis added):

ðu miht wið *III*   and wið *XXX*,
þu miht wiþ attre   and wið onflyge,
þu miht wiþ þa[m] laþan   ðe geond lond færð.

[**You have power against** three and against thirty,
You have power against poison and against flying disease,
You have power against the loathsome one that travels throughout the land.]

The 'ofer ðy' ['over you'] frame directed toward Way-broad similarly reinforces the herb's particular strengths, in this case the power to withstand and persevere (9–10; emphasis added):

ofer ðy cræte curran,   ofer ðe cwene reodan,
ofer ðy bryde bryo- / dedon,   ofer þy fearras fnærdon.

[**Over you** carts creaked, **over you** women rode,
Over you brides trampled, **over you** bulls snorted.]

The addresses to both Mugwort and Maythe also employ anaphora through their repetitions of 'hwæt þu' ['what you'] that highlight the significance of previously mentioned declarations, in both cases linking the *b* half-lines and subsequent *a* half-lines structurally. This frame first appears in the incantation to Mugwort (1–2):

    hwæt þu ameldodest,
hwæt þu renadest

    [what you declared,
what you brought about].

The framing language is then formulaically repeated in the incantation to Maythe (23–24):

> hwæt þu ameldodest,
> hwæt ðu geændadest
>
> [what you declared,
> what you brought to an end].

In both cases anaphora thus serves to emphasize the herbs' respective accomplishments in overcoming adversity. The repetition in the address to Attorlaðe is chiastic rather than anaphoric, but it accomplishes a similar function by employing rhetorical structuring devices to foreground the herb's inherent power. As with the 'what you' frame, the device serves to link the *b* half-line with the following *a* half-line (21–22; emphasis added):

> Fleoh þu nu Attorlaðe   seo læsse ða maran
> seo mare þa læssan,   oððæt him beigra bot sy.
>
> [Put to flight now, Attorlaðe **the lesser, the greater,
> the greater, the lesser** until there is a cure for them both.]

As Pettit observes, the lines are 'metrically problematic, there being no alliteration in this, the traditional, arrangement' and are also 'difficult to understand, clearly being to some extent deliberately riddling'.[48] Once again, though, the structuring device highlights the innate power of the herbs against their respective maladies and demonstrates a nuanced understanding of differing measures or types of herbs needed to effect healing.

While structural repetition is also present within the *Herbarium* incantations, these rhetorical devices emphasize very different elements in the more Latinate environment. Rather than reinforcing the herbs' inherent strengths, these incantations use anaphora instead to foreground the desired outcomes. As with the previously discussed device of apostrophe, the anaphoric structure of the Latinate charm highlights the practitioner's role as supplicant rather than as colleague or ally. Underscoring the collaborative relationship between practitioner and plant, the Old English rendering of the incantation to Ricinum adds a structural repetition to the

Old English not present in the Latin, through 'þæt þu' ['that you'] (emphasis added):

> Ic bidde
> þæt þu ætsy minum sangum 7
> þæt ðu awende hagolas 7 ligræsceas.

> [I ask
> that you be present at my songs and
> that you turn aside hail and lightning flashes.]

Structural repetition addressing the plant as a colleague works similarly in the persuasive speech directed toward Periwinkle, again highlighting the desired outcomes (emphasis and line breaks mine):

> þæt ðu glæd to me cume mid þinum mægenum blowende,
> þæt ðu me gegearwie
> þæt ic sy gescyld 7 symle gesælig 7 ungedered fram attrum 7 fram yrsunge.

> [that you come to me happy with your strengths blooming,
>   that you prepare me
>   that I may be shielded and always lucky and unharmed by poisons and by anger.]

Thus, anaphoric repetition structurally continues the same pattern established by the opening direct address. The Germanic incantations of the 'Nine Herbs Charm' appeal to herbs as collaborators and highlight through repetition the worldly deeds of the already sentient herbs. In contrast, the Latin-derived incantations appeal to the herbs as (initially) absent potential benefactors and highlight through repetition the wishes of the speaker. It is a broadened understanding of metonymy in terms of oral traditional and performance contexts, however, that most meaningfully ties all of these classical and Germanic rhetorical patterns together in a powerful healing hybridity.

Metonymy and 'metonymic referentiality'

Even narrowly defined as a specialized rhetorical trope, metonymy can also be seen as a distinctive feature of the incantations in both collections.[49] The *Herbarium*'s incantation to Periwinkle asks the herb to come with its 'mægnum blowende' ['strengths blooming'], strengths metonymically representing the possessor of strength, the blooming herb. And in the repeated formulaic phrase from the 'Nine Herbs Charm' 'wið þa laþan ðe geond lond færð' ['against the loathsome one that travels throughout the land'] (6, 13, 20[50]), the 'loathsome one' refers not just to one ailment but metonymically references all maladies against which the herb is believed efficacious.

Viewed within the larger healing context, however, the metonymic referentiality of the more Germanically resonant 'Nine Herbs Charm' reaches well beyond its immediate context and activates meaning within multiple registers. Noting the 'rhetorical persistence of traditional forms', John Foley offers a way of understanding metonymy within distinctly oral traditional contexts, one in which the rhetorical device of metonymy is aligned with 'the paratactic, additive impulse as a primary pattern in oral tradition'.[51] Rather than viewing rhetoric as the exclusive domain of classical learning and literate culture, he offers a tradition-dependent and more culturally relative way of understanding such devices as metonymy and anaphora to interpret oral and oral-derived verbal art more productively. This approach is especially fruitful for the genre of medieval healing remedies; while these works survive only in manuscript form, they were explicitly intended for oral performance and, further, were doubtless connected to an ambient oral tradition.

Foley's concept of traditional metonymy even involves a rethinking of anaphora in terms of a broader generic and cultural context:[52]

> As a compositional figure, it [metonymy] underlies the formation and maintenance of the idiom at the level of both generalized structure and specific sequences. From the point of view of metonymic referentiality, each occurrence of any traditional structure would constitute a figure of anaphora, and thus a kind of parallelism, since it would have primary reference not to spatially or temporally contiguous occurrences but to the immanent meaning keyed in performance.

Viewed from this angle, the rhetorical force of 'wið þa laþan ðe geond lond færð' ['against the loathsome one which travels throughout the land'] not only connects lines 6, 13, and 20 within this particular incantation, but also links the herb's power with other herbs in the healing tradition more broadly. Utilizing very similar phraseology, the poem *Ic me on þisse gyrde beluce* (discussed earlier in Chapter 2), for instance, is said to be effective for 'eal þæt lað þe in to land fare' ['all evil which goes in to the land'] (l. 5). The force of this formulaic language reaches even beyond verse incantations to prose remedies as well, and a remedy for travelers found in the *Leechbook* suggests placing mugwort in one's hand or shoe 'wiþ miclum gonge ofer land' ['against much going over land'].[53] These connections invest the individual remedy with the authority of the larger ambient tradition.

On a more thematic level, the 'Nine Herbs Charm', like numerous other Old English healing texts, also employs such traditional metonymy to index a larger heroic tradition that further intensifies the power of the herb as a healing force. For instance, this wider traditional background is what gives deeper meaning and purpose to the commands to 'remember' in the direct addresses to mugwort and the other herbs discussed above; as Judith A. Vaughan-Sterling observes, the 'hearkening back' to unspecific feats in these incantations follows a similar pattern to the poem's later references to Germanic mythology and legend in the allusion to Woden and even Christ, in effect structurally and rhetorically linking the herbs' past accomplishments with heroic, even mythic, feats.[54] Such linkages to heroic registers are employed throughout the Old English medical texts, such as in a remedy against a swarm in MS CCCC 41 where the bees are addressed as *sigewif*, literally 'victory women', or even more directly in the previously discussed *Wið færstice*, where sudden pain is likened to a spear and the practitioner vows to send a spear back in retaliation.[55]

While mythic heroic contexts are invoked with some regularity in the Latin-derived *Herbarium*, such allusions are again situated very differently, and they do not appear in either of the actual incantations directed toward plants. For instance, the entry immediately above *ricinum*, that for *Achillea* (entry 175), reminds readers (presumably practitioners) that Achilles used the herb to cure wounds, and an entry for mugwort (entry 13) recounts that Chiron the centaur once made a remedy from the herb and that he named the plant for Diana, the Roman equivalent of Artemis. In both cases the legendary stories function etiologically, explaining the herb's Latin names, *Achillea* and *Artemisia*. Thus, even though both texts link herbal healing with larger heroic contexts, these linkages also involve contrasts that work hand in hand with the patterned usages we have already seen for other rhetorical devices in these texts. The Germanic mode of healing as reflected in the 'Nine Herbs Charm' assumes a collaborative relationship between practitioner and herb, heroic allies armed against a host of ailments. In keeping with this healing philosophy, the direct addresses remind the herbs of past heroic exploits, and the structural patterning serves to highlight heroic strengths. In contrast, the direct addresses and structural patterning within the two incantations of the *Herbarium* imply a very different type of relationship, that of a supplicant appealing to a distant and supernatural force for specific and much-needed aid.

Still, the fact that such different rhetorical ends could be achieved through the use of shared rhetorical devices and strategies is a testament to the multi-layered and complex world of early medieval healing. The compilers of the *Herbarium* were of course selective in what they chose for inclusion. As Maria Amalia D'Aronco notes, the criteria for inclusion 'are still unclear',[56] but it seems that a certain degree of compatibility with parallel Germanic medicine must have played at least some part. The selection process would have been one of 'merging and adaptation' rather than of slavish translation,[57] and it would be ill-conceived to oversimplify matters and default to classifying the Old English *Herbarium* as 'literary' just because it derives from Latin and thus oppose it to the more vernacular and 'oral' *Lacnunga* remedies. As Van Arsdall explains, the *Herbarium of Pseudo-Apuleius* 'crossed the English Channel in Latin probably well before the reign of King Alfred' and circulated in England, and with this text came a tradition of healing that 'was disseminated orally and in writing'.[58] So by the period when the compilation that we now have was written down, Latinate 'charms, incantations, and magic, as well as written texts' were already very much a part of the Old English healing tradition 'and had been for quite some time'.[59] Sauer suggests that, while the usual pattern was for Old English formations to be translated from the Latin, there is evidence that in some cases the Old English plant-names instead influenced the Latin. *Venenifuga* (literally 'venom-loather'), for instance, may actually be a translation of *attor-laþe*, 'and not the other way round'.⁶⁰ This possibility of mutual influence on something as fundamental as names of the plants themselves points toward a vibrant exchange between Latinate and vernacular medical learning.

Rhetoric and the logic of healing in practice

The nature of the comparisons to be made between these different modes of speech thus teaches us a great deal about the rewards of broadening our scope to encompass 'both oral and written discourse' across 'a broader range of social practices'.⁶¹ At a local level, we can appreciate the subtle nuances underlying the particular incantations of entries 176 and 179 of the Old English *Herbarium* and the 'Nine Herbs Charm' of the *Lacnunga*. But more importantly, we come to a richer understanding of the Old English healing tradition, one flexible enough to simultaneously accommodate multiple healing and linguistic registers in a powerful healing hybridity. These rare glimpses into the plant/practitioner relationship allow us to see *how* healing plants are viewed, even when they are not directly addressed. In the 'Nine Herbs Charm', the direct speech is not sustained, shifting back and forth between second and third person, which seems more natural when we consider the performance context suggested in the prose instructions that follow the poem. Before preparing the herbs into a paste, the practitioner is to 'sing þæt galdor on æcre þara wyrta III' ['sing that incantation over each of the herbs three times']. But the incantation is also to be sung over the afflicted individual: 'ond singe þon men in þone muð and in þa earan buta and on ða wunde þæt ilce gealdor, ær he þa sealfe on do' ['and sing into the mouth of the man and both the ears and on the wound that same incantation, before he applies the salve']. The implied audience of the incantation itself therefore becomes rather fluid—moving between the herbs and also various body parts of the afflicted individual—but the flexible relationship implied by the rhetoric directed toward plants in the charm as a whole demonstrates the collaborative plant/practitioner dynamic in play elsewhere.

Hybridity of rhetoric in Harley 585   151

As the next small step toward this wider appreciation of plant-oriented rhetoric, let me end this chapter by returning to the remedy for a snakebite with which we began and see why it perhaps would not have been a contradiction at all for the medieval practitioner to render the Latin 'canto', most easily translated as 'I sing', as the Old English imperative 'besing', '[you] sing'. The collected medical texts in the Harley 585 have shown us that there was always room in early medieval England for thinking about and engaging with healing plants in quite diverse ways. For instance, in the Latin incantations of the *Herbarium*, plants are not invested with authority in and of themselves. Not inherent in the plant, their powers must be summoned, and, further, those powers must be granted in the name of God, 'naman ælmihtiges Godes'. It thus stands to reason that in the Latin snakebite incantation the plant would not be called upon directly to exert its power of its own accord. In the Old English translation, however, not only the language but also the power dynamic shift to that seen in the vernacular tradition of the *Lacnunga*. In this construct, plants work of their own volition and agency to collaborate with practitioners and can even be persuaded by appeals to a shared heroic past. The imperative 'besing 7 ofercum' ['sing and overcome'] thus translates the Latin incantation into the vernacular healing logic, transferring authority from the human practitioner to the courageous plant (*ellen-wyrt*) itself. Such transference of control away from the healer to a plant that presumably has been invested with power by God also has the added effect of removing the impression that the healer might be exercising powers of enchantment, a healing practice prohibited in a sermon of Ælfric:[62]

> ne sceole we urne hiht on læce-wyrtum besettan, ac on ðone Ælmihtigan Scyppend, þe ðam wyrtum ðone cræft forgeaf. Ne sceal nan man mid galdre wyrte besingan, ac mid Godes wordum hí gebletsian....
>
> [We must not set our hope in healing plants, but in the almighty creator, the one that has given that craft to those plants. One must not sing/enchant a plant with incantations, but with words of God must bless it....]

The literal words might say 'I sing', but the Old English clarifies that the healer is not acting on their own. We don't need to view the translator as being in error or emend a perceived scribal error. The differences between the Latin and Old English can be seen as reflecting the complex diversity of the rhetorical traditions in play.

Finally, our exploration of healing rhetoric in this chapter also provides a much fuller sense of what dynamic would have been in play for those medieval English remedies that call for speech but do *not* provide specific language. *Herbarium* entry 19, for instance, requires the harvester of herbs to explain to *proserpinaca* how it will be used: 'cweð þæt þu hy to eagena læcedome niman wylle' ['say that you wish to take it for a remedy of the eyes']. Entry 24 also asks the harvester to enlist the plant's assistance by sharing the larger healing goal: 'þonne hy man nime cweþe þæt he hy wille wið flean 7 wið eagena sare' ['when one takes it, say that he wishes it against specks[63] and against sore eyes']. While we can't know exactly how a practitioner might have worded these explanations, we can discern that there was likely an underlying logic assuming a shared endeavor and an outcome that could be reached only through the active cooperation of the plants themselves, not by the practitioner's agency alone.

It is with this idea of plant volition and agency in mind that we will now in the next chapter turn to what is perhaps the most famous plant hybrid known in medieval medicine, the mandrake. In probing the differences within the *Herbarium* entry for mandrake as it appears in tenth- and twelfth-century manuscripts, we shall see a subtle but undeniable shift away from the kind of plant/human collaboration found within the Harley 585 as the relationship between these two realms evolved instead toward the quite different model that remains prevalent even today within modern medicine.

Notes

1 All three names appear with the illustration in the MS Cotton Vitellius C.iii, f. 47v.
2 Though scribal error or misreading is always a possibility, the first-person present indicative of *cantare* is *canto*, requiring no emendation whatsoever. The imperative future (the expected form of the future for recipes) would have been something closer to *cantato* or, perhaps if the

verb were understood as a form of *canere*, *canito*. Even if the earlier text had been intended as a future imperative, the form was relatively rare in late medieval Latin and less likely to have been recognized as such by a tenth-century scribe in England, especially when *canto* had a much more straightforward meaning. Many thanks to David Sick for helping me think through these various grammatical possibilities.

3 *DOE*, s. v. *ellen*, sense 1: 'courage, strength'; sense 1.c: 'specifically of ardent feeling or emotion'. Bosworth and Toller, s.v. *wæl*, sense 1.a, 'generally of death in battle'. See also Sauer and Kubaschewski's reading as an alternate form of 'wealh-wyrt', 'foreigner plant, foreigner wort, Welsh plant', *Planting*, p. 259.

4 Many thanks to Tiffany Beechy for noticing this second possibility.

5 See, for instance, Pollington, *Leechcraft*, who translates as 'I charm and overcome all evil wild beasts', p. 331. On the other hand, Cockayne and Van Arsdall both translate in the imperative, 'Enchant and overcome', and de Vriend's edition glosses both verbs as imperative. Cockayne, *Leechdoms*, vol. 1, p. 203. Anne Van Arsdall, *Medieval Herbal Remedies: The Old English Herbarium and Anglo-Saxon Medicine* (New York: Routledge, 2002), p. 190.

6 See, for instance, Jonathan Roper's attempt to identify 'the rhetorical structures and devices typically present in the words of a charm': 'Towards a Poetics, Rhetorics, and Proxemics of Verbal Charms', *Folklore*, 24 (2003), 7–49, at 23. Roper treats Old English charms in particular on pp. 10–11. See also Edward Karshner's exploration of 'the parallel epistemological roles magic and mysticism share with rhetoric and philosophy'; while his goal is to devise terminology applicable to verbal charms cross-culturally, his primary examples draw from ancient Egypt, 'Thought, Utterance, Power: Toward a Rhetoric of Magic', *Philosophy and Rhetoric*, 44 (2011), 52–71, at 53. For a bibliography of scholarship through the mid-1970s addressing the subject of rhetoric in early medieval England, see Luke M. Reinsma, 'Rhetoric, Grammar, and Literature in England and Ireland before the Norman Conquest: A Select Bibliography', *Rhetoric Society Quarterly*, 8 (1978), 29–48. An analysis of Old English poems as political rhetoric can be found in Peter R. Richardson, 'Making Thanes: Literature, Rhetoric and State Formation in Anglo-Saxon England', *Philological Quarterly*, 78 (1999), 215–232. Ursula Schaefer has offered a very insightful treatment of rhetorical structures present in *Beowulf* as well as a history of relevant scholarship on the subject in 'Rhetoric and Style', in Robert E. Bjork and John D. Niles (eds), *A Beowulf Handbook* (Lincoln, NE: University of Nebraska Press, 1997), pp. 105–124. On the adaptation

of classical rhetoric in early medieval England, see further Gabriele Knappe, 'Classical Rhetoric in Anglo-Saxon England', *Anglo-Saxon England*, 27 (1998), 5–29.
7 Martin Camargo, 'Defining Medieval Rhetoric', in Constant J. Mews, Cary J. Nederman, and Rodney M. Thomson (eds), *Rhetoric and Renewal in the Latin West 1100–1540*. Disputatio 2. (Turnhout: Brepols, 2007), pp. 21–34, at 22.
8 Foley, *Singer*, p. 81.
9 Janie Steen, *Verse and Virtuosity: The Adaptation of Latin Rhetoric in Old English Poetry* (Toronto: University of Toronto Press, 2008), p. 3.
10 Louise M. Bishop, *Words, Stones, and Herbs: The Healing Word in Medieval and Early Modern England* (Syracuse: Syracuse University Press, 2007), p. 83.
11 Jennifer Vaught (ed.), *Rhetorics of Bodily Disease and Health in Medieval and Early Modern England* (Farnham: Ashgate, 2010), p. 17.
12 Lisi Oliver and Maria Mahoney, 'Episcopal Anatomies of the Early Middle Ages', in Jennifer Vaught (ed.), *Rhetorics of Bodily Disease and Health in Medieval and Early Modern England* (Farnham: Ashgate, 2010), pp. 25–41, at 25. C. Jan Swearingen and Edward Schiappa likewise encourage scholars to 'attend to the presence of multiple rhetorical models and cultures throughout the world', leading to 'a rich new diversity and revisionism among research methods' and a growing 'movement toward inclusion and comparison', 'Historical and Comparative Rhetorical Studies: Revisionist Methods and New Directions', in Andrea A. Lunsford et al. (eds), *The Sage Handbook of Rhetorical Studies* (Newbury Park: Sage, 2009), pp. 1–12, at 1.
13 The intervening text is the *Medicina de Quadrupedibus* (ff. 101v–114v), a collection of remedies made from animal products that accompanies the *Herbarium* in all four of the *Herbarium*'s extant manuscripts. This text does not include any incantations.
14 The Latin plant name is *Artemisia*. For a discussion of this herb and its nomenclature, see Philip G. Rusche, 'Dioscorides' *De materia medica*', in Biggam (ed.), *From Earth to Art: The Many Aspects of the Plant-World in Anglo-Saxon England* (Amsterdam and New York: Rudopi, 2003), pp. 181–194, at 182–183.
15 Most likely *Plantago major* L., greater plantain, according to Sauer and Kubaschewski, though possibly dock or sorrel, *Planting*, p. 261. The etymology given in the Old English Plant Names database notes the compound of *weg* [road] and *brad* [broad] developed 'because of the plant's habitat [along paths] and the shape of the leaves'. *DOEPN*, http://oldenglish-plantnames.org.

16 Hans Sauer identifies as 'cockspur grass', 'The Morphology of Old English Plant-Names', in C. P. Biggam (ed.), *From Earth to Art*, pp. 161–179, at 166.

17 For discussion of the history of *maythe* as treated in the *Oxford English Dictionary* and its various medieval and modern identifications, see Anthony Esposito, 'Medieval Plant-Names in the *Oxford English Dictionary*', in Biggam (ed.), *From Earth to Art*, pp. 231–248, 243–245.

18 The remedies to be discussed here can be found as follows: *Lacnunga*, 'Nine Herbs Charm', folio 160r ff.; *Herbarium* chapter 176 (*ricinum*) folio 93v ff.; *Herbarium* chapter 179 (*peruica*) folio 96r ff. Quotations from the *Herbarium* follow Jan de Vriend's edition of Cotton Vitellius C.iii, the language of which is virtually identical to that of the Harley 585.

19 Rather than viewing the Latin text as the portion to be recited and the Old English translation as merely clarification, D'Aronco asserts that this 'prayer should be recited twice before picking the plant, first in Latin and then in Old English', 'Anglo-Saxon Plant', p. 143.

20 Chapters 13–85 'are the translation of a choice, whose criteria are still unclear, of remedies derived from two pseudo-Dioscoridean treatises, the *Liber medicinae ex herbis femininis* and the *Curae herbarum*, besides a group of seven chapters of uncertain origin', D'Aronco, 'Anglo-Saxon Plant', p. 134. Chapter 176, for *ricinum* (discussed further below), is one of those of uncertain origin, but it clearly draws from this same Latinate tradition. Chapter 179 (*priapisci* or *peruica* [periwinkle]) closely follows the *Liber medicinae ex herbis femininis*. The remedy as found in MS L. Lucca, Biblioteca Governativa, no. 296, f. 37v is printed in de Vriend, *Old English Herbarium*, p. 225.

21 On the distancing of medieval charms from medical practice in modern scholarship, see Anne Van Arsdall, 'Reading Medieval Medical Texts with an Open Mind', in Elizabeth Lane Furdell (ed.), *Textual Healing: Essays on Medieval and Early Modern Medicine* (Leiden: Brill, 2005), pp. 9–29.

22 Luke E. Demaitre, 'The Art and Science of Prognostication in Early University Medicine', *Bulletin of the History of Medicine*, 77 (2003), 765–788, at 765.

23 Nancy G. Siraisi, 'Oratory and Rhetoric in Renaissance Medicine', *Journal of the History of Ideas*, 65 (2004), 191–211, at 204.

24 Compelling arguments, however, have been made previously for just such a conscious employment of rhetorical devices by vernacular poets. See, for instance, Jackson J. Campbell's description of *The Wanderer* as the work of a 'conscious rhetorical artificer', 'fully cognizant of the

techniques to be learned from the Latin rhetorical tradition as well as the English alliterative tradition'. But the argument put forth in the present study bases no claims on intentionality, leaving open the possibility (and even likelihood) that features shared by vernacular and Latinate texts reflect an overlapping aesthetic that may or may not have been conscious. As Campbell astutely observes, 'Latin learning was far from incompatible with an ability to compose in the formulaic style', 'Learned Rhetoric in Old English Poetry', *Modern Philology*, 63 (1966),189–201, at 201, 194.
25 Steen, *Verse*, p. 19.
26 Ibid., p. 16.
27 Van Arsdall, 'Reading', pp. 18–19. See also John M. Riddle, 'Theory and Practice in Medieval Medicine', *Viator: Medieval and Renaissance Studies*, 5 (1974), 157–184. In Riddle's view, 'when one particular part of an herb, say a root, was found as being effective for some specific action, this information was orally transmitted whenever and wherever men communicated and one generation taught the other. This process takes place independently of literary transmission', p. 165.
28 The rhetorical persistence of apostrophe and personification continued into the early Middle English period, where their uses become more defined and explicit, as both receive fairly extensive treatment as modes of amplification in Geoffrey of Vinsauf's *Poetria Nova*. See Martin Camargo (ed. and intro.), *Poetria Nova*, by Geoffrey of Vinsauf, trans. Margaret F. Nims (Toronto: Pontifical Institute of Medieval Studies, rev. edn, 2010), pp. 27–35.
29 This Old English entry is adapted from the Latin 'herba ricinum precor uti adsis meis incantationibus'. Throughout this chapter, I have used capitalization when discussing the anthropomorphized herbs and lowercase in other contexts.
30 From the Latin 'Te precor uica peruica … ut ea mihi prestes'.
31 For further discussion on direct addresses towards these herbs, see Marie Nelson and Caroline Dennis, 'Nine Herbs Charm', *Germanic Notes and Reviews*, 38 (2007), 5–10.
32 Cf. *AHD*, s.v. *apostrophe*: 'the direct address of an absent or imaginary person or of a personified abstraction'. As will be discussed in more depth below, the extent of personification varies considerably.
33 Jackson J. Campbell, 'Rhetoric in Old English Literature: Adaptation of Classical Rhetoric in Old English Literature', in James J. Murphy (ed.), *Medieval Eloquence: Studies in the Theory and Practice of Medieval Rhetoric* (Berkeley: University of California Press, 1978), pp. 173–197, at 194.

34 Cf. Paxson, who, building from Paul de Man, explains that 'rhetorical apostrophe engenders a prosopopoeia because the linguistic structure of the apostrophic utterance assumes or predicates a responsive human consciousness in inanimate objects'. James J. Paxson, *The Poetics of Personification* (Cambridge: Cambridge University Press, 1994), p. 52.
35 As Steen notes, there is 'no direct evidence' that such rhetorical treatises circulated in early medieval England, *Verse*, p. 9. However, several scholars have noted the presence of rhetorical devices described in the *Rhetorica ad Herennium* in early medieval writing. See, for instance, Campbell, 'Rhetoric in Old English Literature', esp. p. 187. It is also crucial to note that such devices are not limited to classical traditions.
36 'Conformatio est cum aliqua quae non adest persona confingitur quasi adsit, aut cum res muta aut informis fit eloquens, et forma ei et oratio adtribuitur ad dignitatem adcommodata aut actio quaedam'. Quotation and translation from Harry Caplan (ed. and trans.), *Rhetorica ad Herennium*, LCL 403 (Cambridge, MA: Harvard University Press, 1954), pp. 398–399.
37 'Exclamatio est quae conficit significationem doloris aut indignationis alicuius per hominis aut urbis aut loci aut rei cuiuspiam conpellationem', Caplan, *Rhetorica ad Herennium*, pp. 282–283.
38 See Dendle, 'Plants'. Referring to Chapter 79, D'Aronco identifies the incantation as a *precatio*', 'Anglo-Saxon Plant', p. 143.
39 From the Latin 'nomen omnipotentis Dei qui te iussit nasci'. Emily Kesling makes a compelling argument that the diffusion of this text can be attributed to its place within the movement of Benedictine reform, *Medical*, p. 133 *et passim*. Acknowledging the 'diverse background of inherited opinions', she observes that 'it is impossible to say there was a single, comprehensive theology of medicine' in early medieval England and that traditional medical practice should not be seen 'in opposition to faith', p. 154.
40 Being remembered for valor and bravery was central to the heroic ethos of the Germanic *comitatus* in the poetic tradition. When Beowulf appeals to the coastguard for an audience with Hygelac, for instance, he rests his argument in part on the place of his own father, Ecgþeow, in public memory: 'hine gearwe geman / witena welhwylc wide geond eorþan' ['Each of wise men throughout the world continues to remember him'] (*Beowulf* 267–268).
41 I follow Pettit's edition here, which acknowledges the compound, split across a page break.
42 'þa wyrte gesceop witig drihten' ['the wise lord shaped these plants'] (l. 37).

43 'Crist stod ofer alde' ['Christ stood over disease'], *alde* being an alternate spelling of *adl*, *adle* (*DOE*, s.v. *adl*). This Christian element is emphasized through a rudimentary cross inscribed in the left margin, f. 162v. www.bl.uk/manuscripts/Viewer.aspx?ref=harley_ms_585_f16 2v. Accessed 1 August 2021.

44 It is important to note, though, that while anthropomorphized to the point of presumably hearing, the herbs of the incantation are not completely anthropomorphized. The implication here is therefore less an outright personification of the herb than a reciprocal *comitatus* relationship that accommodates both plants and people. The plants are implied to be sentient, to be sure, even to have 'declared' in the past, which would suggest the capacity for communication, yet the plants are very clearly called upon with full regard for their plant-like qualities. This is most clear in the Way-broad invocation, which refers to the herb's growing location in pathways. Not only might the incantation 'illustrate the resilience of the plantain', but it could also 'constitute an aetiological tale accounting for the plantain's (*Plantago major* L.) broad leaves and peripherally flat appearances'. Pettit, *Anglo-Saxon Remedies*, p. 127. The plantain's tendency to grow along roadsides has been well-documented, lending credence to the speaker's reminder of its time spent beneath chariots.

45 As Louise Bishop has observed, 'rhetoric and cosmos run in parallel not only with each other, but with healing words', *Words*, p. 85.

46 'cum eadem dictio bis sæpiusve per principia versuum repetitur'. Text and translation from Bede, *Libri II De Arte Metrica et De Schematibus et Tropis: The Art of Poetry and Rhetoric*, ed. and trans. Calvin B. Kendall (Saarbrücken: AQ-Verlag, 1991), pp. 172–173.

47 A. G. P. Van der Walt, 'Early Medieval Stylistic Rhetoric', *Literator*, 2.3 (1981), 48–61, at 49.

48 Pettit, *Anglo-Saxon Remedies*, p. 132. The consensus view (reflected in Pettit's rendering) is that 'greater' and 'lesser' here refer to two different types of *attorlaðe* and their corresponding impact on greater and lesser poisons. The compound *attorlaðe* literally means 'poison harm' and has therefore been understood as encompassing a range of plants. The sense in Pettit's understanding is thus: 'Attorlaðe the lesser, put to flight the greater poison; Attorlaðe the greater, put to flight the lesser poison'.

49 The *Rhetorica ad Herennium*, for instance, defines metonymy (*denominatio*) as follows: 'Denominatio est quae ab rebus propinquis et finitimis trahit orationem qua possit intellegi res quae non suo vocabulo sit appellata', such as 'aut instrumento dominum' ['Metonymy is that which draws from near and adjoining things an expression by which it

is possible to understand the thing which is called forth not by its own name', such as 'the instrument for the possessor'], Caplan, *Rhetorica ad Herennium*, pp. 334–335.
50 While the first two instances occur within the direct addresses toward Mugwort and Way-broad, the example at line 20 does not appear in an incantation directed towards the herb but in this instance is used to describe the herb Stiðe's power.
51 Foley, *Singer*, p. 13.
52 Ibid.
53 See also Cameron, *Anglo-Saxon Medicine*, p. 133.
54 Vaughan-Sterling, 'Anglo-Saxon', p. 189.
55 On the *sigewif* of MS CCCC 41, see Garner and Miller, 'Swarm'; on *Wið færstice*, see Chapter 3.
56 D'Aronco, 'Anglo-Saxon Plant', p. 134.
57 Ibid., 144.
58 Van Arsdall, *Medieval Herbal Remedies*, p. 74.
59 Ibid., p. 74.
60 Sauer, 'Morphology', p. 171.
61 Camargo, 'Defining Medieval Rhetoric', p. 22.
62 Benjamin Thorpe (ed. and trans.), *The Homilies of the Anglo-Saxon Church*, vol. 1 (London: Richard and John Taylor, 1844), p. 476.
63 De Vriend glosses *fleah* here as 'white speck in the eye', *Old English Herbarium*, p. 359.

5

Of mandrakes and manuscripts: hybridity of being in Harley 6258B

Ðeos wyrt þe man mandragoram nemneþ ys mycel 7 mære on gesihþe 7 heo ys fremful

[This plant that one calls mandrake is great and glorious in sight and it is beneficial]

(Old English *Herbarium*, Cotton Vitellius C.iii)

… what with loathsome smells,
And shrieks like mandrakes' torn out of the earth
That living mortals, hearing them, run mad….

(*Romeo and Juliet*, Act 4, Scene 3)

Quite easy to overlook, in the middle of the page near the middle of an herbal produced early in the Middle English period, an unassuming entry headed *de mandragora* describes how to wring oil from mandrake leaves for the treatment of earaches and headaches and then how to use the powder from the mandrake root in drinks to reduce swelling from gout, lessen the effects of spasms, and treat certain forms of mental illness. (See Figure 5.1.) This entry of Harley MS 6258B begins on folio 20v and continues on 23r, concluding on 23v.[1] As we have seen in previous chapters, the surrounding herbal—typically known as the Old English *Herbarium*—is the first text in a manuscript compilation dedicated exclusively to the practice of medicine and provides an excellent point of access into early medieval healing at the moment of transition from what we now think of as Old to Middle English.[2]

Before proceeding any further, however, I must explain that few, if any, modern readers would be likely to first encounter the Old English mandrake through the Harley 6258B manuscript. Three

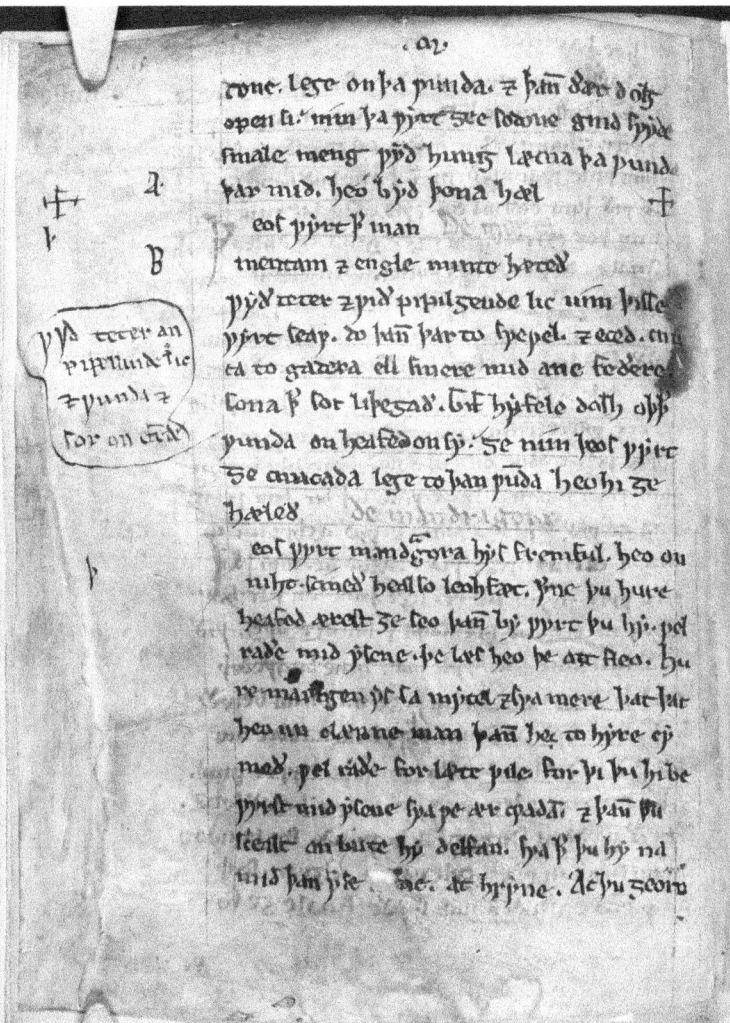

Figure 5.1 Entry for *mandragora*, British Library MS Harley 6258B, f. 20v.

earlier versions of this herbal remedy collection (Bodleian Library MS Hatton 76 [folios 74r–124r], British Library MS Cotton Vitellius C.iii [folios 20r–74r], and British Library MS Harley 585 [folios 1r–101v]) have been given far more authority, falling as they do more solidly in the Old English period, and, of these three, the Cotton Vitellius C.iii is the least damaged and most fully illustrated, thus most typically used as the *Herbarium*'s 'base' text.[3] The starting point for *Herbarium* scholarship is virtually never the twelfth-century Harley 6258B, but rather almost always this much earlier, relatively pristine, lavishly illustrated predecessor. To the extent that its existence is acknowledged at all, the Harley 6258B is described almost exclusively in relation to the Cotton Vitellius C.iii. The British Library's description of the Harley 6258B lists the three earlier copies of the *Herbarium* and the *Medicina de Quadrupedibus*, yet so established is the primacy of Cotton Vitellius C.iii that the Library's description of that manuscript does not even mention any of the other three versions.[4] Modern editions and translations likewise default to Cotton Vitellius C.iii as the base text, with variants provided primarily for comparative purposes.[5]

And regardless of manuscript, the first details most often shared about the mandrake are not focused around its specific healing properties, but rather its elaborate harvesting ritual, requiring a hungry dog to pull it from its roots after its 'head' has been encircled by iron, the plant's raw power too great for any practitioner to handle directly. This emphasis on the risk-reducing ritual is further enhanced by visual images of the mandrake, such as the illustration accompanying the entry in the Cotton Vitellius C.iii depicting a fully anthropomorphized root with sharply defined ribs and muscular arms as well as leafy 'hair'. (See Figure 5.2.) Such images—which are absent from the Harley 6258B manuscript and the other extant manuscripts—have long superseded in the popular (as well as scholarly) imagination the much more routine descriptions of the mandrake's preparation and application within healing remedies.

What I wish to argue is not that we change the default text or that we ignore the fantastical hybridity conveyed in the entry. On the contrary, Cotton Vitellius C.iii has long served as the base text for many excellent reasons. It is written in the dialect most familiar to modern scholars of Old English, it is the most well-preserved

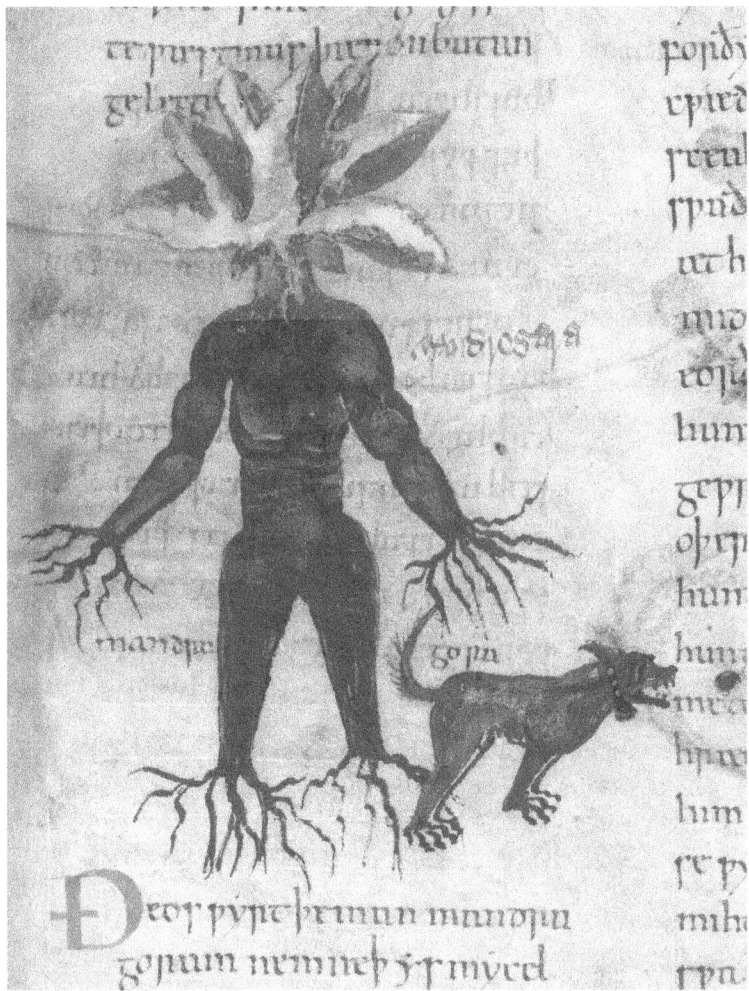

Figure 5.2 Entry for *mandragora*, British Library MS Cotton Vitellius C.iii, f. 57v.

version with the fewest lacunae and is thus more accessible to modern readers, and its beautiful illustrations go far in contextualizing the remedies for us even today. Not being practitioners of medieval medicine, modern readers *need* the clarity provided by what was likely a presentation copy, geared as it was even then toward non-specialists with an interest in healing practice. Rather, what I hope to accomplish here is to show what can be gained at the same time by looking at this anomalous entry completely on its own terms, removed from the restrictions of periodization and the conventional expectations of modern western medicine. Standing (and the humanoid plant is indeed standing) in sharp contrast to the relatively mundane majority of the *Herbarium*'s entries, the human/plant hybrid and its alarming description would doubtless have been conspicuous even in its own time, and, though the *Herbarium*'s mandrake doesn't literally scream (even if a twelfth-century addition to that effect has accompanied the mandrake legend into the modern era) or even speak, it is nonetheless important to consider what it might be telling us about plant healing.

A first step towards this understanding of the mandrake's various manifestations in the manuscript tradition involves recognizing and addressing fundamental prejudices in past approaches. Marginalizing manuscripts such as Harley 6258B as mere context for the pristine presentation copies belies a number of biases, privileging modern ideals and values over those presented in the medieval manuscripts themselves. Similarly, examining the mandrake harvesting ritual without the full (and seemingly uninteresting by comparison) backdrop of the 184 other remedies, we miss much of what the exceptional entry might have conveyed to medieval healers. When we privilege earlier texts over later texts, exceptional texts over routine, human over plant, we put ourselves at a higher risk for projecting our own expectations onto this early medieval text. What I propose here is to explore instead this exceptional entry within an otherwise unassuming text by removing the constraints of rigid periodization and shifting some common default interpretive settings.

With these goals in mind, this analysis begins with examination of the Harley 6258B for what it can show in and of itself rather than simply as a footnote to the 'base' text Cotton Vitellius C.iii. Next, I will examine the mandrake entry in particular within the larger context of medieval medicine and offer a comparative analysis of the mandrake entry in these two manuscript versions. Finally, our exploration will move toward the larger implications of the mandrake's portrayal in this twelfth-century context. An appendix at the chapter's end provides a newly edited text and translation of the mandrake entry in the Harley 6258B, with footnotes offering comparison with the Cotton Vitellius C.iii—a reverse of the typical treatment. Far more than mere superstition or ignorant irrationality, what becomes most salient in this seemingly bizarre entry for *mandragora* is a deep empathy for both human and plant suffering, and thus a space for more compassionate, collaborative healing.

Privilege, periodization, and the Harley 6258B

One result of privileging the pristine and lavishly illustrated Cotton Vitellius C.iii over the later Harley 6258B is a missed opportunity to better understand healing practice as it was understood at the end of the Old English period. Indeed, the very features that have rendered the Harley 6258B manuscript a less desirable object of study—its poor condition, its post-Conquest date, and its radical departures from Latin and earlier Old English antecedents—are the very features that testify to its ongoing importance in twelfth-century medical practice.

'a mean manuscript written upon shreds'

Thomas Oswald Cockayne's nineteenth-century description of Harley 6258B, which he (along with later editors) designated MS O, began a long tradition of relegating this manuscript to side notes: 'MS O is a mean manuscript written upon shreds of vellum'.[6] One of the most distinguishing features of the 'O' manuscript is its reorganization of the *Herbarium*'s plant entries into alphabetical order, but like many who followed, Cockayne saw this alphabetization not as an innovative modification testifying to the text's ongoing practicality, but as a corruption of an original, now 'broken up'.[7] The potential value of Harley 6258B for Cockayne was almost wholly for purposes of linguistic comparison.[8] 'In editing an ancient work', he wrote, one should 'print from the best MS and supply its defects, if any, from the next best'. Towards this goal, 'the three best conspire' (i.e., Cotton Vitellius C.iii, Harley 585, and Hatton 76), but 'the fourth' (i.e., Harley 6258B) 'is not taken into account'.[9]

The subsumption of Harley 6258B into the works simply contextualizing the Cotton Vitellius C.iii continues to the present day.

But it is worth noting that many of the characteristics that make the Cotton Vitellius C.iii so appealing to many today—including its beautiful illustrations and its well-preserved nature resulting from its status as a presentation copy—would have been rare outliers in their own time, and if we wish to understand actual medical practice in early medieval England, it makes better sense to look more and not less closely at the manuscripts that have been adapted the most freely, witnessed the most wear, and shown the longest patterns of use. As Stephanie Hollis has noted, 'What is remarkable about the English vernacular medical tradition is both its durability and its continuing capacity to innovate'.[10] The modifications of Harley 6258B in a new era are indeed a sign of the herbal's ongoing relevance into the post-Conquest period as a dynamic, changeable guide, and, more importantly, a guide that shows signs of active use. D'Aronco notes that all extant copies of the *Herbarium* 'were read, used, and glossed by Englishmen who inserted Old English plant names clearly connected with the Old English botanical lore',[11] but it is arguably the final and least-studied copy in the Harley 6258B that demonstrates its importance to practitioners most compellingly. This particular collection not only made the transition into post-Conquest England, but was important enough to copy even in an era of radically reduced scribal resources. Danielle Maion's thorough assessment of the Harley 6258B manuscript in *The Production and Use of English Manuscripts 1060 to 1220* describes the parchment as 'not good quality with numerous flaws and repairs', 'small-format', and 'economical to produce'.[12] The volume measures 184 x 145 mm with the number of lines per page varying from 21 to 31;[13] in contrast, the leaves of the Cotton Vitellius C.iii are substantially larger at 250–275 x 190mm,[14] and would have been larger still originally, the leaves showing evidence of edges having been burnt in fire and then cut away during repairs.

As early as Cockayne's writing, the Cotton Vitellius C.iii was recognized as having been 'executed at an enormous expense',[15] and D'Aronco asserts that it 'bears comparison with the greatest illustrated herbals from Italy and France'.[16] More concerned with aesthetics than with conserving vellum, the scribe of Cotton Vitellius C.iii wrote the text in columns in the style of Latin manuscripts, 31 lines per page with few exceptions. Such extravagance in the Cotton Vitellius C.iii, combined with the fact that the herbal is preserved in three additional manuscripts, is of course a testament to the *Herbarium*'s popularity; its utility, however, becomes most apparent in the Harley 6258B, whose production seems to have been focused more on practicality than appearance. As Linda Sanborn describes, this manuscript's prickings are 'crude', and the 'scribe's mistakes are never erased, only expunctuated'.[17] The medical remedies in the Old English *Herbarium* were clearly, therefore, deemed important enough to the compilers of 6258B to include despite insufficient resources, but this importance seems specifically to have been related to use. The 'general appearance', Sanborn says of the manuscript, 'is more that of a working handbook', and D'Aronco describes its look as that of 'a small handy copy which could be easily carried in a pouch and shows signs of long usage', features that evidence its having actually been used by a medieval physician.[18]

Though it might seem counter intuitive, the lack of images in Harley 6258B would not have been likely to reduce the manuscript's practicality. As D'Aronco notes, even the most accurate and realistic illustration 'is not always sufficient to permit recognition of the plant under discussion, since different environments can produce significant morphological variation in the same species'.[19] Even within the classical tradition there was doubt regarding the value of illustrations, Pliny the Elder going so far as to describe reproductions of plants as deception (*fallax*), not only on the grounds of imperfections that arose through copying but also because of the impossibility of capturing a plant's appearance in all its diversity and across every stage of its life cycle.[20] The two manuscripts (Harley 585 and Harley 6258B) of the *Herbarium* that include other substantial medical texts as well are the same two that were planned and executed without illustrations,[21] suggesting that at least some medieval compilers saw such images as non-essential for active practitioners.[22] These two manuscripts also align with vernacular practice in their presentation: while the Cotton Vitellius C.iii and Hatton 76 follow the Latin practice of organizing their text into columns, the Harley 585 and Harley 6258B follow the vernacular employment of long lines without columns. I do not intend to suggest, however, that refocusing our attention and analysis upon the Harley 6258B means concomitantly disregarding or discounting the earlier, more pristine Cotton Vitellius C.iii or the context it can provide. That context is indeed rich. For instance, the illustrations that are noticeably absent from the later manuscript are themselves a testament to how important the *Herbarium* itself was. So valued were the remedies copied into the Harley 6258B that the plants in the earlier presentation copy of the Cotton Vitellius C.iii were illustrated in multiple layers.[23] As D'Aronco observes, 'the study of the illustrations is indispensable for the reconstruction of the textual tradition'.[24] Nevertheless, when we flip the traditional scholarly focus, we can see Harley 6258B not simply as a radically diminished and 'imperfect' copy, but rather as a medical workbook that is itself important through its reflection of an impulse to reproduce medical lore that had been highly valued in England for centuries.

'three (or four) manuscripts': beyond periodization

For more than a century, the Harley 6258B has almost always been omitted from standard lists of Old English manuscripts. It is, for instance, nowhere to be found in Neil Ker's *Catalogue of Manuscripts Containing Anglo-Saxon*, and, at least partially on this basis, the Harley 6258B has been treated tangentially ever since. To the extent that the manuscript is acknowledged at all, it is typically with regard to its translation of the *Peri didaxeon*, which exists only in this single attestation, and its *Herbarium* text tends to be regarded only as supplemental to the three earlier texts, all of which can more solidly be placed in the Old English period. Hugo Berberich, noting the limited use of this version even in Cockayne's notes, edited the text in its entirety in 1902 but published it as an example of Middle—not Old—English (*mittelenglischen*), a pattern that for the most part has continued up through present-day treatments.[25] Anne Van Arsdall, for instance, separates 6258B from the other *Herbarium* manuscripts as 'Middle English' and only tentatively counts it among the Old English versions in a discussion of 'how the three (or four) manuscripts' relate to a possible earlier exemplar.[26] On the other hand, de Vriend explains that while 'it is understandable' that the medical texts in Harley 6258B 'have been regarded as early ME', there is abundant evidence from statistical analysis of linguistic features that 'its language is not ME but late OE'.[27] Inconveniently produced unequivocally in neither Old nor Middle English, the remedies of Harley 6258B have thus largely fallen through scholarly cracks, mere footnotes to the 'Old English' majority.

The time is now right to remove such periodizing labels and the restrictions they create. Recent calls in medieval studies to critically examine our notions of categorization and identity have opened a space for recovering voices long marginalized, including those omitted due to rigid standards of periodization. Elaine Treharne has long fought against the sharp divide that has traditionally separated periods of English history, and her points are worth restating. She argues that '[t]he division of literary history into ever more precise and specific periods and interests is a familiar, and perhaps inevitable consequence of the politicization of university curricula, professional associations and academic subject areas';[28] such a 'superficially imposed division of English literary and linguistic development', she observes, does 'identify broad historical differences' but has also resulted in an unfortunate 'gap'.[29] 'Teleological' interpretations of 'Old English' ending in October 1066 risk a gross 'misreading', 'but one that has been so often repeated that the supposed death of English literature after the Norman Conquest has become an accepted part of literary history recounted by most standard analyses of the period'.[30] In reality, the vernacular texts that continued to be produced can tell us a great deal, if only we remove the constraints that have kept us from bringing them into the conversation.

This overdue reassessment is especially important in the case of medical literature, and there is much to be gained from bringing texts previously seen as liminal like the Harley 6258B more firmly into the conversation. D'Aronco has shown that although the late-eleventh through the thirteenth century 'can appear almost marginal in the history of medicine in England since the medical production was mostly written in Latin or in French', the twelfth

170   *Hybrid healing*

century saw in England and in Europe at large not only an increase in the availability of medical texts but also a 'proliferation of healers'.[31] Though a minority, Old English medical texts such as the *Herbarium* were a significant part of this growth and attest to continual use of vernacular texts and modes of healing across the Conquest. Debby Banham describes a 'new medicine' that arrived in England in the eleventh century, an 'international medicine which was much more learned than had been available in England before' in contrast to the medicine of early medieval England, which 'appears to have developed largely in isolation from Continental Europe'.[32] Yet, through manuscripts such as the Harley 6258B, the Old English *Herbarium* made it through this transition, testifying to its continued importance in the new post-Conquest millennium.[33] While the dramatic linguistic and cultural shifts render the text's transmission into the twelfth century remarkable in and of itself, the subtle changes and adaptations distinguishing the tenth- and twelfth-century versions witness a more subtle and ongoing cultural change connected with an increasing role of texts and literacy within medical practice.

'The original work has been broken up': restructuring thought in the Harley 6258B

As has been true for other aspects of this manuscript, assessment of the Harley 6258B's structure has also been determined based on its comparison with the earlier three manuscripts. Cockayne's early description of the later *Herbarium* as merely a 'broken up' version of the unadulterated 'original' text—a perception that has followed the Harley 6258B ever since—overlooks the insights to be found in what are actually fascinating innovations, adaptations, and omissions within this twelfth-century manuscript. The omissions and changes from the earlier tenth- and eleventh-century translations of the *Herbarium* to the later 6258B connect with larger cultural patterns such as those involving a shift toward greater literacy, and it is helpful to view these modifications from the perspective of twelfth-century medics rather than as a process of devolution. For instance, although the standard edition by Jan de Vriend is a wonderful resource for comparison of parallel entries of the Cotton Vitellius

C.iii and Harley 6258B manuscripts with its facing-page renderings, without consultation of the actual manuscripts this editorial choice of prioritizing parallelism between the texts still creates the somewhat misleading impression that the Cotton Vitellius C.iii and Harley 6258B are more alike than they actually are—with the differences consistently pointing toward perceived deficits in the later text. But the reasons for such differences are often much more complicated, and in a number of ways.

For one, these alterations suggest a growing influence of writing and literacy on medical text production, most notable in the later manuscript's reorganization of entries into alphabetical order, with letters and texts becoming the primary organizing principle.[34] But the more particular choices in *how* to alphabetize, especially when the items to be classified might be referred to by multiple different names, can be quite telling. In general, the entries of the Harley 6258B are organized according to the plants' Latin names—which often appear alongside their English counterparts as headers to each entry. And there is a tendency toward this Latinate organization even when the Latin version does not appear in the header itself, as is the case with *hæwenhudela* (*hæwenhydele* in Cotton Vitellius C.iii), where the Harley entry header is in English, but its placement is with the *b*'s, presumably according to its Latin name *brittanica*, which is included as an alternate name only within the text of the entry in both manuscripts: 'þa Grecas bryttannica 7 Engle hæwenhudela nemneð' ['which the Greeks call *brittanica* and the English *hæwenhudela*'].[35] In such ways, the alphabetization and reliance on Latin point towards a subtle but undeniable shift away from the spoken vernacular in this later copy of the Old English *Herbarium*.

Returning to the Harley 6258B's mandrake entry, we find that inserted within that entry are two slips of vellum with entries for other herbs alphabetized under *m*: *menstrasus* (horsemint) and *merce* ('march', or wild celery). The placement of *menstrasus* of course adheres to the rules of alphabetization by Latin name, but the inclusion here of *merce* by its English nomenclature overrides the usual organizing principle, even though the Latin name appears in that entry's header: *de apio*.[36] De Vriend observes that *apium* here is 'inserted out of place'[37] according to the otherwise alphabetical arrangement, and by way of explaining the perceived error suggests that this entry 'was probably originally inserted under *a* and afterwards moved to *m* on account of the OE name *merce*'.[38]

But this entry for *merce* is only 'out of place' if we expect complete compliance with a default organization and view the compilers of the Harley 6258B as merely re-creating a (perhaps defective) version of an earlier text. If, though, we switch our perspective to that held by those who would have actually utilized this text, we can understand that *merce*'s alphabetization under its English rather than Latin name provides important information about how the herb was likely referenced in actual usage, the compiler placing it exactly where medical practitioners would be most likely to look for it. Though admittedly rare, this phenomenon is indeed seen in herbs other than *merce*. *Temolum*, too, is indexed with the *s*'s, according to its vernacular name, *singrene*, rather than its Latin form.[39] Breaking apart literally as the compound 'always green', the name *singrene* could have been an incredibly practical designation in connection with year-round harvesting possibilities.[40] Further, the choice reminds us of the linguistic hybridity of the medical tradition during this period, emerging simultaneously out of Latin learning and vernacular English tradition. And returning to the larger context of the encapsulating mandrake entry itself, we can also see that the Harley 6258B text did not seem to privilege the mandrake remedy as exceptional and had no problem interrupting the text with not just one but two inserted leaves. All of this insight is lost if we see Harley 6258B as a mere supplement to the earlier 'base' text found in Cotton Vitellius C.iii.

One other distinctive feature of the Harley 6258B that demonstrates both this shift to the visual rather than spoken word but also to the practical usefulness of the manuscript is that the margins of its entries often index common usages of herbs, presumably for ease of reference. In the mandrake entry, for instance, we see Latin marginalia indicating its uses 'ad dolorem capitis et sompnum', 'ad morbum aurium', 'ad morbum pedum', and 'ad demoniacos' ('for head pain and sleep problems', 'for ear disease', 'for foot disease', and 'for demons'). This boiling down of remedies to two or three words indexed in the margins signals what uses and elements of the remedies were viewed in the twelfth century as most important. No such guides are provided in the manuscript preferred by modern scholars, the Cotton Vitellius C.iii. These marginal glosses also provide further insights into how early medieval practitioners distinguished among ailments, *morbum* implying belief of an underlying disease as opposed to *dolorem*, indicating instead pain unattached to a specific cause. De Vriend explains that even though the marginal additions are in Latin, 'it is very unlikely that they were copied from a Latin original',[41] thus suggesting that the marginal notes may have already had an established history as part of the Old English textual tradition even before the production of this particular manuscript.

'highly imperfect with many chapters missing': on the loss of lore

The British Library's description of Harley 6258B as 'highly imperfect with many chapters missing, omitted or abbreviated'[42] again follows the patterns established by Cockayne of measuring the manuscript's value in relation to the earlier three texts, with differences disparaged as 'omissions' from a more perfect original. While the modifications made to earlier versions were, as has been frequently noted, almost always in the direction of reduction rather than expansion, it is important to bear in mind that the manuscript's twelfth-century audiences would not have encountered the manuscript in this comparative way; it would have been a rare healer—if any such existed at all—with the means to consult both the Harley 6258B and the lavish Cotton Vitellius C.iii. Thus, even though it is indeed helpful for us today to understand the patterns of modification and omission by comparing different manuscripts, it is also worthwhile to pause and reflect upon the effects of those changes and deletions for the healers who actively used the information that was made available to them through this stripped-down twelfth-century text without the ability for any such comparison.

As might be expected, some omissions, such as the Harley 6258B's abbreviated introduction to the entry for *dictamnus* (dittany), reflect considerations of resources. If one were conserving precious vellum, information about where precisely in Crete dittany might grow would seem to be an easy cut. Other omissions involving entries that were not just reduced but omitted entirely seem to reflect early stages in an increasing separation of folklore and legend from the herbal aspects of medicine—a pattern that will be discussed at more length below. While missing pages from the Harley 6258B make it difficult in some cases to discern whether particular entries would have been included on those pages, de Vriend has identified twelve entries that would have been expected to appear (based on alphabetical ordering) in undamaged portions of the manuscript and that can reasonably be understood as never having been included at all.[43] Of these twelve, at least three are firmly grounded in folklore and legend. As mentioned earlier, Cotton Vitellius C.iii's entry 13 for mugwort or *artemisia*, absent in the Harley 6258B, attributes the discovery to Diana and claims that the centaur Chiron first prescribed it medicinally and named it after Diana (Artemis). Also absent from the Harley 6258B is entry 58 for *polion*,[44] which requires the leaves and roots to be wrapped in cloth and hung from the neck as a talisman against *monoðseoce* ['moon sickness', or 'lunacy'].

Most relevant to our present exploration of *mandragora*, though, a healer consulting Harley 6258B would likewise not have found an entry for *gorgonion*, which appears as entry 182 in the Cotton Vitellius C.iii. In many ways the text and illustration for this entry are closer than any other to the *mandragora* entry. Like *mandragora*, *gorgonion* is described in terms of bodily features: 'be (þyss)e wyrte is sæd þæt hy(re) wyrttruma sy gea(nlicud þæ)re n(ædran) heafde ðe man g(or)gon nemneð, 7 ða telgran habbað, þæs ðe eac is sæd, ægðer ge eagan ge nosa ge næddrena hiw' ['About this plant it is said that its root looks like the head of a snake that is called a gorgon, and that the branches, so it is also said, have the color, the eyes, and nose of snakes'].[45] Additionally, in the Cotton Vitellius C.iii, the illustration accompanying the *gorgonion* entry shares with the mandrake a highlighting of bodily features, in this case sharply defined eyes, eyebrows, nose, and a mouth. Further, the Gorgons in classical mythology most typically had snakes for hair, and the secondary roots in the Cotton Vitellius C.iii *gorgonion* illustration indeed appear very snakelike. (See Figure 5.3.)

Hybridity of being in Harley 6258B

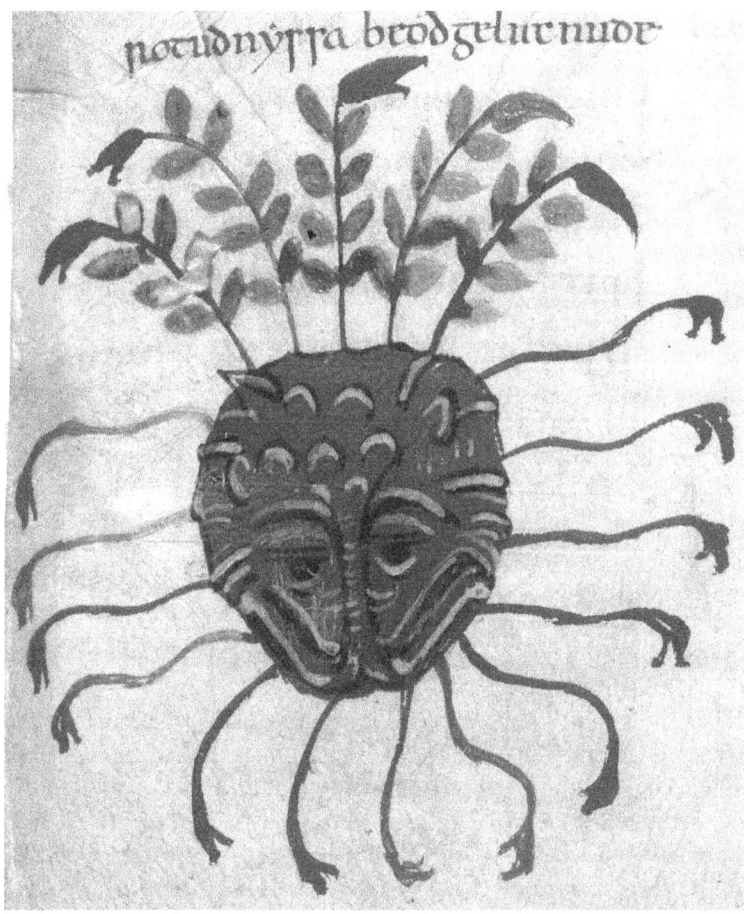

Figure 5.3 Entry for *gorgonion*, British Library MS Cotton Vitellius C.iii, f. 73v.

Further, as with the mandrake entry, there are elaborate instructions for harvesting, due to the plant's alleged power:

> 7 þonne ðu þas wyrte mid hyre wyrttruman niman wylle, ðonne warna þu þæt hy na sunne bescine, ðy læs hyre hiw 7 hyre miht sy awend þurh ðære sunnan beorhtnysse; forceorf hy þonne mid anum wogan 7 swyþe heardon iserne; 7 se þe hy corfan wylle, ðonne sy he

fram awend; for ðy hit nys alyfed þæt man hyre wyrtruman anwealhne geseon mote.

[And if you want to pick the plant with its roots, be careful that the sun does not shine on it, lest its color and strength be changed by the sun's brightness. Cut it only with a curved and very hard iron tool; and whoever intends to cut it must turn away from it because it is not permitted that anyone see its entire root.]

Of course, a clear practical component underlies these seemingly superstition-related requirements of the harvesting instruction: Light does in fact impact the strength of the root, iron is an effective cutting implement, and the cautions serve as a warning of the root's essential power; the story of the Gorgon's head, which can't be seen directly without incurring grave danger, becomes metaphorically linked to an allegedly powerful root. While cutting the Gorgon's 'head' would not turn one to stone as in the myth, the text tells us that harm would come nonetheless in the lessening of the root's potency. The lore surrounding the root thus serves as a powerful reminder to keep the plant away from light during harvesting and to be aware of its capacity for harm if not handled as directed.

To the extent that practical elements can be separated from ritual, mnemonic, or other functions at all, embedded legends and rituals such as those associated with the mandrake or *gorgonion* are actually exceedingly rare in Old English medical texts and especially so in the *Herbarium*. Renée Trilling's systematic analysis of Old English medical texts shows beyond doubt that the types of remedies leading to the false impression of pervasive superstition-driven healing practices in truth constitute only a relatively small percentage of early medieval remedies, and an even smaller minority within the *Herbarium* in particular. According to her statistics, only a tiny .36% of the remedies in the *Herbarium* include charms or incantations, and only 2.87% provide remedies for supernatural afflictions.[46] While Trilling's analysis does not explicitly address anthropomorphized plants, the omission of *gorgonion* clearly helps bring the Harley collection into alignment with this tendency even more closely than do its predecessors. The deletion of this entry, along with the other modifications and omissions discussed above,

Hybridity of being in Harley 6258B 177

might thus make it easy to take it at face value that the compiler of the Harley 6258B was simply less interested in medicinal practices drawing from mythology. However, the continuing—even increasing—prominence of the mandrake shows the issues involved to be rather more complex. As Trilling argues, the approach most respectful of the tradition is 'not to separate the magical or mystical elements' from the practical, but 'rather to investigate how the overlap among these types of remedies allows us to rethink' medieval categories of healing.[47] Thus, my goal in investigating the *mandragora* entry is to understand the Harley 6258B's version of the Old English *Herbarium* on its own terms.

The *mandragora* tradition and the Harley 6258B

If the general pattern in the Harley 6258B was to make this centuries-old medical text more practical—providing marginal indexes, reorganizing for ease of reference, and omitting entries such as the *gorgonion* that appear to demonstrate more affinity with mythology than medicine—one might reasonably expect the *mandragora* entry itself to have been omitted or, at the very least for its seemingly mystical harvesting ritual to have been cut. And to an extent, the mandrake entry does exhibit some of these overarching tendencies. For instance, the Harley 6258B leaves out the final possible use of the mandrake, where it is to be employed against general evil in the home, 'yfelnysse on his hofe', while retaining the rest of the more specific medical ailments it can remedy, including headache, earache, and gout. Yet not only does the Harley 6258B retain the ritual instructions for harvesting the mandrake root, it also relies on the same bodily language amplified by the Cotton Vitellius C.iii's illustration. The section for use of the roots in the fourth remedy in the entry instructs the healer to take three pennies' weight from the *lichoman*, an Old English term that means specifically the body of a person.[48] The root's description in terms of a 'body' has the practical effect of helping a practitioner select the right section and correct portion for medical use. The mandrake entry, which also describes the plant as having hands and feet [*hænde*, *fet*] and mandates surreptitious capture lest the powerful plant escape, is therefore precisely the kind of text that has sustained long-standing perceptions of medieval medicine as grounded more in superstition than in medical science, yet the mandrake's human/plant hybridity is retained even as similar elements are cut elsewhere in the same manuscript. It is thus worthwhile to ask how these impulses that are seemingly in conflict came to bear on the mandrake entry and what this remedy might have meant in its new twelfth-century context. The answers, I argue, are complex and multifaceted, having to do with matters of authority, utility, and—above all—empathy.

Authority in legend

The mandrake, *mandragora*, was emblematic of healing practice long before the Old English *Herbarium*. In the first century, Dioscorides included in his *De materia medica*—a five-volume work on medicinal uses of plants, animals, and minerals that became the standard reference on herbal healing in the ancient world—a description of the mandrake and its uses that remained the basis for countless botanists and writers on botany for years afterward.[49] And even though Dioscorides' text did not mention the harvesting ritual involving the dog,[50] so connected to the mandrake was this ritual that by the sixth century a frontispiece to an illuminated manuscript of this text depicts Dioscorides as he is offered a distinctly human-shaped mandrake root, held out to him by Heuresis and attached to a dog by a thin rope.[51] So one might naturally wonder how the personified mandrake became an image so prominently connected with a work of medical science, and I would argue that it was the mandrake's hybridity that was crucial in pre-modern eras for its capacity to mediate human and plant subjectivities—a capacity that remains important even today.

It is not at all clear precisely when various aspects of the mandrake legend coalesced into the form we see in the Old English *Herbarium*. While Pliny and Dioscorides both include detailed accounts of the mandrake, only Pliny provides the gathering ritual, which involves digging three circles around the root, a detail shared with the *Herbarium*:[52] 'effossuri cavent contrarium ventum et tribus circulis ante gladio circumscribunt' ['the diggers avoid facing the wind, first trace round the plant three circles with a sword'][53] Most of the elements included in the Cotton Vitellius C.iii and after had already appeared at least by the ninth century, but interestingly some of the elements that were firmly attached to the mandrake legend by the Middle Ages were not clearly tied to the mandrake in earlier periods and were instead attributed to other plants altogether. For instance, embedded in Flavius Josephus' *The Jewish War* (c. 70 CE) is an account of an unnamed plant (identifiable only by its location in Baaras) that shares several distinctive features of the mandrake as it is presented in the Old English *Herbarium* and its Latin predecessor. 'Towards the evening', Josephus says, 'it sends out a certain ray like lightning', a detail that closely parallels the *Herbarium*'s description of mandrake as an herb that shines at night like a lantern. '[C]ertain death to those that touch it', this plant, like that described in the *Herbarium* mandrake entry, must be harvested with the aid of a dog. One should 'tie a dog to it: and when the dog tries hard to follow him that tied him, this root is easily plucked up'.[54] And similarly to the mandrake, this plant is said to 'quickly driv[e] away those called demons'.

Even closer to the Old English *Herbarium* entry is the Roman author Aelian's third-century account of the peony. Just as the Old English mandrake shines like a lantern, Aelian's peony 'shines out like a star', and, also like the mandrake, the peony is said to destroy anyone who touches it. The protective gathering ritual is remarkably similar to that seen in the *Herbarium*:

> And so they bring a strong dog that has not been fed for some days and is ravenously hungry and attach a strong cord to it, and round the stalk of the Peony at the bottom they fasten a noose securely from as far away as they can; then they put before the dog a large quantity of cooked meat which exhales a savory odour. And the dog, burning with hunger and tormented by the savour, rushes at the meat that has been placed before it and with its violent movement pulls up the plant, roots and all.[55]

A version of this ritual appears in the composite known as the *Herbarium of Pseudo-Apuleius* that was in circulation by the fifth and sixth centuries, but by this point the dog seems to have been firmly attached to the mandrake in particular,[56] part of an emerging pattern wherein rituals practiced in connection with a wide range of plants in earlier periods become more rare, thus leaving the mandrake as a magnet for such rituals, an increasingly lonely representative of earlier healing lore.

As a potent plant with an already long and extensive history of use in the ancient world, the mandrake had by the Middle Ages accumulated much traditional wisdom surrounding its harvesting, medical properties, and use. But its gathering rituals were relatively unremarkable during earlier stages in the history of medicine, and mandrakes were known first and foremost 'as medicinal plants, primarily discussed as such in pharmaceutical literature'.[57] Nevertheless, as Anne Van Arsdall, Helmut Klug, and Paul Blanz note in their extensive study on the history of the mandrake in medical lore, 'mythic powers have been attributed to the root since prehistoric times', 'undoubtedly because of its anthropomorphic shape, but even more because of its toxic properties, which are more highly concentrated in the root than in leaves and fruits'.[58] *Mandragora*, they explain, belongs to the *Solanaceae* family, and the effect of its 'alkaloids on humans is toxic and healing alike, depending on the concentration, and how they are applied'.[59] It therefore makes sense that practices surrounding its harvesting and use would promote caution and care, and over time the mandrake's medical potency and its gathering ritual gradually became closely linked—and even emblematic of—healing lore more broadly. And as counterintuitive as it might seem, the more fantastical elements associated with the mandrake were the ones that came to be most fully invested with the authority of a long-standing classical tradition of herbal healing practice.

A not dissimilar situation arose in connection with another medieval text whose fantastical elements are frequently overemphasized, Marco Polo's *Description of the World*. Though obviously from a very different genre than the medical compilations, this text includes through its account of the Andaman Islands an especially illustrative example of how such a sense of authority can accrete via unusual elements.[60] Sharon Kinoshita explains that imaginary creatures and fantastical elements are 'exceedingly rare' in this text and that typical entries work to 'demystify the most clichéd examples of medieval credulity'.⁶¹ This pattern thus renders all the more shocking—to modern readers at least—a description of island inhabitants as humans with dog heads, a fact underscored with claims of truth: 'Now know in complete truth that all the men of this island have heads like dogs and that they are all like the heads of great mastiffs'. Kinoshita notes that 'strikingly, the dog-headed people are nowhere described as a "wonder" or a "marvel"',⁶² as one might expect in a text that circulated at a later stage under the title *Book of Marvels*. In fact, the very next line returns us immediately to the relatively mundane world of merchants, of which Marco Polo's family was a part: 'They have a lot of spices'. Kinoshita argues compellingly that this passage, which jumps out to modern readers as most shocking and unexpected, marks what 'most closely conforms to the discursive expectations of its world'.⁶³ As Kinoshita demonstrates, Marco Polo's account follows in a long literary tradition of dog-headed occupants of the Andaman Islands, and, though it might seem illogical to modern readers, this element in the description would have lent the surrounding text the authority of classical tradition. The *mandragora* entry functions similarly, the single seemingly out-of-place entry metonymically reinforcing the *Herbarium*'s connection to longstanding and widely accepted medical tradition through its repetition of ancient legend and ritual.

Finally, contributing to the mandrake's stability across the transition into post-Conquest England (and modern tradition more generally) was the fact that it was not as commonly used as many other herbs employed in medieval healing practice and were therefore subject to adaptation through common use. Although the mandrake carried the full force of classical authority and was unlikely ever to drop out of the tradition altogether as the *gorgonion* entry did, at the same time it was not used frequently enough to warrant practical innovations. 'Despite its wide geographic distribution', Van Arsdall, Klug, and Blanz explain, '*mandragora* does not occur commonly'.⁶⁴ Part of what lent the mandrake its sense of mystery was doubtless its rarity relative to other medicinal plants, and its lack of familiarity combined with its authority has sustained its place in popular imagination even to the present day.

Utility in ritual

A second reason the elements of the mandrake entry that don't neatly align with modern medicine might have persisted has to do with practical horticultural knowledge. Perhaps the most clearly utilitarian instructions in the Harley 6258B *Herbarium*'s entry are those related to the digging up of the plant:

> þu hi bewyrst mid ysene swa we ær cwadan; 7 þanne þu scealt onbute hy delfan swa þæt þu hy na mid þan, ysene athryne. Ac þu ʒeorn/lice mid ylpenbænenan stæfe ðe eorðan delfan.

> [You mark around it with iron, as we said before, and then you must dig around it so that you do not touch it with the iron. But you dig the earth strenuously with the ivory staff.]

Anne Van Arsdall's work with the mandrake invites us to 'deconstruct' this gathering ritual, proceeding from 'an initial assumption' that 'the reasons behind the ancient ritual in classical texts may have originally been practical and not magical'.[65] In particular, the potentially toxic nature of the root would have made it 'dangerous to pull or dig up numbers of mandrake roots at one time', the ritual thus effectually limiting the number of roots to which a gatherer would be exposed. And though this harvesting ritual might stand out as anomalous by the Old English period, it likely would not have been seen as unusual in earlier periods, 'where gathering rituals were commonly described for many plants'.[66] Even in the Old English *Herbarium*, the mandrake's gathering ritual is not a wholly isolated practice. For instance, the entry for *proserpinaca* requires the practitioner to seek the plant just before sunrise or sunset and mark around it with a gold ring ('gyldenan hringe'), then return to it three days later to harvest it. Such rituals could serve important utilitarian functions. Van Arsdall notes, even 'a little common sense' would suggest that these instructions would serve 'simply to loosen the soil so that the root could be taken whole' and that special care 'must be taken when handling toxic plants'.[67]

Regarding the dog—among the most stable of the elements in pre-modern accounts of the ritual—Van Arsdall considers the possibility that 'root gatherers in ancient and medieval eras may have had trained dogs to help them find the mandrake roots, so that they could do their collecting over a period of time and perhaps in unfamiliar locales, just like using pigs and dogs to find truffles'.[68] 'It would behoove the specialists', she notes, that 'not everyone can do this kind of gathering, and that a ritual was involved as well'.[69] Additionally, she suggests that the ritual—which would limit gathering rights to those who have the resources and knowledge to follow it—could also have helped herbal practitioners 'protect their territories'.[70] This added function of marking territory in an era with less distinct written boundaries has been suggested for other rituals as well. The incantation of the Old English swarm charm, for instance, which calls upon a beekeeper to recite a poem directed toward the bees themselves, has been connected to the more recent ritual of 'tanging', the banging of pots and pans to help calm a swarm. Beekeeper Richard Underhill believes that 'the communication was not actually banging the pots and pans to tell the bees to settle the swarm down but the banging of pots and pans was to declare to your neighbor that you were claiming that swarm—because a swarm is valuable'.[71] The ritual associated with the mandrake would doubtless have drawn attention and potentially served a similar function of claiming digging rights.

Just as elements of the ritual likely contributed to successful harvesting, the description—found in all four versions of the Old English *Herbarium*—of the mandrake as a plant that 'shines' (*scineð*) also has an arguably practical value. The added detail of 'like a lantern' contributes to the impression of its preternatural properties, but modern-day guides to identifying plants often describe its leaves and fruit in similar terms. Colin Clair's *Of Herbs and Spices* describes the European mandrake as 'a native of Syria', with 'glossy' leaves and 'shiny' fruit.[72] And in his blog post on locating mandrake plants for medicinal purposes, Richo Cech advises readers to look for the following: 'The leaves part to show a cluster of nascent flowers, already *glowing* distantly purple' (emphasis added).[73] The Pacific Bulb Society describes the leaves of the European mandrake (*mandragora officinarum*) as having 'something of a metallic cast',[74] and the 'ground-hugging rosette of large shiny green leaves' described for *Mandragora* in

First Nature's plant identification guide could also evoke images of the Old English *Herbarium*. The compound *leohtfæt* is typically translated as 'lantern' or 'lamp', though its application to elements in nature is less metaphorically oriented when we break it apart into its literal components, 'light' and 'vessel' (*fæt* developing into modern *vat*).[75] The shape, too, could be evocative of light vessels or lamps such as those found specifically in early medieval England. The clustered grouping of small bright flowers centered on a bed of broad, flat, shiny leaves would not be unlike a candle centered on a hemispherical bowl of the sort found in archaeological sites of this era.[76] It is only when we entirely divorce metaphor and subjectivity from medicine and science that these elements in the entry become reduced to superstitious fancy.

Empathy in personification

A third—and easily overlooked—reason why the mandrake harvesting ritual persisted even as other signs of 'superstition' were slowly eradicated is that the entry is not actually as much at odds with the rest of the *Herbarium* as it might seem to modern readers. On one hand, of course, the high degree of personification within the mandrake entry stands in sharp contrast to the relatively mundane majority of plant descriptions in the *Herbarium*. Even the Cotton Vitellius C.iii's *mandragora* illustration with its distinctly humanoid body and that of the *gorgonion* with its root rendered as a disembodied head were rarities within the herbal tradition, and, as noted earlier, the *gorgonion* falls out of the *Herbarium* by the twelfth-century Harley 6258B. Nonetheless, there is arguably important overlap between this type of personification within the healing tradition and the mode of thinking that underlies the entire collection of plants described in the volume. In standing out amongst the more commonplace herbal entries, such personifications powerfully reify what they share with the larger body of healing remedies, a notion of plants as sentient beings. Entries such as those related to the *mandragora* and *gorgonion* disrupt the potentially misleading sense of familiarity offered by the almost 99% of the *Herbarium*'s largely unassuming entries, and even if they are inexplicit and unstated, the implications of plant agency foregrounded in these atypical entries draw our attention to a potency assumed as typical of *all* plants. Exploring the changes between modern and pre-modern conceptions of plants, Michael Marder argues that 'contemporary biotechnology' has in effect 'disrupted the hybrid relational ontology of the human and the vegetable'.[77] And in his compelling contribution to the rapidly emerging field of critical plant studies, Matthew Hall has explicitly linked this shift in 'plant ontology' to the transition from oral tradition to literate culture:[78] The 'rejection of traditional poetry, story, and ritual', he suggests, 'heralded a shift away from a society focused on maintaining respectful relationships with nonhumans',[79] and '[a]lthough we are limited to the literary documentation of oral tales', myths and stories 'perhaps provide the best sources for exploring plant-human relationships within Europe'.[80] Similarly, in *Essays on Extinction*, Claire Colebrook notes stark consequences resulting from this fundamental shift in how humans have come to understand themselves in relation to the natural world: 'the pre-modern space of knowledge had distributed beings in relations of analogy, such that the universal order of things was reflected in each living being'.[81] 'What is lost', she argues, 'is any sense of the earth as a living whole as bearing a life and temporality of its own, within which human beings are located and towards which they ought to pay due respect and care'.[82] Connections once forged through stories and rituals become severed with categorization schemes that separate human from non-human, sentient from non-sentient, effectively othering a natural world once viewed within a construct of kinship. But the 'otherness' of plants in this paradigm has been incremental. As we shall see below, the subtle differences between the three heretofore privileged manuscripts of the *Herbarium* and the liminal Harley 6258B reflect a shift away from plant agency and volition. Though in most regards the text itself is the 'same', the twelfth-century *Herbarium* deserves to be viewed on its own terms in its own historical moment, a distinct text within a plurality of Old and early Middle English *Herbaria*.

Critical plant studies, medieval mandrakes, and Old English herbaria

As has been often noted, the differences between the twelfth-century *Herbarium* and its three predecessors are—from one perspective at least—admittedly small. However, a close focus on the mandrake entry suggests that these subtle differences collectively mark early stages in a fundamental shift towards 'the dualism of humans and nonhumans'.[83] Offering an interesting lens through which to view the mandrake entry in the Old English *Herbarium* and its transition into the twelfth century, Matthew Hall's work in critical plant studies argues that the 'human marginalization of plants' within a 'general, Western view of plants as passive resources' can have significant ecological consequences and encourages readers to become more aware of 'human-plant continuities'.[84] Similarly, Michael Marder notes that plants have been relegated to the backdrop of human existence, resulting in a common 'incapacity of humans to recognize elements of ourselves in the form of vegetal being'.[85] However, he goes on to suggest that rather than confronting plants as 'still-murky objects of knowledge', we can instead encounter them interactively and attempt to discover traces of the human in the vegetal and vice versa; thus we diminish the gap between the two types of being and employ a 'vegetal philosophy' as we put ourselves 'in the plants' shoes, or rather roots'.[86] I would suggest that the *Herbarium* does for its own readers what Marder does for us, forcing humans to confront the subjectivity and agency of herbs and plants, the 'non-conscious intentionality of vegetal life'.[87] And a crucial first step in bridging that gap is to recognize our inherited and potentially harmful default assumptions.

Mandrakes in motion

The first of these problematic assumptions has to do with plants and their (in)ability to move. As Marder demonstrates, our privileging of movement as one of the most defining aspects of life goes all of the way back to the philosophers of early Greece, who 'associated life with motion' so that herbs and plants, defined 'by their incapacity to move, by their rootedness in the soil that renders them sedentary',[88] therefore fell outside of 'life', instead being relegated to 'thinghood'.[89] This mode of thinking that interprets plant life as 'qualitatively weak as verging on inanimate existence' forces vegetal life 'into retreat, puts it on the run'.[90] While Marder evokes the image of flight here metaphorically as a way of underscoring the 'distance between philosophy and vegetation', the mandrake entry in the *Herbarium* enacts the metaphor quite graphically.[91] At the beginning of the entry in both the Harley 6258B and the Cotton Vitellius C.iii, the harvesting ritual requires that one mark the plant quickly around the 'head' (*heafod*) so that it does not 'flee' (*attfleo*[92]), and in both manuscripts the mandrake is invested with subjectivity in its explicit desire for escape. Interestingly, however, the plant's agency with regard to motion is lessened ever so slightly between the two versions, as the plant 'wants' simply to 'leave' in the later Harley 6258B ('Forlæte wile') manuscript rather than more actively 'flee', as in the Cotton Vitellius C.iii ('Forfleon wyle'). This reduced sense of motion is also reflected in a later subtle difference within the harvesting ritual. In the Cotton Vitellius C.iii, the dog must 'wyrte up abrede' ['snatch up the plant']; in contrast, the Harley 6258B requires only that the dog 'have' the implicitly more passive plant in its possession: 'wyrte habbe' ['have the plant']. From the perspective of the one 'snatched', the force implied by the verb 'abrede' could be quite significant.

A much more noticeable difference between the Cotton Vitellius C.iii and the Harley 6258B is the omission of the mandrake entry's final two remedies in the latter manuscript. The fifth remedy, for an ointment blending the mandrake with oil to be applied for nerve spasms, could be seen as duplicating earlier advice in the entry for mixing with oil for application against various types of pain. The deletion of the last remedy, though, marks yet another clear shift away from a model of plant agency; in the Cotton Vitellius C.iii it reads thus:

Gyf hwa hwylce hefige yfelnysse on his hofe geseo genime þas wyrte mandragoram onmiddan þam huse, swa mycel (sw)a he þonne h(æbbe), ealle yfelu (heo) yt anyd(eð).

[If anyone perceives any grievous evil in the home, take the mandrake plant to the center of the house—as much as one has of it—and it will expel all the evil.]

This remedy's omission implicitly rejects the notion of the plant as a talisman, which was an increasingly common use of the mandrake into the late medieval period.[93] Perhaps even more importantly, however, the omission shifts how one might see the mandrake's agency in active protection, with the power to 'expel evil'. No longer explicitly aligned against 'evil' by the time of the later text, the mandrake is one step closer to the ambiguous or even ominous being of later portrayals such as those seen today.[94]

Encountering the mandrake

Several seemingly small words and phrases that by the twelfth century have been modified or deleted from the mandrake entry collectively mark a gradual lessening of what Marder calls an 'encounter'. 'When instrumentalizing plants, we do not yet encounter them', he argues. 'Still, the uses to which we put vegetal beings do not exhaust what (or who) they are but, on the contrary, obfuscate enormous regions of their being'.[95] The subtle changes between the earliest versions of the Old English *Herbarium* and the twelfth-century Harley 6258B attest to this gradual 'instrumentalizing' and the corresponding 'obfuscation' of the mandrake's very essence.

The Cotton Vitellius C.iii describes the harvester's approach: 'þonne þu to hyre cymst' ['when you come to it']; this language is absent altogether from the Harley 6258B. Further, the earlier version includes several references to the harvester's senses and reactions that are not present in the later Harley 6258B. Where the Harley 6258B employs the name *mandragora* objectively and without qualification, the Cotton Vitellius C.iii acknowledges that the name is projected onto the plant by speakers, 'þe man mandragoram nemneþ' ['which one calls mandrake']. The plant's description orients readers similarly in terms of human perception. The Cotton Vitellius C.iii tells a reader that the plant is perceived by humans ('*ongist* þu hy' ['you will *perceive* it']), that it is experienced through the sense of sight ('on *gesihþe*' ['in *sight*'], 'sona swa þu geseo' ['as soon as you *see* (it)']), and that its healing properties have been transmitted through human speech ('be þysse wyrte ys sæd' ['about this plant it is *said*']). These references to human perception—references that implicitly acknowledge the plant's subjectivity by way of human experience—are the very ones that fall out in the reduced Harley 6258B.

The most poignant example of this shift, however, lies in the literal reduction of 'wonder' in the later manuscript. The first two remedies provided beneath the harvesting ritual in the early manuscripts assert that '*þu wundrast hu* hrædlice se slæp becymeþ' ['*you will wonder* at how quickly sleep will come'] and '*þu wundrast hu* hrædlice he byþ gehæled' ['*you will wonder* at how quickly he will be healed']. Devoid of any promised wonder, the Harley 6258B simply states the anticipated outcomes: 'hrædlice slapeþ' ['sleep will come quickly'] and 'hrædlice he byð ȝehæled' ['quickly he will be healed']. Similarly, even those herbal traits themselves that might evoke such wonder are also reduced in the later manuscript, and with the mandrake being portrayed in terms of its utilitarian value to humans without conveying its capacity to inspire awe in and of itself. The Cotton Vitellius C.iii offers three adjectives in the entry's opening: *mycel* ['great' or 'large'], *mære* ['glorious' or 'famous'], and *fremful* ['beneficial']. The Harley 6258B, however, omits the first two and retains only the adjective that conveys the plant's utilitarian aspect as 'beneficial' for humans. These changes toward plant objectification are paralleled by other phraseological shifts as well. The Cotton Vitellius C.iii instructs practitioners to harvest the mandrake 'þyssum gemete' ['in this manner'], and the mandrake itself is said to deceive 'þam sylfan gemete' ['in this same manner']. These phrases might seem like fillers, but they implicitly acknowledge *other* ways in which healers might harvest and *other* ways in which hallucinogenic plants might affect one's thoughts; their omission in the later Harley 6258B thus in effect eclipses even the possibility of variation, the very hallmark of traditional, collaborative healing as it was normally practiced at earlier points.

As Jacqueline Fay has observed, 'plant potency' in early medieval England can be understood in part as 'an emergent force resulting from an encounter with texts, words, tools, and the human body itself'.[96] In this 'ritual approach to agriculture',[97] encounters between plants and humans assume some degree of equivalence, and there is acknowledgment of at least the potential for a 'participatory, consensual role' for plants as they are used within human culture.[98] By putting the previously neglected Harley 6258B into the foreground, we can see the beginnings of a subtle but undeniable shift away from such plant subjectivity and agency. This shift is more than simply a move away from 'superstition' and instead marks a fundamental change in conceptions of herbal healing. In an earlier context, what looks like straightforward anthropomorphism in the Cotton Vitellius C.iii—though it is of course this, too—can be read simply as an acknowledgment of the personhood of plants, of the overlap uniting human and plant modes of being. What seems like human/plant hybridity can be understood instead as simply a shared existence as beings that are living and alive. The field of critical plant studies offers us a way to think through how the mandrake—and plant life more generally—then lost this subjective status (among humans at least), a shift reflected subtly through minor adaptations in the Old English *Herbarium*.

Suffering and empathy

Marder's aforementioned point about vegetal life being put on the run and violated by a mainstream Western medical tradition is meant at the philosophical level;[99] however, as we have seen, the mandrake's literal wish to 'flee' confronts us with this violation in a very direct way. Marder describes the plant's status as a 'fugitive state of being', 'fugal'.[100] In psychiatry, 'dissociative fugue' involves sudden flight during a dissociative state, usually associated with trauma,[101] and, though projecting such a diagnosis onto a medieval plant would obviously be anachronistic even if we fully accepted the mandrake as a 'person', the phrasing in the Cotton Vitellius C.iii does suggest an awareness of the trauma inflicted by the ritual. By the time of the later Harley 6258B, though, the subtle but clear acknowledgment of the ritual's implicit violence moves towards erasure through the seemingly minor shifts from *forfleon* to *forlæte*, and from *abrede* to *habbe*. The verb *niman*, also among the words included in the Cotton Vitellius C.iii but absent from the Harley

6258B, is another term that draws attention to the potential for harm against the plant, its semantic range including the relatively innocuous 'take' but also meanings much more charged with violence: 'to catch', 'to take forcibly', 'to seize', to 'take away', 'to carry off'.[102]

Such subtle changes to the language evidenced in Harley 6258B also effectually erase the mandrake's potential for suffering, taking the plant world another small step away from kinship and personhood. Regarding suffering, Hall argues that 'expressing its existence engenders the respect and consideration that is potentially lacking if plants are assumed to be insensitive to human action'.[103] A view of 'plants as persons' allows us to see plants as beings 'capable of flourishing and of being harmed',[104] the two potentialities more entangled with one another than we might care to admit. 'As in a human context', he argues, 'knowledge of this subjectivity alone does not preclude the infliction of damage or death, but it is a fundamental for the construction of respectful relationships'.[105] The three earliest manuscripts of the Old English *Herbarium* acknowledge this potential for suffering in the mandrake's desire to flee and its seeming passivity even while being violently uprooted; their visual and verbal images of the more fully personified mandrake allow the 'mediation of a fictional consciousness' that serves as a bridge between plant and human, breaking down the 'dualism of humans and nonhumans'.[106]

But a careful reading of the Harley 6258B entry must also acknowledge that the retained wording of the original might nonetheless have acquired different connotations by the twelfth century, especially within the context of changes away from plant agency and subjectivity. In both the Cotton Vitellius C.iii and the Harley 6258B the mandrake must be captured because of what it *wyle/wile* to do ('flee' and 'leave' respectively). The verb *willan* in the late Old English period had multiple senses, but the dominant sense, as given in Bosworth and Toller, involves volition: 'to will, wish', with the primary definition expressing a clear sense of subjectivity and agency 'to will, to exercise the faculty of willing'.[107] The second sense also explicitly involves subjectivity: 'where the will of the subject determines his own action, to will, purpose, think, mean intend'. The verb's use 'as an auxiliary for the future' in the sense of 'will, shall, to be about to' appears only as sense IX, and the *Oxford English Dictionary* shows this use of the verb as an 'auxiliary expressing mere futurity, forming (with pres. inf.) the future' to be a later development, first attested only in the late Old English period.[108] However, the word's transition towards its current sense would have been well underway by the Middle English period, and the sense of volition implied by *wile* would quite likely have been accordingly less pronounced for readers of the Harley 6258B.

The violence, trauma, and conquest inscribed in the mandrake entry serve as a potent reminder of the subjectivity of plants across the collection, plants whose benefits for human use in healing practice inevitably depend upon the violation of the plants themselves. But the powerful image of a plant with its own desires opens a space for a more 'collaborative, mutualistic relationship between plants and humans'.[109] This 'kinship' dynamic described by Hall in his exploration of ancient and medieval traditions thus aligns closely with the *comitatus* ideal reflected in much Old English heroic verse. 'In a similar way to a kinship relationship', Hall observes, the ideal plant/human relationship involves 'the need for reciprocal care and responsibility'.[110] The violent, martial aspects of *comitatus* culture are typically favored over the kinship elements, but both are clearly operative in this mandrake entry and in the healing tradition more broadly.

The mandrake unleashed

For all of these reasons, the Harley 6258B marks a pivotal moment in the history of herbal medicine, and the mandrake entry bears witness to this fundamental shift. Two significant developments in the twelfth century help explain how the exact same image can be used in such contradictory ways: at precisely the same time that medieval medicine was intentionally distancing itself from anything perceived as superstition, legends and beliefs involving plantlife were rapidly proliferating. While most 'superstitions' involving plants were falling away in early post-Conquest England, the mandrake endured. However, now largely untethered from science, divested of subjectivity and volition, it was arguably but a small and inevitable step for the mandrake legend to become the symbol of magical healing that it has since become for many. The differences that we see between the Cotton Vitellius C.iii and the twelfth-century Harley 6258B thus attest to the objectification of plants at the very same moment that the mandrake in particular was becoming a symbol of supernatural—and increasingly ominous—power. It is in the twelfth century, for instance, that the now-famous perilous scream entered the mandrake legend.[111] Van Arsdall, Klug, and Blanz trace the scream back to twelfth-century vernacular bestiaries, especially Philippe de Thaon's medieval French *Bestiary*; this text, which also includes the now familiar and well-established gathering ritual involving the dog, cautions that the mandrake can 'send forth a cry' so horrific that it would kill anyone who heard it immediately.[112]

It is in this context of the twelfth century's rapidly evolving mandrake lore that we must therefore see the Harley 6258B as more than a mere supplement to the earlier versions and bear in mind that while the *text* of the later manuscript may be virtually identical, the *context* in which it would have been read had shifted quite radically. The scream was not the only element to be added after the twelfth century. While, as we have seen, in late classical and early medieval medical texts, the mandrake was discussed 'largely in terms of its medicinal effects', the 'full-blown mandrake legend' seems to have developed *after* the Old English period.[113] This more expansive legend includes substantially more in the way of 'supernatural' elements, not only the gathering ritual requiring the root to be encircled with iron and a hungry dog to pull the mandrake root from the ground, as well as the scream that can kill anyone who hears it but, in some versions, a root that 'enables witches to fly, provokes hallucinations in humans, grows best in soil under gallows where men are hanged, and, when kept as an amulet wards off evil'.[114] It is also probably not surprising that the twelfth century also saw the greatest proliferation of medieval 'foliate heads', human/plant hybrids that were immensely popular in sculpture of the period.[115]

Against this backdrop of an increasingly fantastical portrayal of the mandrake, it becomes especially interesting that the Harley 6258B moves in the direction of objectification. The omission of the entry's remedy aimed at warding off an abstract and generalized evil, and also the omission of the *gorgonion* entry, point towards more modern scientific notions of healing. Jacqueline Fay describes the Old English *Herbarium* as representing a 'watershed moment for vernacular herbals located between a high point of Latin production on the Continent in the ninth century and the resurgence of the Anglo-Latin tradition of medical writing after the Conquest'.[116] I would add that what she says here of the *Herbarium* generally becomes especially true for the outlier twelfth-century Harley 6258B, produced at the precise historical moment where science and 'superstition' seemingly part ways. For the mandrake plant, the implications are particularly far-reaching. The increasing objectification of medicine witnessed in the twelfth century in effect leaves lore such as that of the mandrake largely disconnected from science, resulting in an explosion of unchecked permutations and embellishments. The precariously positioned *Herbarium* simultaneously occupies both eras as a product of Old English medicine, in which folklore and healing operate more in tandem, and, thanks to the Harley 6258B, of post-Conquest practice which tends to separate the two.

The mandrake's hybridity thus extends beyond its simple personification and manifests itself in ways that still carry important meanings for modern readers today. As but one example, Jeffrey Jerome Cohen's thoughtful and sensitive edited volume *Animal, Vegetable, Mineral: Ethics and Objects* features the plant's image on its cover.[117] Though Cohen's volume never discusses the mandrake explicitly, the mandrake image does quite effectively comment upon the volume's most central question: 'what happens when we cease to assume that only humans exert agency'?[118] Perhaps this wholeness is what the mandrake has always represented. Through its disruptive hybridity, the mandrake mediates the plant and the human, implicitly challenging harmful assumptions that from the twelfth century onward have marginalized plants as a mere means to human ends. But what is the impact of such disruption within the broader context of Old English remedies, most of which do *not* involve such dramatic hybridity? Such is the subject of the next chapter.

Appendix

De mandragora entry, Old English *Herbarium*
Harley 6258B (twelfth century)

Text and translation

The text and translation on the next page reflect the goal of the preceding chapter, namely, to decenter the conventional base text and allow the *mandragora* entry in the twelfth-century text to be read on its own terms. Where typically the Harley 6258B has been presented as auxiliary to the Cotton Vitellius C.iii,[119] this edition and translation reverse the pattern, offering details from the earlier manuscript in comparative footnotes. To convey the linguistic hybridity of the text, the Latin phrases that are circled and written in the margins of the manuscript are here indicated with a hanging indent, to preserve the original effect of organizing information and drawing the eye. These Latin glosses do not appear in the Cotton Vitellius C.iii or in any of the other Old English manuscripts and thus are typically not encountered by modern readers.[120] Translation choices reflect the analyses of the preceding chapter, and footnotes are provided for choices that depart markedly from past treatments.

De mandragora[121]	Of mandrake
Þeos wyrt mandragora hys fremful;[122] heo on niht scineð healso leohfæt; þanne þu hure heafod ærest ʒeseo þanne bywyrt þu hy wel raðe mid ysene þe læs heo þe ætfleo.	This mandrake plant is beneficial; it shines at night just as a light vessel; when you first see its head, then mark around it quickly with iron lest it flee from you.
Hure maenʒen ys sa mycel 7 swa mere þat heo unclænne man, þanne he to hyre cymeð, wel raðe forlæte[123] wile; forþi þu hi bewyrst mid ysene swa we ær cwadan;[124] 7 þanne þu scealt onbute hy delfan swa þæt þu hy na mid þan, ysene athryne. Ac þu ʒeornlice mid ylpenbaenenan stæfe[125] ðe eorðan delfan; 7 þane þu hyre hænde 7 hyre fet yseo, þane ʒewyrt þu hy; nim þanne þane oðerne ende 7 ʒewyrt to anes hundes swyran ða þæt hund hungri sy; wyrp him seððam mete toforen þa þæt he hyne aracen ne mæʒe bute he mid hym þa wyrte habbe[126], for yt ys ysæd be þisse wyrt[127] þæt heo habbe swa micelle myhte þæt hwylce þing hi up atihð þæt hit sona scyle[128] beon beswicen.	Its power is so great and so powerful that from an unclean person, when he comes to to it, it wants to leave quickly. Therefore, you mark around it, as we said before, with iron; and then you must dig around it so that you do not touch it with the iron. But you must eagerly with an ivory staff dig the earth; and when you see its hands and its feet, then you fasten them; take then the other end and fasten to the neck of a dog when that dog is hungry; next, throw meat before him so that he is not able to reach it unless he has the plant with him; for it is said about this plant that it has such great power that each thing that pulls it up soon must be deceived.
Ac þane[129] heo up abroden sy 7 þu hyre ʒeweald hæbbe, ʒenim hy sona on handa swa, anwelce 7 ʒewyrnʒ þæt wos of hure leafen on ane glæsene ampulle, 7 þanne þe neod beo þæt þu hwylcon men þarmid helpen wylle, þane do him þissum ʒemete.	But when it is snatched up and you have power of it, take it soon into your hand so, roll and wring the juice from the leaves into a glass vessel, and then when there is need that you wish to help anyone with it, then do for him in this way.
Ad dolorem capitis et sompnum[130] Wið heafodece 7 wið þæt man slapen ne mæʒe nim þat wos, smire þane anwlitan; 7 seo wirt swa some san silfan ʒeme[te] þane heafodece ʒeliþeʒað 7 hrædlice slapeþ[131].	*For head pain and sleep* Against headache and for the one not able to sleep, take the juice, smear on face; and, in the same way, the plant relieves the headache and one sleeps quickly.

Ad morbum aurium Wið earena sare nim þisse wyrt wos, meng mid ele þe si of nardo, ʒeot on þa earan,[132] hrædlice he byð ʒehæled.

Ad morbum pedum Wið fotadle, ðeah heo hefigust si, nim of þara swyrðran handa 7 of þara wynstran hænde[133] þysse wyrt, of æʒre handan ðreora peneʒa ʒewhyta, wyrc to dust. Sile drincan on wine seofan daʒas, heo byð ʒehæled; no þæt þat an þæt ʒeswel ʒeset, ac eac sara[134] sina toʒunge to hæle ʒelædeð 7 þæt sar þara abuta wunderlice ʒehæled.

Ad demoniacos Wið ʒewitleaste—þæt is wið deofolseocnesse—ʒenim of þan lichama þisse wyrt[135] þreora peneʒa ʒewihte, syle drincan on wyrme wætera swa he eaðelicost mæʒe, sona he bið ʒehæled.[136]

For sickness of ears Against soreness of ears, take the juice of this plant mixed with the oil that is from nard,[137] put in the ears; quickly he will be healed.

For sickness of feet Against foot disease, though it be severe, take in the right hand and the left hand this plant, in either hand, three pennies' weight, work into dust. Give to drink in wine for seven days. He will be healed, not only so that the swelling goes down, but it also leads spasms of sore sinews to health and wonderfully heals both pains.

For demons Against insanity—that is, against devil-sickness—take from the body of this plant three pennies' weight, give to drink in warm water as easily as he is able, soon he will be healed.

Notes

1. Inserted between 20v and 23r are two small flyleaves contemporary with the rest of the manuscript containing entries for *mantrastro/ mentrarum* and *de apio*.
2. The *Herbarium* is followed by the *Medicina de Quadrupedibus*, a medical compilation with remedies employing animal sources, and a third medical compilation known as the *Peri didaxeon*.
3. As Anne Van Arsdall notes in her translation of the Old English *Herbarium*, the Cotton Vitellius C.iii 'has always been the preferred manuscript to study because of its illustrations of many of the plants and its generally good condition', *Medieval Herbal Remedies*, p. 102.
4. Digitised Manuscripts, Cotton Vitellius C.iii, www.bl.uk/manuscripts/FullDisplay.aspx?ref=Cotton_MS_Vitellius_C_III. Accessed 8 July 2021. The website Production and Use of English Manuscripts 1060 to 1220 follows this same pattern, the cross-referencing moving in only one direction, with Harley 6258B clearly subsidiary to Cotton Vitellius C.iii. See Danielle Maion's description of Harley 6258B at www.le.ac.uk/english/em1060to1220/mss/EM.BL.Harl.6258B.htm #EM.BL.Harl.6258B-objectDesc. Accessed 8 July 2021. The project's description of the Cotton Vitellius C.iii (by Orietta Da Rold) can be found here: www.le.ac.uk/english/em1060to1220/mss/EM.BL. Vite.C.iii.htm. Accessed 7 July 2021.
5. See, for example, de Vriend on Cotton Vitellius C.iii as 'the basic OE text' for what has become the standard edition, *Old English Herbarium*, p. lxxxv.
6. Cockayne, *Leechdoms*, vol. 1, p. lxxxiv.
7. Ibid.
8. Ibid., p. lxxxv.
9. Ibid., p. lxxvi.
10. Stephanie Hollis, 'Anglo-Saxon Secular Learning and the Vernacular: An Overview', in László Sándor Chardonnens and Bryan Carella [who now publishes under the name Kristen Carella] (eds), *Secular Learning in Anglo-Saxon England* (Amsterdam: Rodopi, 2012), pp. 1–43, at 39.
11. Maria Amalia D'Aronco, 'Anglo-Saxon Medical and Botanical Texts, Glosses and Glossaries after the Norman Conquest: Continuations and Beginnings. An Overview', in Patrizia Lendinara, Loredana Lazzari, and Claudia Di Sciacca (eds), *Rethinking and Recontextualizing Glosses: New Perspectives in the Study of Late Anglo-Saxon Glossography* (Turnhout: Brepols, 2012), pp. 228–248, at 241.

12 Maion, 'London, British Library, Harley 6258B Medical Treatises'.
13 de Vriend, *Old English Herbarium*, p. xxxi.
14 Ibid., p. xvii.
15 Cockayne, *Leechdoms*, vol. 1, p. lxxv.
16 D'Aronco, 'Anglo-Saxon Medical', p. 238.
17 Linda Sanborn, 'An Edition of British Library MS. Harley 6258B: Peri Didaxeon' (unpublished doctoral thesis, University of Ottawa, 1983), p. 6.
18 Ibid., p. 242.
19 Maria Amalia D'Aronco, 'Gardens on Vellum: Plants and Herbs in Anglo-Saxon Manuscripts', in Peter Dendle and Alain Touwaide (eds), *Health and Healing from the Medieval Garden* (Woodbridge: Boydell Press, 2008), pp. 101–127, 104.
20 *Nat. Hist.*, xxv, 8. qtd in D'Aronco, 'Gardens', p. 105.
21 While the Cotton Vitellius C.iii is the only version with illustrations, the Hatton 76 has spaces allotted for the reproductions, which were never filled in.
22 Harley 6258B includes not only the *Herbarium* and the *Medicina de Quadrupedibus* (which are included together in all four manuscripts), but also the only extant copy of the *Peri didaxeon*. Similarly, the Harley 585 includes the Old English collection known as the *Lacnunga*.
23 On the skill and technique required, see D'Aronco, 'Gardens', p. 114.
24 Ibid., p. 115.
25 Hugo Berberich, *Das Herbarium Apuleii nach einer frühmittelenglischen Fassung* (Heidelberg: Carl Winter's Universitätsbuchhandlung, 1902).
26 Van Arsdall, *Medieval Herbal Remedies*, p. 103.
27 de Vriend, *Old English Herbarium*, p. xxxi.
28 Treharne, *Living*, p. 2.
29 Ibid., pp. 2–3.
30 Ibid.
31 D'Aronco, 'Anglo-Saxon Medical', pp. 229, 235.
32 Debby Banham, 'England Joins the Medical Mainstream: New Texts in Eleventh-Century Manuscripts', in Hans Sauer and Joanna Story (eds), *Anglo-Saxon England and the Continent*. MRTS Essays in Anglo-Saxon Studies, 3. Tempe: ACMRS (2011), 341–350, at 350.
33 See further Banham, 'A Millennium in Medicine? New Medical Texts and Ideas in England in the Eleventh Century', in Simon Keynes and Alfred P. Smyth (eds), *Anglo-Saxons: Studies Presented to*

Cyril Roy Hart (Dublin: Four Courts Press, 2006), pp. 230–242, esp. pp. 232–238.
34 Walter Ong follows a related line of thinking in *Orality and Literacy: The Technologizing of the Word* (London: Routledge, 1982), at 122–123.
35 Harley 6258B f. 7. Cf. 'ðe Grecas brittanice 7 Engle hæwenhydele nemneð' in Cotton Vitellius C.iii, f. 31.
36 See Sauer and Kubaschewski, *Planting*, p. 173, entry 614, which gives *merce* as Old English, perhaps 'related to *mere* (sea)', corresponding to Latin *apium, apio*.
37 de Vriend, *Old English Herbarium*, p. xxxvii.
38 Ibid., p. xxxiv.
39 The alphabetization scheme in the Harley 6258B does not go beyond the first letter. *Temolum/singrene* appears between *stauis agria* and *saxifraga/sundcorn*. See Berberich, *Das Herbarium*, p. 130, entries 126–128.
40 Cf. Old High German *singruen*. Sauer and Kubaschewski list common periwinkle, houseleek, and barren privet as modern equivalents, *Planting*, p. 213.
41 de Vriend, *Old English Herbarium*, p. xxix.
42 British Library, Digitised Manuscripts Home, www.bl.uk/manuscripts/FullDisplay.aspx?ref=Harley_MS_6258_B and www.bl.uk/manuscripts/FullDisplay.aspx?ref=Cotton_MS_Vitellius_C_III. Accessed 8 July 2021.
43 de Vriend, *Old English Herbarium*, p. xxxiv.
44 Identified by Van Arsdall as sage-leaved germander. *Medieval Herbal Remedies*, p. 175.
45 de Vriend, *Old English Herbarium*, p. 228; trans. Van Arsdall, *Medieval Herbal Remedies*, p. 228.
46 Renée Trilling, 'Health and Healing in the Anglo-Saxon World', *Studies in Medieval and Renaissance History*, 13 (2016), 41–69.
47 Ibid., p. 57.
48 Bosworth and Toller, s.v. *lic-hama*.
49 Anne Van Arsdall, Helmut W. Klug, and Paul Blanz, 'The Mandrake Plant and its Legend', in Peter Bierbaumer and Helmut W. Klug (eds), *Old Names—New Growth: Proceedings of the 2nd ASPNS Conference* (Bern: Peter Lang, 2009), pp. 285–346, at 286.
50 Dioscorides' entry for mandrake appears in Book 4, entry 76, *De materia medica*, Vienna, Österreichische Nationalbibliothek. This text includes the references to male and female mandrakes and the plant's use as a love potion (alongside uses for eye drops and as an anesthetic prior to surgical procedures). See Robert T. Gunther (ed.),

The Greek Herbal of Dioscorides (New York: Hafner Publishing, 1968), pp. 473–474.
51 *De materia medica*, Cod. Med. Gr. 1, fol. 4v. On this frontispiece, see also John M. Riddle, *Dioscorides on Pharmacy and Medicine* (Austin, TX: University of Texas Press, 1985), pp. 186–188.
52 This detail goes back as far as Theophrastus (9.8.4–8). For an early but nonetheless thorough account of references to *mandragora* in Greek and Latin texts, see Charles Brewster Randolph, 'The Mandragora of the Ancients in Folk-lore and Medicine', *Proceedings of the American Academy of Arts and Sciences*, 4.12 (1905), 487–537. For an account of medieval developments, see Anne Van Arsdall, 'Exploring What was Understood by "Mandragora" in Anglo-Saxon England', in Peter Bierbaumer and Helmut W. Klug (eds), *Old Names—New Growth: Proceedings of the 2nd ASPNS Conference* (Bern: Peter Lang, 2009), pp. 57–74.
53 Pliny, Book 25.94.
54 *The Jewish War*, Book VII, chapter 6.3 in Josephus, *Works*, trans. William Whiston (London, 1737), http://penelope.uchicago.edu/josephus/. Accessed 18 July 2021.
55 A. F. Scholfield (trans.), *Aelian: On the Characteristics of Animals*, vol. 3, Books XII–XVII (Cambridge, MA: Harvard University Press, 1959). Van Arsdall notes that Aelian's work may not have been known directly in the Middle Ages, but nonetheless this entry suggests a gathering ritual that was not yet limited specifically to the *mandragora*, 'Exploring', p. 64 n. 8.
56 Van Arsdall, Klug, and Blanz, 'Mandrake', p. 300.
57 Ibid., p. 286.
58 Ibid., p. 290. This study of both pharmaceutical and folkloric history of the mandrake serves as a long-overdue replacement of and corrective to C. J. S. Thompson's *The Mystic Mandrake* (New Hyde Park: University Books, 1934), which, while offering a useful historical account in many ways, nonetheless revels in the idea of the plant's 'magical character', 'mysterious rites and customs', and 'secret ceremonies', p. 19.
59 Van Arsdall, Klug, and Blanz, 'Mandrake', p. 290.
60 Chapter 172.3 (F Text), in Sharon Kinoshita (trans.), *Marco Polo: The Description of the World* (Cambridge: Hackett Publishing, 2016).
61 Sharon Kinoshita, 'Traveling Texts: De-Orientalizing Marco Polo's *Le Devisement du monde*', in Gesa Mackenthun, Andrea Nicolas, and Stephanie Wodianka (eds), *Travel, Agency, and the Circulation of Knowledge* (Waldkirchen: Waxmann, 2017), pp. 223–246, at 238.
62 Ibid., p. 238.

63 Ibid., p. 240.
64 Van Arsdall, Klug, and Blanz, 'Mandrake', p. 289.
65 Van Arsdall, 'Exploring', p. 67.
66 Van Arsdall, Klug, and Blanz, 'Mandrake', p. 286.
67 Van Arsdall, 'Exploring', pp. 67–68.
68 Ibid., p. 67.
69 Ibid.
70 Ibid.
71 Qtd. in Garner and Miller, 'Swarm', p. 371.
72 Colin Clair, *Of Herbs and Spices* (London: Abelard, 1961).
73 Richo Cech, 'Growing Mandrake—Beyond the Basics', https://blog.strictlymedicinalseeds.com/growing-mandrake-beyond-the-basics/. Accessed 26 July 2021.
74 *Mandragora*. www.pacificbulbsociety.org/pbswiki/index.php/Mandragora. Accessed 12 March 2021.
75 www.first-nature.com/flowers/mandragora-autumnalis.php. Accessed 26 July 2021. This entry for *mandragora autumnalis* lists *mandragora officinarum* as a synonym. Another member of the nightshade family (*Solanaceae*) is the plant known as 'Chinese lantern' (*Physalis species*) due to its enlarged calyx, which results in a lantern-shaped covering over its fruit. However, the *mandragora officinarum* and *mandragora autumnalis* do not share this particular feature.
76 The British Museum collections include a number of such lamps, such as the iron tripods with rounded bowl found at Sutton Hoo and Clobb's Row (Essex) (museum numbers 1010.166 and 1216.15).
77 Michael Marder, *Plant Thinking: A Philosophy of Vegetal Life* (New York: Columbia University Press, 2013), p. 101.
78 Matthew Hall, *Plants as Persons: A Philosophical Botany* (New York: SUNY Press, 2011), p. 5.
79 Ibid., p. 19.
80 Ibid., p. 125.
81 Claire Colebrook, *Death of the Posthuman. Essays on Extinction*, vol. 1, Critical Climate Change series (London: Open Humanities Press, 2014), p. 68. The creation of the earth from the literal flesh and blood of the giant Ymir in Norse mythology is but one example of this type of connection.
82 Ibid., p. 68.
83 Hall, *Plants*, 2.
84 Hall, *Plants*, pp. 5, 4, 6.
85 Ibid., p. 4. This inability is far from inevitable, and Marder notes that 'non-Western and feminist philosophies contain a wealth of venerable

traditions much more attuned to the floral world than any author or mainstream current in the history of Western thought', *Plant Thinking*, p. 6.
86 Ibid., pp. 8–9; pp. 9–10.
87 Ibid., p. 12.
88 Ibid., p. 19.
89 Ibid., p. 24.
90 Ibid., p. 27.
91 Ibid.
92 Cotton Vitellius C.iii, *atfleo*.
93 See, for instance, Van Arsdall, Klug, and Blanz, 'Mandrake', p. 335.
94 An especially extreme example of the mandrake as emblematic of sentient (and evil) plantlife is the 2010 *Mandrake* movie, filmed in Louisiana. In the film's painful 90 minutes, there is not a single mandrake plant of any variety, and the word 'mandrake' is not uttered once during the entire movie. Instead, the plot involves an unnamed 'dormant plant creature—part plant, part animal, and all bloodthirsty' (film synopsis, https://louisianaentertainment.gov/projects/film/details/Mandrake-Unearthed, accessed 18 July 2021)—the monstrous hybridity having become synonymous with the mere idea of the mandrake.
95 Marder, *Plant Thinking*, p. 4.
96 Fay, 'Farmacy', 201.
97 Ibid., p. 196.
98 Ibid., p. 188.
99 Marder, *Plant Thinking*, p. 27.
100 Ibid., p. 28.
101 On the technical diagnosis of dissociative fugue, see Dean Haycock et al., 'Dissociative Fugue', *The Gale Encyclopedia of Mental Health*, vol. 2, ed. Brigham Narins (Farmington Hills, MI: Gale Publishing, 4th edn, 2019).
102 Bosworth and Toller, s.v. *niman*.
103 Hall, *Plants as Persons*, p. 127.
104 Ibid., p. 10.
105 Ibid., p. 127.
106 Ibid., p. 2.
107 Bosworth and Toller, s.v. *willan*, sense I.
108 *OED*, s.v. *will*, sense 14.a
109 Hall, *Plants as Persons*, p. 35.
110 Ibid., p. 35.
111 An especially well-known example of the mandrake's simultaneous power and danger in the modern imagination is found of course

in the world of Harry Potter. In the second volume of the series, Hogwarts herbology students must wear ear coverings to protect themselves from the mandrake's screams. J. K. Rowling, *Harry Potter and the Chamber of Secrets* (New York: Scholastic, 1998), p. 92 and following.

112 Van Arsdall, Klug, and Blanz, 'Mandrake', pp. 311–312.
113 Van Arsdall, 'Exploring', p. 58.
114 Ibid., p. 61.
115 Numerous twelfth-century examples can be seen in Tina Negus, 'Medieval Foliate Heads: A Photographic Study of Green Men and Green Beasts in Britain', *Folklore*, 114.2 (2003), 247–261.
116 Fay, 'Farmacy', p. 197.
117 The image is taken from the *Tacuinum Sanitatis in Medicina* manuscript, ca. 1390.
118 Publisher's summary: https://punctumbooks.com/titles/animal-vegetable-mineral-ethics-and-objects/. Accessed 1 August 2021.
119 Berberich's 1902 edition of *Das Herbarium Apuleii* is a notable exception, though it has received little attention in scholarship on Old English, likely because it labels the text as Middle English, *mittelenglischen*, in its subheading.
120 In de Vriend's edition, these marginal notes are included in parentheses, a choice that risks indicating that these passages are less visually salient, rather than more so.
121 Cotton Vitellius C.iii: 'mandragora, mandregara' (no Latin *de* as in Harley 6258B).
122 This entry's opening in the Cotton Vitellius C.iii is more expansive. The sections not appearing in the Harley 6258B are presented here in bold: 'Ðeos wyrt þe man mandragoram nemneþ ys mycel 7 mære on gesihþe 7 heo ys fremful; ða þu scealt þyssum gemete niman, þonne þu to hyre cymst, þonne ongist þu hy be þam þe ...' ['This plant **that one calls mandrake is great and glorious in sight and it** is beneficial; **when you encounter it, you must take it in this way; when you come to it, then you perceive it because ...**']
123 Cotton Vitellius C.iii, *forfleon* ['flee'].
124 Oddly, this clause, 'as we said before', is omitted from Van Arsdall's translation even though it appears in all four manuscripts.
125 This line is the first on its page, f. 23r. As such, there is room above for the following Latin gloss: 'cum eburneo baculo' ['with an ivory stick']. Translations such as Pollington's as 'wand' add to the sense of magic, when the actual text simply denotes a stick or staff.
126 Cotton Vitellius C.iii, 'up abrede' ['snatch up'].

127 Cotton Vitellius C.iii, 'be þysse wyrte ys sæd' ['about this plant it is said'].
128 Cotton Vitellius C.iii, followed by 'þam sylfan gemete' ['in the same manner'].
129 In place of 'Ac þane', the Cotton Vitellius C.iii reads 'for þy sona swa þu geseo ...'. ['Because of this, as soon as you see ...'].
130 These Latin designations indicated here in parentheses appear in the margins of the Harley 6258B, circled, beside their respective remedies. These Latin glosses do not appear in the Cotton Vitellius C.iii nor in any of the other Old English manuscripts.
131 '7 hrædlice slapeþ' extends into the right margin of the page. Cotton Vitellius C.iii: '7 eac þu wundrast hu hrædlice se slæp becymeþ' ['and you will wonder at how quickly sleep comes'].
132 Cotton Vitellius C.iii, followed by 'þu wundrast hu ...' ['you will wonder how ...'].
133 The Cotton Vitellius C.iii does not repeat 'hand': 'genim of þære swyþran handa þysse wyrte 7 of þære wynstran' ['take in the right hand or the left'].
134 In place of the adjectival *sara* ['sore'], the Cotton Vitellius C.iii has only the demonstrative *þæra*.
135 Cotton Vitellius C.iii: 'ylcan wyrte mandragore' ['same mandrake plant'].
136 Two additional entries follow in the Cotton Vitellius C.iii:

'Eft wið sina togunge genim of ðam lichoman þysse wyrte anre ynsan gewihte, cnuca to swyþe smalan duste, gemencg mid ele, smyre þonne þa þe ðas foresprecenan untrumnysse habbað.
  Gyf hwa hwylce hefige yfelnysse on his hofe geseo genime þas wyrte mandragoram onmiddan þam huse—swa mycel (sw)a he þonne h(æbbe)—ealle yfelu (heo) yt anyd(eð)'.

['Again, for tugging of sinews (nerve spasms), take one ounce by weight from the body of this plant, pound it into small dust, mix with oil, then smear it on one who has the previously mentioned condition.
  If anyone perceives any grievous evil in his home, take the mandrake plant to the middle of the house—as much as one has of it—it will expel all the evil'.]

137 Spikenard, *Nardostachys jatamansi*. See Sauer and Kubaschewski, *Planting*, p. 181.

6

On health and hearing: hybridity of environment in *Bald's Leechbook*

Before the arrival of print and film, both hearing and Deaf cultures were 'oral' in that they were based on live, face-to-face interaction. . . . Writing in Deaf and medieval European cultures influenced but did not obviate their strong manual/oral aspects.

(Christopher Krentz, in *Signing the Body Poetic*)[1]

Ða se ellengæst   earfoðlice
þrage geþolode,   se þe in þystrum bad,
þæt he dogora gehwam   dream gehyrde
hludne in healle.

[Then the powerful spirit[2] grievously[3]
suffered a time, the one who dwelled in darkness,
that he heard joy each day,
loud in the hall.]

(*Beowulf*, ll. 86–89)

Before moving forward, I want to pause here and explicitly acknowledge the fact that most of the remedies treated thus far as 'hybrid' are exceptional within the corpus of Old English healing. The personification of the mandrake (Chapter 5), the remedies calling for direct speech to plants (Chapter 4), the poetic battle narrated in the *Lacnunga* remedy against sudden pain (Chapter 3), the protective poem for travelers (Chapter 2), and the elaborate ritual for poor crops (Chapter 1) all seem to have been relatively novel forms emerging in their own present moment from crossings of diverse cultural and linguistic traditions, yet their singularity renders them from another perspective anomalous. But what of healing in the everyday, if such a word can even be applied? In truth, the vast majority of Old English remedies do *not* exhibit the more extreme examples of hybridity seen in the preceding chapters, and it thus remains to examine more precisely how such extraordinary examples of 'hybrid' texts intersect and interact with the preponderance of more typical, arguably *non*-hybrid, remedies.

In nature, as in culture, hybrids that lead to speciation are relatively rare, 'normal in the plant kingdom' but only 'occasional or sporadic'.[4] But these exceptions contribute importantly to the overall diversity and health of the larger ecosystem. Studies on 'hybrid habitats' have shown that the 'high species richness' found in 'hybrid ecosystems' 'contributes greatly to conservation of local biodiversity'.[5] A similar pattern holds in literary texts, the richness of the stand-out 'hybrids' facilitating and fostering a culture of rich diversity. The impact of hybridity, however seldom, should thus not be understated, and particularly relevant for our present exploration of medieval English medical texts is the potential of hybridity to mediate. Biological hybrids 'obscur[e] the discontinuities' that distinguish the biological species from which they originate.[6] As a result, taxonomic categories of species 'break down in practice', just as genre categories too rigidly applied fail to account for the diversity of early medieval texts produced in a 'hybrid ecosystem'.

As in biology, metaphorically hybrid texts have the potential to mediate—and often obfuscate—difference. This mediation within a 'hybrid ecosystem' can expose and begin to mitigate bias, even when dealing with seemingly mundane texts. But to understand such mediation, a hybrid methodology is also required, a fundamentally new and interdisciplinary way of thinking that accounts for subtle nuances and differences across texts and remedies. Where Chapter 5 demonstrated how the hybrid mandrake entry in the *Herbarium* implicitly challenged the human/plant hierarchy that became increasingly pronounced across the later medieval period, this chapter turns to a different type of bias, one closely tied to matters of orality/aurality, traditionality, performativity, spoken rhetoric, and oral transmission treated in previous chapters: the faculty of hearing itself. This chapter brings a hybrid methodology that draws from what might seem an unlikely combination—oral theory and Deaf studies—to bear on remedies for hearing loss. This perspective not only exposes the implicit privileging of hearing and aurality within oral tradition studies but also demonstrates what early medieval medical texts can still teach with regard to common modern default—and often ableist—assumptions that frequently underlie interpretations of seemingly straightforward texts. As with the mandrake entry and other texts treated in previous chapters, close attention to the language of a seemingly straightforward entry in *Bald's Leechbook* elucidates subtle patterns that point the way toward alternative ways of understanding adversity, bodies, and subjectivity in medieval and modern contexts.

Orality, aurality, and the faculty of hearing

The famous *Hwæt* that opens the Old English epic *Beowulf* and numerous other Old English texts in the heroic style is often translated as 'listen', understood as an idiomatic marker of an utterance meant to be heard, words that even on the manuscript page suggest connections to an ambient oral tradition.[7] It has long been acknowledged that contexts of performance and orality are ever-present in both the poetry and prose of the period, such as during the feast at Hrothgar's hall, when 'scop hwilum sang / hador on Heorote' ['a poet sang, clear-voiced in Heorot'] (ll. 496–497). Even at the moment of his death, Beowulf himself recalls hearing the recitation of 'syllic spell' ['strange/wonderful stories'] (l. 2109). We also know that early medieval English laws were likewise 'preserved by a tradition of oral transmission' and that the written laws that survive 'stand boldly at the watershed between orality and literacy', showing 'traces of their spoken past as they move into the literate future'.[8] However, access to the oral/aural culture of early medieval England would undoubtedly not have been the same for everyone, and to assume so is to participate in what Lennard Davis has referred to as 'one of the foundational ableist myths of our culture'.[9] Maren Tova Linett places the growth of 'these cultural biases in favor of hearing and speech' as reaching their height 'during the modernist period',[10] and indeed in early medieval England we find a situation with arguably less imbalanced assumptions. Law codes from the period provide particular guidance for indicted individuals born deaf and also dictate highly specific recompense for victims of violence that resulted in hearing loss later in life.[11] And the Old English poetic record suggests that even hearing itself was not always beneficial but could be associated with pain and torment, since in *Beowulf* it is of course the unendurable sounds from the hall that draw Grendel's wrath: 'he dogora gehwam dream gehyrde / hludne in healle' ['heard joy each day, loud in the hall'] (ll. 88–90), sounds endured *eorfoðlice* ['grievously, bitterly, painfully'] (l. 86). Frequently referred to as a 'hybrid' creature,[12] Grendel manifests this hybridity in part through a seemingly human faculty of hearing that remains at odds with what is understood as typical human desire, a situation that draws attention to suffering and implicitly challenges modern preconceptions of medical ideals. Clearly the experience of hearing was not perceived as a monolithic one in early medieval England, and the surviving Old English medical record, which offer remedies for a wide range of ailments affecting hearing and sensory perception, can help us develop a more nuanced understanding of the actual sense of hearing as experienced and conceptualized in the largely oral/aural culture of early medieval England.

Remedies for various changes to hearing survive in all of the major medical texts—the so-called *Leechbooks* (BL, Royal 12 D.xvii), the *Lacnunga* (Harley 585), and the Old English *Herbarium* (Harley 585, Hatton 76, Cotton Vitellius C.iii, Harley 6258B)—but it is *Bald's Leechbook* in particular that offers the most sustained consideration of hearing anywhere in the medical corpus or, for that matter, in any work surviving from the period. This text, deriving from a mid-tenth-century manuscript with marginal additions that indicate its ongoing use into at least the eleventh century,[13] tends to be organized more by the affected part of the body and ailment (rather than by herb, as in the *Herbarium*)[14] and thus offers a unique opportunity within the Old English medical texts to examine the faculty of hearing. After entries 1 (on ailments of the head) and 2 (on remedies for eyes), entry 3 (ff. 14v–16r),[15] which focuses on the ears, implicitly conveys awareness of a broad range of hearing experiences as recognized, categorized, and treated within the early medieval healing tradition. This entry includes twenty-five[16] remedies all devoted to different kinds of ailments that could impact the ears and hearing. The contents page alone delineates numerous distinct hearing-related ailments (f. 1r):

Læcedomas wið eallum earena ece 7 sare; wiþ earena deafe; 7 wiþ yfelre *hlyste*; 7 gif wyrmas on earan syn 7 wiþ earwicgan; 7 gif earan dynien 7 ear sealfe ælces cynnes.

[Remedies against all aches and soreness of ears; against deafness of ears; and against poor hearing;[17] and if worms are in ears; and against and if ears din; and ear-salves of every kind.][18]

The compiler's choices illustrate that not all hearing loss was the same, with some conditions ascribed to insects that caused 'dinning' ears, possibly some form of tinnitus. Together, the remedies in entry 3 clearly show that polarized concepts of hearing and deafness alone are insufficient for understanding the broad range of sensory perceptions that seem to have been widely recognized in early medieval England, yet these distinctions among auditory sensory experiences—which would have been crucially important within a culture heavily reliant on spoken communication—have nonetheless been largely overlooked within the field of oral theory. The analysis that follows thus first examines ways that approaches in medieval studies drawing from oral theory can benefit from a deeper awareness of work in Deaf studies, then probes *Bald's Leechbook* I.iii for the insights it can offer into the sense of hearing, and finally moves into larger implications of these findings in connection with other records of early medieval England, including law codes, burial sites, historical accounts, and theological texts.

Deaf studies and oral theory

Developed as an academic discipline in the 1970s around the centrality of Deaf culture rather than around a view of deafness as physical deficit, the burgeoning and innovative field of Deaf studies has challenged many preconceptions about not only the experience of deafness but also what it means to be hearing. And while a great deal of scholarly attention has been devoted to concerns of orality and aurality in Old English texts, very little of this work has yet incorporated the tremendous insights gained in recent years from Deaf studies. An unfortunate result of these omissions is that longstanding assumptions about the sense of hearing itself have remained largely unexamined within the corpus of Old English medical texts, yet several overlooked questions concerning hearing and deafness are crucial for a thorough understanding of oral/aural culture in early medieval England. How, for example, did those in early medieval England understand the faculty of hearing? What would it have meant to be deaf or hard of hearing in a society that relied as heavily as it clearly did on orality and the spoken word? What range of sensory experiences along the spectrum of hearing and deafness were recognized, and how were these various experiences perceived and addressed? Complete answers to at least some of these questions are likely impossible, but recent scholarship emerging from various philological, sociological, and even medical areas of inquiry can help us begin to understand the complexities of hearing and deafness in the early medieval period.

As shown in preceding chapters, with the technology of literacy limited to a small minority of the population, the world as experienced by many or most in early medieval England would necessarily have been a predominantly oral and aural one, though one impacted increasingly by writing and literacy. Far from binary concepts, 'orality' and 'literacy' would have been linked inextricably in the early medieval period, and previous scholarship has demonstrated unequivocally that—even allowing for the vexed question of what constitutes 'literacy'[19]—'illiterate' individuals were still often profoundly influenced by literate culture, and conversely even the period's most 'literate' individuals continued to engage texts in distinctly aural/oral ways. The Old English medical texts attest to this complex matrix, since remedies written on the manuscript page frequently call for oral performance, and, in turn, rituals accompanying healing practice rely on writing and inscriptions alongside spoken incantations.

The semantic range of vocabulary related to hearing and deafness offers some insight into this complexity but can also be potentially misleading. The verb *hyran* shows us that the sense of hearing was implicitly linked not only with the physical perception of sound ('to hear') and the acquisition of orally conveyed information (to 'hear of'), but also with the very social fabric of early medieval culture; through extension of the sense 'to listen to', secondary meanings for the verb include 'follow', 'serve', 'obey', 'be subject to', and even 'belong to'.[20] And at the opposite end of the hearing spectrum, the semantic range of the Old English *deaf* also includes the similarly sound-independent meanings 'unproductive' and 'barren' so that, for instance, in Alfred's translation of Gregory's *Pastoral Care*, land that is not producing grain ('corn') is lamented as being 'deaf' (l. 20; *DOE*, s.v. *deaf*, sense A.2).[21] On the surface, these usages might seem to suggest that being hard of hearing would render one unfit to lead or follow, thus outside the fabric of early medieval social structure and as unproductive as a barren field. Yet work by disability scholars reminds us not to be too quick in assuming that hearing differences would automatically have led to ostracism.

Tory Pearman stresses the understanding of disability instead as socially constructed and 'historically located', and Christina Lee has written extensively on the risks of projecting modern notions of disability in general onto early medieval contexts, rightfully noting that it is 'wrong to assume that impaired people are automatically disabled in their societies'.[22] In fact, Lee draws important parallels within modern culture to illustrate this point, noting how many individuals within the Deaf community opt not to have cochlear implants because they 'do not see themselves as disabled, but as a language minority', using American Sign Language (ASL) rather than spoken English.[23] In some medieval cases as well, she demonstrates, 'impairment is seen as a blessing or advantage and not as a disability'. In texts such as Ælfric's *Lives*, for example, 'paralysis is not a punishment or a state that needs intervention from a saint' but rather an enhancement of 'the "natural" abilities of these women to intercede on behalf of others', the limitations of physical movement allowing them to 'pray even more fervently'.[24] Deafness, too, has been occasionally aligned with power in medieval narrative beyond England. In a discussion of memory in medieval Irish narrative, for instance, Joseph Falaky Nagy draws our attention to the late medieval collection *Feis Tighe Chonáin* ('Feast of Conán's House'); within this collection, memory acquires mystical associations in a wondrous story where a deaf warrior is said to have a vast repertoire of oral stories committed to memory.[25] In this narrative, the sense of hearing is clearly distinct from storytelling performance or acquisition, and deafness is not presented as a spiritual or even physical deficiency; it prevents neither the man's service as a warrior nor his capability as a storyteller. Quite the contrary, he is presented as a vital part of the warrior band, and his deafness enables a miracle of memory.

Before continuing, I want to clarify that these differences observed between medieval and modern modes of thinking about disability and deafness should not be taken as any unqualified endorsement of medieval thought or practice. Pearman has responsibly drawn attention to the all too common 'innate desire on the part of scholars to "rescue" the Middle Ages from assumptions that construe medieval society as intolerant of and even cruel toward people with physical and mental impairments',[26] a tendency that sometimes 'comes dangerously close to supplanting a monolithic view of the Middle Ages as intolerant with an equally monolithic view that borders on nostalgic'.[27] As she notes, many medieval discourses (including those of early medieval England) did in fact 'stigmatize physical and mental impairments as markers of sinfulness and/or Otherness' and 'should not be ignored'.[28] I thus follow Pearman's goal here in taking conflicting views within the medieval world into account, 'conceding the sometimes negative connotations surrounding the impaired body in the Middle Ages while also acknowledging medieval society's frequent acceptance of and care for the impaired'.[29] In the Old English texts discussed below, for instance, deafness is sometimes explicitly used as a metaphor for spiritual lack, within the same culture that just as clearly acknowledged and accepted a far greater diversity of hearing experience than we often see today. Crucial first steps to understanding these texts on at least something closer to their own terms involves recognizing and actively resisting assumptions emerging from the now deeply entrenched 'medical and rehabilitation models' of disability that 'focus on the "restoration" of a disabled body to a socially constructed "norm"'.[30]

The rapidly growing body of scholarly work in Deaf studies has been especially powerful in countering such potentially harmful medicalized notions of the body. H-Dirksen Bauman, for instance, advocates 'disowning an imposed medicalized identity and developing an empowered identity rooted in a community and culture of others who share similar experiences and outlooks on the world'.[31] Demonstrating the importance of this approach with regard to medieval texts in particular, Christina Lee cautions against imposing this type of 'medical model of disability' onto pre-modern cultures.[32] A rather large stumbling block in changing this scholarly default with regard to medieval oral-connected texts, however, has been the implicit assumption that hearing was a universal experience, an unexamined view frequently perpetuated in oral theory, even though Deaf studies itself has long employed approaches from oral tradition scholarship.

For decades, scholars within Deaf studies have drawn many important and insightful connections to oral traditions and modes of storytelling. In a discussion of deafness and the arts, Neil Glickman, for example, notes that 'the major literary form of Deaf culture has been its "oral" tradition of storytelling'.[33] Approaching the subject from the angle of rhetoric, Brenda Jo Brueggemann describes ASL as 'an "oral" language in that it exists primarily outside of writing when two living beings are communicating with each other in the immediate present':

> 'orality' rings in my ears when I consider sign language. Writing removes us from the present. Writing disembodies. Writing provides a synonym for literacy. Orality does not; sign language does not. In these ways, then, sign language is the 'same but different' in its relation to our two dominant locations for locution—orality/speech and writing. An understanding of that relation, and thus our investigation of sign language itself, can radically revise our thinking about literacy.[34]

Thomas Holcomb makes similar connections in urging that 'Deaf lit[erature] needs to be embraced for what it is—a strong "oral" tradition presented in a visual manner'.[35]

One of the most fully developed and deeply insightful applications of oral theory to Deaf studies has been Kristen Harmon's fascinating analysis of ASL poet Gilbert Eastman's protest performance of a self-described 'epic'; Eastman's performed narrative poem related events in the 'Deaf President Now' movement at Gallaudet University, where student and alumni leaders gathered in 1988 to organize a call for the institution's first Deaf president. Expanding upon earlier theoretical models of John Foley, Harmon addresses the shift in focus from a 'text-based, and thus fixed, understanding of epic composition to a dynamic and fluid, yet structured, sense of epic composition'. She explains that 'we now understand epic as performed by a poet using culturally determined formulaic structures to aid in composing' and demonstrates that, as with oral epic, the ASL poem's power derives largely from its production 'within culturally determined parameters of performance through the use of genre-specific structural formulas and registers'. The process, she explains, is similar to ways that oral traditional poets in spoken languages 'compos[e] in and throughout performance before a knowledgeable audience'.[36]

Even the Old English *Beowulf* has made its way into these important conversations. In his contribution to *Signing the Body Poetic*, Christopher Krentz compares the impact of manuscript culture on early medieval oral traditions to the influence of film on poetry composed and performed in ASL. 'Before the arrival of print and film', he argues, 'both hearing and Deaf cultures were "oral" in that they were based on live, face-to-face communication'.[37] The technology of film provided the potential to fix visual performances in the same way that print has the effect of fixing spoken language. Krentz demonstrates that in spite of these radical changes in performance medium, ASL poetry continues to exhibit—even depends upon—many of the elements from person-to-person exchanges, much as *Beowulf* depends upon an oral poetics for meaning within the new medium of writing and textuality.[38]

Yet, to our detriment, while Deaf studies has embraced models found in oral theory for decades, deafness in oral tradition scholarship has remained largely unaddressed and is even used as a metaphor for missing the connotations of orality. For example, in well-intentioned and important efforts to shift our defaults away from literacy-mindedness to make room for a better understanding of dynamic oral traditions, readers are cautioned not to be 'deafened by epistemology and time',[39] warned that by encountering oral narratives in print 'we'll be deaf to a telltale shift of loudness or intonation',[40] and advised that 'the ear of the outsider is deaf to the subtlety and the allusions' of traditional language.[41] Similarly, we are told that 'writers can be dumb and readers deaf as long as literacy is imagined to exist on a plane of signs, above, outside of, or apart from the agitations of voice'.[42] This line of thinking develops from what Lennard Davis has called the 'deafened moment', that is, the 'dialectical moment in the reading/critical process, that is defined by the acknowledgment on the part of the reader/writer/critic that he or she is part of a process that does not involve speaking or hearing'; Davis notes that 'many of our assumptions about writing, about language, about communication are based on the premise that language is in fact sonic, audible, vocalized'.[43]

In this construct, sign language and deaf culture are 'othered' as not *written* but also not *oral*. Such omissions and oversights inevitably result not only in missed opportunities but also in significant misunderstandings. We need to take into account a third, vital modality, one that is silent *and* visual. Leslie Arnovick suggests that a 'deaf spot', analogous to the idiomatic 'blind spot', must be kept in mind when we consider oral poetics';[44] I would like to suggest here that we follow this important advice but shift our concept of a 'deaf spot' away from the perception of deficit to become instead an awareness of possible gain.[45] To this end we might consider Edna Edith Sayers' use of deafness as a positive descriptor within oral tradition studies, which appeared in the wonderfully collaborative electronic symposium titled 'Deafness and Orality', published in *Oral Tradition* in 1993.[46] As part of a larger discussion on ways that ASL 'rewards study by oral traditional scholars', Sayers praises scholarship within the field of oral theory that 'looks deaf to me', clarifying this description as 'a compliment to all concerned'.[47]

On the other hand, in an effort to correct flawed assumptions and overgeneralizations that have been perpetuated within medieval studies, Sayers also exposed a number of such misconceptions as early as 1997 in the *Journal of Deaf Studies and Deaf Education*. The main difficulty, she explained, is that scholarship 'has developed in two separate disciplines among two distinct sets of scholars', namely scholars of medieval studies and those of deaf history. In addition to arguing, for instance, that the term 'monastic sign language' is, in particular, potentially misleading since the finger alphabets and sign systems of the period provided more of a lexicon than a language with its own syntax and grammar,[48] Sayers also pointed out the quite problematic nature of the oft-made assumption that 'the deaf were mercilessly persecuted as defectives in the

"Dark Past" until the rise of Deaf Education rescued them from this "Dread and Despair"'.[49] Along these same lines, Sayers additionally cautioned against a strong tendency 'to retroject modern assumptions about deaf people ... onto antiquity and the Middle Ages' and the impulse to view the deaf as 'defective: pitiable objects of charity or pathological specimens', reminding readers that 'the medical model of deafness (and disability, too) is a modern and culture-specific construct'.[50] Still, even though Sayers published these concerns over twenty years ago, the impact has yet to be fully felt in medieval studies scholarship.

As Emily Cockayne noted in an article on deafness in sixteenth- and seventeenth-century England, part of the difficulty here is that most scholarship addressing pre-modern deafness has actually focused on only the late eighteenth century and afterward, which has led to potentially reductive claims about deafness in the medieval world itself.[51] Jonathan Rée's study of the history of deafness, for example, is quite informative and nuanced in its treatment of later periods, but the early ones are dismissed in a few short paragraphs as brutal eras of 'uncomprehending cruelty' of 'the so-called "deaf and dumb"'.[52] While Rée's claims may certainly be true of some locations, such assertions risk generalizations that do not apply equally to all pre-modern cultures in all parts of the world. But focusing more narrowly on early medieval England— and on a particularly useful text within that period—can help us begin to move beyond such vast overgeneralizations. Let us turn, then, to *Bald's Leechbook*, chapter iii, a text that describes not only a broad range of sensory experiences that existed along the hearing spectrum but also an equally diverse set of responses to deafness and hearing during this period, a diversity that could not only be accommodated but even thrive as part of a hybrid environment.

Old English medical texts and the BL, Royal 12 D.xvii

As discussed earlier, while all of the major medical texts surviving from early medieval England demonstrate a range of hearing experiences, it is only *Bald's Leechbook* that delineates various ailments in relation to one another by structuring them through a connected presentation of a fairly extensive range of treatments.

Additionally, Emily Kesling has observed that BL, Royal 12 D.xvii, the manuscript containing *Bald's Leechbook*, 'boasts the most complex organisational structure'[53] of all the medical texts, and, as such, this structure warrants our close attention. To that end, Table 6.1 illustrates three important organizational structures that emerge within entry iii of *Bald's Leechbook*: manuscript divisions, distinctions of individual recipes and remedies, and general

Table 6.1 Rhetorical structure of *Bald's Leechbook* (I.iii)

C	D	Text	Translation
		Introduction	
1		Læcedomas wið eallum earena sare 7 ece 7 wið earena adeafunge. 7 gif wyrmas on earan synd oþþe earwicga. 7 gif earan dynien. 7 earsealfa fiftyne cræftas.	Leechdoms against all soreness and ache of ears and for deafening of ears. And if worms are in ears or earwigs. And if ears din. And ear-salves. Fifteen crafts.
		Remedies primarily for aches and soreness	
2	1	Wiþ earena sare 7 ece …	Against soreness and ache of ears …
	2	Eft wiþ þon ilcan …	Again against the same …
	3	Wiþ earwærce 7 wið deafe …	Against ear pain and against deafness …
	4	Wiþ þon ilcan …	Against the same …
	5	Wiþ þon ilcan …	Against the same …
3	6	Wiþ þon ilcan …	Against the same …
4	7	Wiþ þon ilcan …	Against the same …
5	8	Wið þon ilcan …	Against the same …
	9	Wiþ earena sare …	Against soreness of ears …
		Remedies primarily for changes to sense of hearing	
5 (cont.)	10	Wiþ earena deafe …	Against deafness of ears …
6	11	Wiþ þon ilcan gif earan willen adeafian oþþe yfel hlyst sie …	Against the same if ears wish to deafen or if hearing be poor …

Table 6.1 (Continued)

C	D	Text	Translation
7	12	Wiþ þon ilcan gif yfelne hlyst ...	Against the same if hearing be poor ...
8	13	Eft ...	Again ...
	14	Wiþ þon ilcan ...	Against the same ...
	15	Eft wiþ þon ilcan ...	Again against the same ...
9	16	Wiþ ðon ilcan ...	Against the same ...
	17	Viþ earena adeafunge eft ...	Against deafening of ears again ...
	18	Eft wiþ þon ilcan ...	Again against the same ...
10	19	Eft wið þon ilcan ...	Again against the same ...
11	20	Wiþ þæt ilce ...	Against the same ...
		Remedies for insects and noise in ears	
11 (cont.)	21	Gif wyrmas on earan syn ...	If worms are in ears ...
	22	[no condition identified]	—
	23	Wiþ þon gif earan dynien ...	Against a case if ears din ...
12	24	Eft wiþ þon ilcan ...	Again against the same ...
	25	Wiþ earwicgan ...	Against earwigs ...

groupings by conditions to be treated. The left column of the table indicates the divisions as they appear in the manuscript itself (see Figure 6.1), where they are marked in the folios by an extension of the text into the left margin and the placement of three triangulated dots at the end of the previous section. These manuscript divisions are retained in Cockayne's edition and are thus labeled here as *C* as an aid for those using Cockayne's numbering. The second column provides the numbering of the individual remedies in succession, typically signaled through 'wið' ['against'], 'eft' ['again'], or 'gif' ['if']; Doyle's numbering follows these divisions, and accordingly I have here designated the column as *D*. The third structural pattern—with the remedies grouped according to the general condition to be treated—is more nebulous, but it is arguably the most important for a nuanced understanding of hearing as presented in this text. Thus, general groupings are labeled in italics. The early

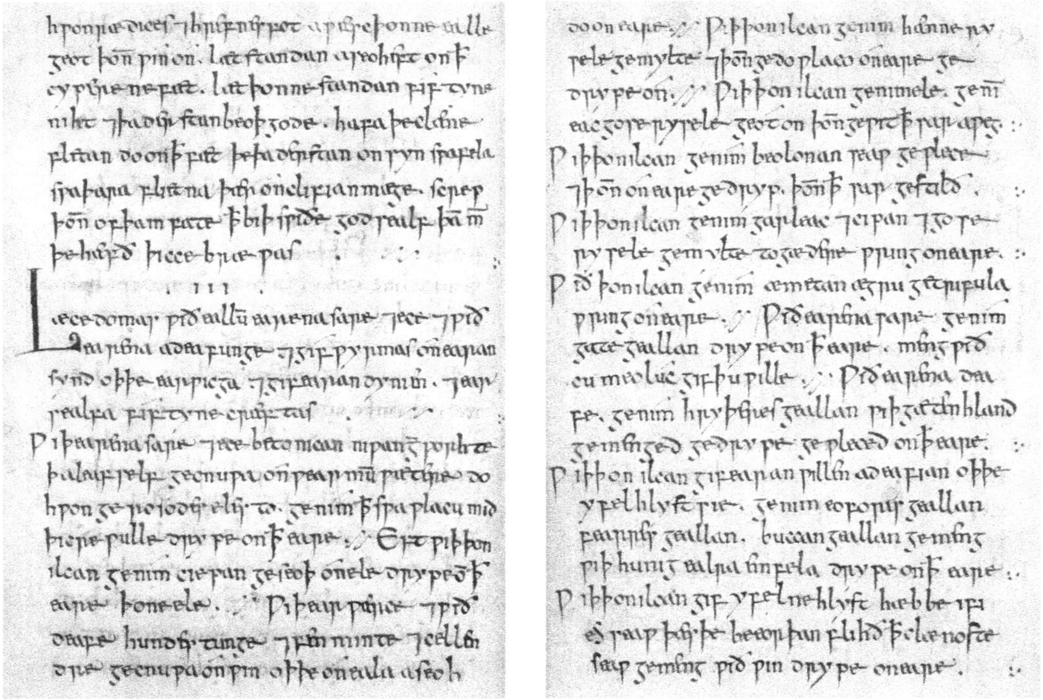

Figure 6.1 *Bald's Leechbook* (I.iii), British Library MS Royal 12 D.xvii, f. 14v–15r.

remedies can be loosely categorized as having to do with pain and soreness, with changes in hearing mentioned only secondarily, followed by remedies that deal more explicitly with the faculty of hearing, and finally remedies for perceived insects or sounds within the ear. Since my purpose here is to underscore the groupings and identification of conditions to be treated, the specific preparations and recipes are omitted, but full texts and translations can be found in both Cockayne (vol. 2) and Doyle (vol. 2).

Ear pain associated with changes in hearing

Before providing its series of specific remedies, the general introduction to entry iii offers several important insights into medieval English perceptions of hearing:

> Læcedomas wið eallum earena sare 7 ece 7 wið earena adeafunge.
> 7 gif wyrmas on earan synd oþþe earwicga.
>
> [Leechdoms against all soreness and ache of ears and against deafening of ears. And if worms or earwigs are in the ears.]

The most significant word here is *adeafunge*, 'deafening'—not a noun such as 'deafness', or an adjective 'deaf', or even a past participle 'deafened', any of which would denote a completed and essentially passive state. Instead, we see a present participle, 'deafening' (or, as the *DOE* renders, 'growing deaf'), denoting an active process of change, as it might exist at any point along an ongoing continuum. Just as importantly, for both *adeafunge* and *adeafian* further below, the agent of that process is not a 'deafening' sound, as we might assume based on modern English usage, but rather the ears themselves. The modern sense of 'deafen' as 'to make deaf, to deprive of the power of hearing', a sense that renders the 'deafened' individual as victim rather than subject, is actually not attested in English until the seventeenth century (*OED*, s.v. *deafen*). Rather, the Old English sense of what it means to 'deafen' projects a concept of hearing that is varying and variable, and the processuality of 'deafening' ears challenges modern notions of a 'hearing line', 'that invisible boundary separating deaf and hearing people'.[54]

Though there is obvious overlap between the sense of hearing and pain of the ears, the ordering of entries and the itemization of ailments tend to separate such pain from hearing itself. Remedies 1–8 all involve remedies for ear pain and soreness. Remedy 1 (a recipe for eardrops made from betony) and 2 (eardrops from onion) open 'Wiþ earena sare 7 ece' and 'Eft wiþ þon ilcan' respectively ['against soreness and ache of ears', 'also for the same']. Remedy 3 (a recipe for eardrops made from several herbs mixed with wine or ale) does include deafness, but only secondarily after ear pain: 'Wiþ earwærce 7 wið deafe' ['Against ear pain and against deafness[55]']. Remedies 4 and 5 (both recipes for eardrops made from animal fat) open with 'Wiþ þon ilcan' ['Against the same'], leaving it ambiguous as to whether the remedies are for pain or hearing in particular; however, iii.5 closes with the promise that 'þonne gewit þæt sar aweg' ['then that pain will be gone'], clarifying the primary focus on pain. The Latin analogue offers further support that *pain* is the referent, 'ad *dolore* aurium' ['for *pain* of ears'].[56] Remedies 6–8 (all recipes for eardrops) likewise make no explicit mention of hearing, 'Wiþ þon ilcan' presumably again referring back to *sar*, soreness or pain.[57] Remedy 9 continues in like manner, 'Wiþ earena sare' ['against soreness of ears'].

Variable experiences of hearing

It is beginning with remedy 10 and continuing through to 25 where the entry more consistently references the faculty of hearing directly. These remedies specifically for changes to hearing are distinct from those for earaches prioritized in remedies 1–9, which can, of course, impact hearing, but are categorized here as a fundamentally different condition. Remedy 10 offers a recipe for drops made from ox gall and goat's urine[58] as a treatment 'wiþ earena deafe' ['against deafness of ears']; remedy 11, involving drops from animal gall mixed with honey, is declared 'wiþ þon ilcan' ['against the same'] but with greater specificity: 'gif earan willen adeafian oþþe yfel hlyst sie' ['if ears may wish to deafen or if there is poor hearing']. The phrasing 'willen adeafian' here has puzzled some editors and translators, in particular its implications of volition.[59] As we saw with the mandrake in the preceding chapter, however, volition could be precisely what is implied, and the verbal construction should be accepted at face value. The use of *willen*, the subjunctive plural of *willan*, ever so slightly shifts the source of agency towards ears that 'may wish' or perhaps 'seem to wish'. The implied agency granted to non-humans in the healing process—to herbs and plants and even to disease itself—opens a space for recognizing more subtle implications of volition and agency for what they are.

The modern reluctance to render the subjunctive *willen* in terms of volition reflects a fundamental difference in thinking about the faculty of hearing in early medieval and modern medicine. Rather than viewing the person experiencing changes to hearing in terms of a lack, as is more typical in the modern medical model, with a 'loss' of hearing, the Old English text instead posits that the ears themselves have agency and 'wish' to change by becoming deaf. The verb *adeafian* here, too, is telling. As we have seen, *adeafian* means not 'to *be* deaf' but rather 'to *grow* deaf' or '*become* deaf',[60] thus implying a process of hearing change instead of a single, monolithic state of sensory experience, and reinforcing a much less passive concept of hearing and hearing loss than that which dominates in modern English. And lest we think that the compiler was simply eccentric or in error by employing this grammatical construction, Audrey Meaney has identified a parallel remedy from the BL Cotton Otho B.xi transcribed by Lawrence Nowell (following the Cotton fire in 1731): 'Gis [for Gif] earen willen adeafian'.[61] Though the relationship between this manuscript and *Bald's Leechbook* is close,[62] as Meaney's analysis shows, the entries are not always duplicates, and the process of inclusion was furthermore selective. The phrasing 'willen adeafian' was logical and apparently worth preserving for both compilers.

The opening of remedy 12, 'Wiþ þon ilcan gif yfelne hlyst' ['against the same if hearing be poor'], repeats 'yfelne hlyst' ['poor hearing'], which appears in remedy 11 within the clause immediately following 'willen adeafian.[63] This remedy and the one that follows it (where it starts off simply with 'Eft …' ['Again …']) have close parallels in the *Herbarium*. Remedy 12 includes a recipe for eardrops made from ground ivy mixed with wine, similar to *Herbarium* entry 100 for *eorðyfig* [earth-ivy], which also blends wine with the plant's juice. Remedy 13, which calls for drops from juice of ribwort mixed with warm oil, is analogous to *Herbarium* entry 98 for *ribbe* (ribwort), where the herb is to be blended with oil after being pounded.[64] More importantly for our understanding of medieval views toward hearing, though, these *Herbarium* entries and those of *Bald's Leechbook*, as well as its analogue in the BL Cotton Otho B.xi, follow similar patterns of pairing conditions in ways that once again reinforce the notion of hearing as a range of experiences:

Bald's Leechbook (I.iii.11):
... gif earan willen adeafian oþþe yfel hlyst sie ...

[... if ears wish to deafen or if hearing is poor ...]

Herbarium 98.3 (ribwort):
Wiþ ðæra earene unnytlicnysse 7 wið ðæt man wel gehyran ne mæge ...

[Against unusefulness of ears and against when one is not able to hear well ...]

Herbarium 100.7 (ground ivy):
Wið þæra earena unnytlicnysse 7 wið þæt man ne mæge well gehyran ...

[Against unusefulness of ears and against when one is not able to hear well ...]

BL Cotton Otho B.xi (from Nowell transcript):
Gis [for Gif] earen willen adeafian an oþþe yfel hlist sie ...

[If ears wish to deafen or if hearing is poor ...]

In each case, one condition of the ears—either a wish to deafen or unusefulness—is connected by a coordinating conjunction to another in which hearing is partially affected, collectively indicating a substantial range of hearing experiences.

Of particular importance here is the *Herbarium*'s employment of *unnytlicnysse*. The most common gloss for this noun is 'uselessness', the term followed in numerous translations of the collection, such as Cockayne's[65] and Pollington's[66] and the only definition offered in de Vriend's standard edition.[67] To break *unnytlicnysse* down into morphemes, *nyt*, defined in Bosworth and Toller as 'use', 'advantage', 'profit', is prefixed by *un-* and followed by the adjectival *-lic* and finally the nominalizing *-nysse* (modern *-ness*). An alternate translation, therefore, as 'unusefulness' or even Cockayne's 'unprofitableness'[68] comes much closer to the literal, and less pejorative, meaning of the term.[69] Though 'useless' and 'unuseful' might be seen as synonymous, and the difference in translation inconsequential, the connotations are actually decidedly different. The 'un-' prefix added to a positive trait in English typically evokes more neutral connotations than the 'less' suffix: for instance, 'joyless' versus 'unjoyful', 'lawless' versus 'unlawful'. And as we have seen already, the parallel collocation from *Bald's Leechbook*—'willen adeafian'—was not necessarily a pejorative one, indicating that we should refrain from pressing such negative connotations onto *unnytlicnysse* as well. 'Unprofitable' ears do not denote a simple lack of faculty but rather leave open infinite possibilities for other strengths and assets beyond mere utilitarian concerns. These differences matter.

Remedies 14–16, then, offer various animal- and plant-based eardrops for presumably the same pairing of conditions, each opening 'Eft wiþ þon ilcan' ['Again against the same']. The same processuality we saw with *adeafian* in remedy 10 is similarly implied in a recipe in remedy 17 for eardrops made from the juice of pounded alder branches to aid 'earena adeafunge' ['deafening of the ears'], the present participle allowing for infinite gradations that a static adjective would not. Remedies 18–20 continue in this same vein, opening with 'eft' ['again'] and 'Wiþ þæt ilce' ['against the same']. Quite clearly, then, rather than being limited solely by external events that happen to the ears, the faculty of hearing is instead presented in Old English medical texts as one where ears actively participate in the sensory experience and can do so in ever-shifting capacities and environments. The understanding of the body as an entity with a single, unified subjectivity shifts in this construct, raising the possibility that different elements of the body might also manifest different wants from one another. As in the remedies explored in previous chapters, the body once again becomes a site of potential conflict, and the medical texts again subtly imply a need to negotiate balance, rather than simply to find a 'cure'.

'Dinning' of the ears

Where remedies 9–20 addressed conditions involving the ears' ability to hear external sounds, remedies 21–25 shift their focus toward sounds and ailments perceived as originating inside the ear. For instance, remedy 21 is prescribed 'gif wyrmas on earan syn' ['if worms be in the ear'], which would seem to represent quite a different circumstance from the 'poor hearing' and ears that 'wish to deafen' of the several previous entries. However, this well organized entry does indeed include a logical transition. While remedy 20 does not itself deal with a condition caused by parasites, it almost anticipates the shift by including as part of its treatment a solution made from insects: 'do þon*ne* on eare þara readena æmetena hors' ['then put those red horse/worker ant eggs into the ear'].[70] It is perhaps worth mentioning that such parasites, or *wyrmas*, are actually one of the more common ailments mentioned in Old English medical texts. As Karen Jolly explains, worms account for a variety of mysterious illnesses as creatures of Germanic folklore, though at the same time 'illnesses caused by tapeworms or other known worms were common', 'not surprising from the experience of modern medicine in areas of poor sanitation'.[71] Following Charles Singer, Godfrid Storms views such 'worms'—alongside elfshot and 'flying venoms'—as supernatural sources of disease within the Germanic tradition.[72] But Jolly's discussion reminds us that actual parasites would inevitably have been a disruptive part of life for many and therefore should not be understood purely in supernatural terms, especially given the juxtaposition of these harmful 'wyrmas' in remedy 21 and the previous remedy's employment of healing ant eggs from the natural world. Though perhaps not as powerful as mythological dragons, small *wyrmas* still posed very real dangers. Remedy 22 then continues by offering a new remedy but no new ailment and is thus seemingly intended for a similar problem involving parasites. Later, remedy 25 offers the final remedy of this chapter in *Bald's Leechbook*, 'wiþ earwicgan' ['against earwigs'], calling for a *windelstreaw* (a thin dried stalk of grass) to remove the insects.[73]

These particular entries do not directly address hearing; however, sandwiched between the remedies against such creatures are two that more explicitly do involve the faculty of hearing and suggest connections across the section. First, in remedy 23's very simple treatment to be used 'gif earan dynien' ['if ears din (make noise)'], oil is applied to the ear with wool held in place while sleeping. Entry 24, 'eft wiþ þon ilcan' ['again for the same'] employs steam from wormwood boiled in water to create a healing vapor for the ears. The inclusion of these two remedies between those against *wyrmas* and *earwicgan* indicates that the conditions they treated were perhaps experienced in somewhat similar ways, as sounds created inside rather than outside of the ears. Yet, as with *adeafian*, the verb *dynien*, which possibly indicates a form of tinnitus, still imbues ears with agency, the capability to make noise.[74]

Through its organizational logic and especially its subtly nuanced phrasing, *Bald's Leechbook* thus calls attention to our own largely unexamined patterns of modern usage, which often tend toward polarizing what should instead be understood as a broad range of auditory experiences. As Kristen Harmon notes in a compelling discussion of modern terminology connected with hearing and deafness, 'to use one description over another is to sanction a particular ideology', yet 'where one fits in a spectrum of sensory difference is always defined in relation to hearing, a much more powerful partner in that binary'.[75] Harmon further describes the tendency to focus 'on the sheer profundity of loss' as 'obsessive shortsightedness', noting that 'the simple *deaf*' 'is largely descriptive of social, political, and biological categories and processes and distinct from the jarring emphasis on the flattening and aggregating technicalities of hearing loss, as seen in *profoundly deaf*'.[76] And while Old English medical writings certainly can't be seen as a model of sensitivity and to posit such would be inherently anachronistic at best, it is worth noting that *Bald's Leechbook*, the medical text most widely acknowledged for its connection to practical medicine in early medieval England, consistently employs terminology that allows space for a tremendous diversity of experience and therefore includes fewer 'pathologizing binaries enclosing a Deaf person in a hearing world'.[77]

Finally, there is one auditory condition that receives much less attention than might be expected in *Bald's Leechbook*: because the entries focus on factors that might change one's capacity for hearing, little is said about congenital deafness. But Irina Metzler's research on perceptions of deafness in the central Middle Ages indicates that congenital deafness was relatively rare.[78] Given, then, that *Bald's Leechbook* focuses on the faculty of hearing as a range of perception rather than as something that one either possesses or lacks, and also the fact that in this period there would have been little to be treated in connection with congenital deafness, its relative omission here is hardly surprising. Evidence outside the medical texts, however, suggests that such deafness was met, at least in some documented instances, with compassion and acceptance.

Beyond *Bald's Leechbook*

The insights from *Bald's Leechbook* offer meaningful context for references to hearing and deafness outside the medical texts as well. As we shall see, early medieval law codes, for instance, show support for those experiencing deafness or changes to hearing, and comparison of the language describing deafness in the medical texts with the language used in theological and other literary contexts suggests that pejorative metaphors of deafness as a spiritual lack were not paralleled by actual practice. Additionally, archaeological evidence from graves of deaf and hard of hearing individuals does not indicate social marginalization or perceived inferiority of these individuals, with their lived experience being perhaps at least somewhat closer to the situation described in Brenda Jo Brueggemann's poignant discussion of identity as one of 'betweenity'.[79]

Deafness and access: laws of Alfred, cap. 14

In the same work where Kristen Harmon points out the problematic nature of modern usage patterns around hearing and deafness, she also powerfully advocates for language that 'goes beyond disability', for a framework in which 'ability is no longer the contested site; language use and access are'.[80] 'To some', she explains, 'this suggestion might feel like yet another semantic exercise about perception and self-identification, but beyond breath and water there is little more that is fundamental to being human than communication'.[81] I would here like to apply this line of thinking to early medieval law, especially the laws of Alfred, where access to justice is, at least for some rulers, conveyed as the ultimate goal. As a general pattern, early medieval law codes mention deafness not as a marker of deficiency, but most frequently to allow financial compensation for changes in hearing due to violence or accidental injury.[82] As with the healing remedies, the law codes also suggest that deafness later in life was far more common than deafness from birth. The laws of Alfred, however, include a very rare and deeply insightful reference (cap. 14) to deafness from birth.

> Gif mon sie dumb oðð̄e deaf geboren, þæt he ne mæge [his] synna onsecggan ne geandettan, bete se fæder his misdæda.
>
> [If anyone is born unspeaking or deaf, so that he can neither deny nor confess his wrongdoings, his father shall pay compensation for his misdeeds.]

In keeping with patterns that we saw in *Bald's Leechbook*, nothing in the language here marks deafness as a fundamental flaw or deficit, though this lack of judgment can be easy to miss since the phrasing is very close to modern 'deaf and dumb', wording that the National Association of the Deaf describes as 'a relic from the medieval English era', 'the granddaddy of all negative labels pinned on deaf and hard of hearing people'.[83]

But these hearing-biased interpretations and translations that perpetuate stigmatizing views need to change. I have thus translated the Old English *dumb* throughout this discussion as 'unspeaking' because the adjective *dumb* did not carry its current intensely negative connotations until centuries after the Old English period. The OED shows *dumb* in the sense of 'inexpressive, meaningless' as unattested until as late as the sixteenth century (s.v. *dumb* 7.a), and its appallingly pejorative sense of 'foolish, stupid, ignorant' as not appearing until the mid-eighteenth century. If we therefore extricate the law code's usage from later stigmatizing and harmful developments and view it instead in the auditory context understood in the medieval medical texts, what we see is an attempt at addressing the need for alternate ways to navigate a legal system still heavily reliant upon oral/aural language. In an era of only newly emerging literacy—one heavily dependent upon language as spoken and heard—such access to legal justice would have indeed been a crucial concern. The Old English tract known as *Swerian*, for example, includes an oath explicitly assuming the capacity to hear: 'On ælmihtiges Godes naman ... swa ic hit minum egum oferseah 7 minum earum oferhyrde þæt him mid sæcge' ['In the name of the almighty God ... so I with my eyes oversaw and with *my ears overheard*, that which I say'] (II. 8, emphasis added).[84] The exact same formula—'eagum oferseah ond earum oferhyrde'—recurs in the later law codes of Cnut.[85] But even though speech was required to testify and hearing was required to witness, the particular law under Alfred offers legal protection for those who cannot speak or hear, allowing one's father to pay compensation on a child's behalf. The issue at stake in Alfred's law, then, is primarily one of access rather than ability.

The particular wording of the law code—'Gif mon sie dumb oððe deaf geboren' ['If one is born unspeaking or deaf']—also aligns with the range of hearing experiences seen in *Bald's Leechbook*. The employment of 'oððe' ['or'], for instance, rather than *ond* ['and'] signals acknowledgment and validation of varying experiences with both speech and hearing. The more usual phrasing in the Old English corpus is 'dumb *ond* deaf' ['unspeaking *and* deaf'; emphasis added]. So common is the phrasing with *ond*, in fact, that F. Liebermann's edition states that *oððe* should be translated in this case as 'and', in line with the more usual collocation (II. 8).[86] However, the fact that the law does go against the more conventional formula, which would have presumably been easiest and most natural for an author or scribe, would seem to indicate that the 'or' was important enough to override formulaic convention and should thus be accepted at face value.

Additionally, a closer look at the 'dumb *ond* deaf' formula across the Old English corpus shows that it most often appears not in the medical texts and law codes where it would apply to (often specific) hard of hearing and deaf individuals—where it would thus likely reflect perceptions and behaviors from actual lived experience—but rather in theological and other literary contexts where the inabilities to speak and hear are evoked metaphorically. In the heroic hagiography *Juliana*, Juliana refuses to give tribute to 'dumbum ond deafum deofolgieldum' ['unspeaking and deaf idols'] (l. 150).[87]

And in 'Soul and Body I', the soul berates the body for being 'dumb ond deaf' (l. 65),[88] while in the *Old English Life of St. Margaret* the virgin martyr twice tells her enemies that their god is 'dumb and deaf'.[89] These usages for the most part convey abstract and less subtle notions of deafness and speechlessness. In contrast, Alfred's law, which is presumably designed to address actual, living people, leaves open the possibility that one could be deaf and speaking or, conversely, hearing and unspeaking. What is emphasized as most crucial in the law code is the capacity for (or lack of) language sufficient to confess or deny wrongdoings, the law applying 'if anyone is born unspeaking *or* deaf', not necessarily both.

The ordering of the words in the Old English formula, with 'unspeaking' (OE *dumb*) followed by *deaf*, also runs counter to what in later centuries became the more usual formula of of 'deaf and dumb', the Old English predating the fixity of this particular phrasing. Ursula Schaefer suggests this change to a 'collocation that in modern English has survived as *deaf and dumb*' is due to a shift in physiological knowledge, where 'we know that muteness may be a secondary consequence of deafness, and that the relation between the pair *deaf-dumb/mute* is that of cause and effect' (emphasis added).[90] But this logic assumes that the texts' composers and compilers did not themselves understand the relationship and that the ordering must always have been based on cause and effect, when the ordering perhaps more logically might have instead been based simply on the order of observation. Deafness itself is invisible, and the lack of speech is often noticed before a lack of hearing.[91]

Christian Laes' study of deafness in classical antiquity notes that there were *some* who seem to have believed that deafness proceeded from an inability to speak—that both were caused by an obstruction that impeded the tongue and the ear—and he cites evidence of medical remedies for deafness that involved surgery on the tongue; however, he notes that even in antiquity this belief seems to have been a minority view. He argues that ancient authors referred more directly to speechlessness 'not because of their ignorance of the hearing impairment', but because the lack of speech had 'the more important consequences in an oral culture'.[92] Such was likely the case in early medieval England as well. As Lisi Oliver and others have convincingly argued, the Old English laws that survive 'are brought from an era of oral transmission into the written law'.[93] She explains the situation thus:

> That Germanic law must have been passed down orally in the pre-literate era is inferable from several indicators. First, both common sense and anthropological parallels in other illiterate societies dictate that law is not an invention introduced concomitantly with literacy. Second, the early Germanic laws recorded in Latin contain certain similarities [that] ... may be attributed to a common source. And third, we find throughout the Germanic territories a figure whose job was the oral proclamation of law'.[94]

Levi Roach has similarly argued that 'literacy and orality were working hand-in-hand: written law codes facilitated the dissemination and oral promulgation of royal decrees to audiences beyond those present at the original royal assembly'.[95]

Even more significantly, law in early medieval England was *practiced* within a largely oral context, as even our modern concept of a legal 'hearing' suggests—the guilt or innocence of the accused depending to a great extent upon evidence conveyed orally and received aurally. Matthias Ammons has likewise observed that legally binding agreements—formalized through the giving of pledges—were in this period mostly 'of an oral nature'.[96] With one's very fate determined by oral skills, it thus stands to reason that an inability to speak would register a greater urgency—and primacy in formulaic expression—than the ability to hear. In all these ways, the surviving tracts and law codes point not toward deafness as a personal deficit but to an urgent need for access to communication in legal contexts.

Speech and deafness in Bede's Ecclesiastical History, *Book 5, Ch. 2*

Recognizing the primacy of speech implicit in the 'unspeaking and deaf' collocation as an effect of social impact rather than as a reflection of a medical condition with a cause-and-effect relationship can also help clarify what might seem a striking omission from Bede's account of John of Beverley, which describes how the bishop restored speech to an 'adulescens mutus' ['an unspeaking youth'] (Book 5, Ch. 2).[97] Even though the child's hearing is never mentioned explicitly in the story and he is healed by a sign made over his tongue, it has been widely assumed that the child was also deaf. The portion of the story that has had the greatest impact is not the miracle of speech, but the kindness of the bishop in offering the boy—even before he had been cured—a modest lodging 'in quo manens cotidianam ab eis stipem acciperet' ['in which the youth might receive from them his daily alms']; several British organizations devoted to the deaf—such as the St. Bede's Centre for Deaf People in London—have embraced Bede as a patron and advocate, in large part due to this story. The British Deaf History Society volume *Venerable Bede* asserts that Bede's 'story of how Bishop John of Hexham taught speech to a dumb boy via the alphabet and his description of the world's first recorded fingerspellings system showed also that he had no prejudice which confined the message to a particular modality' and goes on to say that 'it is a source of great credit to the Christian Churches of Britain today that they have rarely wavered from the fine example of the Venerable Bede and have ministered to the deaf members of their congregations'.[98] And in *Deaf Liberation Theology*, Hannah Lewis explains that St. John of Beverley had been adopted by the Deaf church by at least the late nineteenth century.[99] As but one of many examples of more recent veneration, the entry for 25 October—John of Beverley's feast day—in the *Miniature Lives of the Saints* describes the bishop as 'the special patron of the deaf and dumb'.[100]

Because Bede and the bishop whose story he relates have both been held up by so many as advocates for the Deaf, it might seem strange to modern readers that Bede never actually mentions the youth's deafness. But just as we've seen to be true within early medieval England more generally, even in a religious context the lack of speech would have been more salient than an inability to hear, even in cases where deafness had been the ultimate cause of speechlessness. Miranda Wilcox has offered extensive evidence for the importance of oral confessions of belief for salvation in early medieval Christianity; such confessions served as speech acts that 'qualified a Christian for meriting eternal life after death as well as for receiving sacramental grace'.[101] Focusing more specifically on the role of speech in this particular narrative, Irina Dumitrescu has convincingly argued that the 'tongue's loosening' offers 'an escape from the impediments of physical disability' and 'a figurative deliverance from the bonds of pagan sin'.[102] In this allegorical context, it simply makes sense that Bede's story would privilege the restoration of speech above that of hearing, whether or not the boy had been deaf. Thus, as with the 'deaf ond dumb' idols mentioned above, it is important not to overgeneralize about medieval attitudes toward actual deafness based on miracle stories that are often didactic or allegorical. Religious texts from early medieval England at times convey attitudes toward disability that—as inherently harmful and stigmatizing as they undoubtedly are—in many ways do run counter to evidence in medical texts, law codes, and archaeological research. Christina Lee thus advocates caution with regard to such 'patristic sources', noting that 'homiletic and hagiographical texts often contain a stock image of the afflicted' in which 'transgressions of the soul are visible on the body'.[103]

Surveying tendencies in medieval Europe more widely, Aude de Saint-Loup maintains that miracle stories and saints' lives can nonetheless provide valuable insights into the deaf experience. Observing that 'it was generally the religious orders that took responsibility for the education of deaf children and adults', she argues that many miracle stories implicitly attribute the deaf with important capabilities for learning through the teaching of others:

> Putting aside the strictly miraculous aspect of these narratives, we can speak of cases in which the deaf are taught to read, speak, and write. Admittedly, this is not a common phenomenon, but why should it be in a society where the vast majority was illiterate? At the same time, it shows that there was no doubt about a deaf person's ability to be educated.[104]

The story of John of Beverley teaching the unspeaking youth to speak would seem to be an example of such a case. At the very least, Bede's story, like Alfred's law, implicitly supports, and encourages kindness toward individuals lacking the ability to speak—and to possibly hear—rather than ostracism or abuse.

Burial practices

Finally, archaeological evidence from the period offers additional insights into what the social experience might have been for an individual whose condition was described in terms such as Bald's Leechbook's *deafe*, *adeafunge*, and *adeafian*, and suggests that deafness would not have been as socially marginalizing as has been sometimes been maintained. As with the medical texts and law codes, the archaeological record indicates conditions that would have been accompanied by gradual changes to hearing across a range of auditory experiences. One such condition is otosclerosis, a middle-ear disease 'in which proliferative new bone fixes the footplate of the stapes into the oval window, causing deafness'.[105] One study of 1,164 temporal bones of individuals dating from the fourth through seventeenth centuries indicated that the disease affected 0.9% of the population, a prevalence comparable to modern populations.[106] The impact would, however, have been greater than today due to lack of modern treatments, such as hearing aids and, in more severe cases, a surgical procedure known as a stapedectomy.[107] With the age of onset typically between 15 and 45 and very seldom before age 5[108] —and with the change in hearing itself being gradual—deafness resulting from otosclerosis would almost always have been post-lingual, with less direct impact on one's capacity for speech, which—as noted before—was crucial in numerous religious and legal contexts.

Otosclerosis identified from skeletal remains has been determined in a number of graves dating to early medieval England itself, with important social implications. An examination of ear bones in the Castledyke Cemetery at Barton-on-Humber, for instance, revealed otosclerosis in a woman aged between 17 and 25. While only one ear of the remains was intact enough to undergo examination, otosclerosis typically affects both ears, and the woman was most likely completely deaf at the time of her death.[109] Her deafness, however, does not seem to have impacted her social standing negatively in the community, at least with regard to burial practices. Her grave was in the midst of others, not on the fringes of the cemetery, and her grave goods were generous, including a wooden box, knife, beads, and valuable copper objects.[110] D. M. Hadley cites a similar burial at Tanners Row, an adult male buried in the usual manner in the churchyard, with compacted bone in his ear that would have caused deafness.[111] To the extent that early medieval burial practice reflects the social fabric of daily life, such evidence would seem to suggest that deafness in itself was not viewed as cause for ostracism or marginalization.

The language of the Old English medical texts alongside all of the other available evidence from the period affirms that early medieval England did not base identity on a 'hearing line' existing between hearing individuals and the deaf. Ears could hear, but ears could also 'deafen' and 'din'. It was also understood that one could be in the process of 'deafening' and that there was space for hearing as well as 'unhearingness'. Bringing oral theory into closer alignment with the tremendous work in Deaf studies opens up the possibility for us to more fully appreciate these subtle distinctions as they were at work in Old English medical texts and as they were lived in early medieval life. Taken together, medical, legal, historical, and archaeological evidence from early medieval England shows us a world in which there were many known causes of deafness and hearing loss—not only deafness from birth, but also acquired deafness, infection, middle ear disease, tinnitus, earworms, violence, and accidental mutilation, just to name a few. The view reflected in Old English medical texts is thus quite similar to that of 'a *deaf spectrum*—or "deafnesses"—that has replaced the deaf/hearing binary' in much modern biomedical and cultural thought.[112]

Further, we discover that this diversity of experience was accompanied by a diversity of attitudes towards deafness and hearing loss: contrary to some overgeneralizations we see in overviews of deafness in the medieval period,[113] practitioners in early medieval England did in fact distinguish deafness as distinct from an ability to speak, and evidence from early medieval England affirms that the deaf and hard of hearing were provided with medical remedies, legal accommodations, and fairly lavish burial customs as well, even as theological texts continued to employ deafness as a metaphor for spiritual lack. This diversity could be easy to miss when approached through the lens of modern medicine but becomes more salient when examined in light of the diversity and variance fostered within the larger hybrid healing tradition.

Finally, and most importantly, examining the medical texts within larger social contexts and through the dual approaches of oral theory and Deaf studies helps us begin to remediate against certain kinds of audism implicit in much oral tradition scholarship, work that has often tended to privilege the voice as the ideal medium of traditional narrative and knowledge.[114] Oral theory has long been utilized in Deaf studies, and our understanding of oral traditions has much to gain from a more genuinely two-way dialogue. We can achieve a richer, more nuanced understanding of medieval texts when we are able to recognize simultaneously both the connectedness of many medieval texts to dynamic oral/aural traditions and the inherent diversity of the aural experience through which these traditions would have been received. When, for example, we read the famous opening of *Beowulf* that includes 'we have heard' ['we ... gefrunon'], we should thus bear in mind that the physical act of hearing could not then, and cannot now, be understood as a universally shared experience. Not everyone in early medieval England could hear, and not everyone who could hear heard in the same way. Just as modes of language and performance varied, so too did experiences and perceptions of hearing. In the next chapter, we'll continue this exploration of diversity in bodily experience and the ways such awareness can expand our understanding of Old English literature and culture beyond the medical texts alone. In the ring composition so common in oral narrative, we will now return to where this study began, with the tormented speaker of an Exeter Book riddle who laments a lack of healers who might otherwise ease an endless suffering. Though healers in poetry, like healers in this speaker's *folc-stede*, are conspicuously absent, we can now see deep and meaningful ways that the Old English healing tradition can nonetheless significantly impact our understanding of hybridity in early medieval literature and culture more broadly.

Notes

1 Christopher B. Krentz, 'The Camera as Printing Press: How Film Has Influenced ASL Literature', in H-Dirksen L. Bauman, Jennifer L. Nelson, and Heidi M. Rose (eds), *Signing the Body Poetic: Essays on*

American Sign Language Literature (Berkeley: University of California Press, 2006), pp. 51–70, at 53.
2 Though the compound *ellengæst* is often translated to emphasize Grendel's monstrosity as something closer to 'demon spirit' (the second of two possibilities given in the *DOE*), *ellen* means simply 'courage, strength' (*DOE*, sense 1), a positive trait attributed to heroes past as early as the third line of *Beowulf*, and *gæst/gast* has the primary sense of neutral 'spirit' or 'life', ultimately deriving from the sense of 'breath' (*DOE*, senses 1, 3). These lines arguably invite us to empathize with Grendel's hardship, suffering that unambiguously results from hearing. On empathy with Grendel with regard to healing and medicine, see further Chapter 3.
3 *Earfoðlice* is another word frequently translated so as to demean Grendel, such as 'impatient' (e.g., Raffel) or 'angrily' (e.g., Gordon, *Anglo-Saxon Poetry*); however, the primary senses as given in the *DOE* would evoke instead empathy, suggesting 'difficulty' (*DOE*, s.v. *earfoþlice*, sense 1) and even physical 'pain' (sense 3). Burton Raffel (trans), *Beowulf* (New York: Penguin, 1963).
4 Grant, *Plant Speciation*, p. 197.
5 Kasari Liis, et al., 'Hybrid ecosystems can contribute to local biodiversity conservation', *Biodiversity and Conservation*, 25.14 (2016), pp. 3023–3041, at 3026.
6 Grant, *Plant Speciation*, p. 68.
7 Noting that *hwæt* in this position as an opening interjection occurs most typically in conjunction with verbs of speaking or hearing, John Foley uses what he calls the '*hwæt* paradigm' as an especially compelling illustration of the way that oral traditional structures would have remained 'the only pathways to a referential world beyond the reach of purely textual signals for some time after the advent of the written word as an instrument for composition and reception', *Immanent Art*, p. 215.
8 Oliver and Mahoney, 'Episcopal', pp. 35, 36.
9 Lennard J. Davis, *Enforcing Normalcy: Disability, Deafness, and the Body* (London: New Left Books, 1995), p. 15.
10 Maren Tova Linett, *Bodies of Modernism in Transatlantic Modernist Literature* (Ann Arbor, MI: University of Michigan Press, 2017), p. 89.
11 See below on law codes involving injuries to hearing.
12 E.g., Martyn Hudson's description of Grendel as 'animalistic and hybrid', *Visualizing Worlds: World Making and Social Theory* (Abingdon and New York: Taylor and Francis, 2021), digital edition,

Hybridity of environment in Bald's Leechbook   239

n. p.; Almudena Nedo's discussion of Grendel as 'a hybrid man-monster', 'In the Form of a Man: Grendel's Changing Form in Film Adaptations', in Frank Jacob and Verena Bernardi (eds), *All Around Monstrous: Monster Media in Their Historical Contexts* (Wilmington, DE: Vernon Press, 2019), 97–126, at 109.

13 The BL, Royal 12 D.xvii, dated to the mid-tenth century, contains three distinct books unattested elsewhere in the Old English corpus, written in the same hand. Though each of the three books includes its own table of contents (ff. 1r–6v, 58v–54v, and 109r–111r respectively), a colophon at the end of the second book (folio 109r) has led to the modern appellation of the first two collectively as *Bald's Leechbook*: 'Bald habet hunc librum …' ['Bald has this book …']. The text now known as *Leechbook III* seems to have been based on a separate exemplar. On sources of *Bald's Leechbook*, see especially J. N. Adams and Marilyn Deegan, 'Bald's "Leechbook" and the "Physica Plinii"', *Anglo-Saxon England*, 21 (1992), 87–114; M. L. Cameron, 'Bald's "Leechbook" and Cultural Interactions in Anglo-Saxon England', *Anglo-Saxon England*, 19 (1990), 5–12. Like the Harley 6258B discussed in the previous chapter, the BL, Royal 12 D.xvii is devoted exclusively to medical texts, and it is a remedy added to the margins of *Bald's Leechbook* in the eleventh century (f. 49r) that evidences its ongoing use as a medical text.

14 See Kesling on the structure of *Bald's Leechbook*, including its '*a capite ad calcem*' organization, *Medical*, p. 25.

15 Entry numbers here and throughout refer to the explicitly numbered sections as designated within the BL, Royal 12 D.xvii.

16 The entry's introduction announces that there will be 'fiftyne cræftas' ['fifteen crafts'], though only eleven divisions are marked in the manuscript, through the text being extended into the left margins. This system of division is followed by Cockayne, *Leechdoms*. Because the more precise subdivisions by Doyle's recent edition are better suited to analysis of the range of ailments, I follow his system of numbering here. Quotations also follow Doyle unless otherwise noted. Conan Doyle (ed.), *Anglo-Saxon Medicine and Disease: A Semantic Approach*, 2 vols (doctoral thesis, University of Cambridge, 2017).

17 The *DOE* also cites this particular passage as an example of 'yfel hlyst', 'poor hearing', which occurs three times in the *Leechbook*. Doyle reads as *hlyfte* (the manuscript page is faded, but the character does look quite like an *f*), and he translates accordingly as 'air' without comment. Since *hlyste*, 'hearing', does appear multiple times in the entry itself and makes much more sense in the context of

remedies for hearing, I have here followed the *DOE*. That said, the character in question could indeed be an *f*, and it is perhaps possible that poor 'air' in the context of a remedy for ailments of the ears could refer to ear pain brought about by wind, moisture, and the elements. Alternatively, *air* might indicate an awareness that sound travels through air.

18 Doyle, *Anglo-Saxon*, vol. 2, 7; cf. Cockayne, *Leechdoms*, vol. 2, p. 2. Except where otherwise noted, translations are my own.
19 See, for instance, Katherine O'Brien O'Keeffe, 'Literacy', in Michael Lapidge, John Blair, Simon Keynes, and Donald Scragg (eds), *The Blackwell Encyclopedia of Anglo-Saxon England* (Oxford: Wiley-Blackwell, 1999), pp. 289–290, at 289.
20 Bosworth and Toller, s.v. *hyran*, p. 582. For an examination of syntactic and semantic relationships among Old English verbs of hearing in these various senses, see Eulalia Sosa Acevedo, 'Exploring Semantic and Syntactic Relations within the Old English Verbs of Hearing', in M. Brito and M. Martín González (eds), *Insights and Bearings: Festschrift for Dr. Juan Sebastián Amador Bedford* (La Laguna: Universidad de La Laguna, 2007), pp. 317–330.
21 Henry Sweet (ed.), *King Alfred's West-Saxon Version of Gregory's Pastoral Care*, vol. 2 (London: Early English Text Society, 1871), p. 411.
22 Pearman, *Women and Disability* , p. 3; Christina Lee, 'Disability', in Jacqueline Stodnick and Renée R. Trilling (eds), *A Handbook of Anglo-Saxon Studies* (London: Wiley-Blackwell, 2012), pp. 23–38, at 29.
23 Lee, 'Disability', p. 28.
24 Ibid.
25 Qtd. in Joseph Falaky Nagy, 'Orality in Medieval Irish Narrative: An Overview', *Oral Tradition*, 1 (1986), 272–301, at 290.
26 Pearman, *Women and Disability*, p. 4.
27 Ibid., p. 5.
28 Ibid.
29 Ibid.
30 Ibid., p. 2.
31 Bauman, 'Introduction: Listening to Deaf Studies', in H-Dirksen L. Bauman (ed.), *Open Your Eyes: Deaf Studies Talking* (Minneapolis, MN: University of Minnesota Press, 2008), pp. 1–34, at 9.
32 Lee, 'Disability', p. 29.
33 Neil Glickman, 'The Development of Culturally Deaf Identities', in Neil S. Glickman and Michael A. Harvey (eds), *Culturally Affirmative Psychotherapy with Deaf Persons* (New York: Routledge, 1996), pp. 115–154, at 124.

34 Brenda Jo Brueggemann, *Lend Me Your Ear: Rhetorical Constructions of Deafness* (Washington, DC: Gallaudet University Press, 1999), pp. 185–186.
35 Thomas K. Holcomb, *Introduction to American Deaf Culture* (Oxford: Oxford University Press, 2013), p. 134.
36 Kristen Harmon, '"If there are Greek epics, there should be Deaf epics": How Protest Became Poetry', in H-Dirksen L. Bauman, Jennifer L. Nelson, and Heidi M. Rose (eds), *Signing the Body Poetic: Essays on American Sign Language Literature* (Berkeley, CA: University of California Pres, 2006), pp. 169–194, at 171.
37 Christopher B. Krentz, 'Camera', p. 52. Krentz notes that 'my use of *oral* in this context may run up against objections, and with good reason. First, the very term *oral* seems a misnomer in connection with the Deaf community. After all, ASL is quite different from speech. *Oral* also echoes *oralism*, the movement spearheaded by Alexander Graham Bell to eradicate sign language, stop deaf intermarriage, and in effect quash Deaf culture. Perhaps *manual* better indicates how Deaf people passed on their stories, folklore and poetry through sign', 'Camera', pp. 52–53.
38 Ibid., p. 54.
39 Arnovick, *Written Reliquaries*, p. 245.
40 Foley, *How to Read an Oral Poem*, p. 139.
41 John D. Waiko, '"Head" and "Tail": The Shaping of Oral Traditions among the Binandere in Papua New Guinea', *Oral Tradition*, 5 (1990), 334–353, at 351.
42 Johannes Fabian, *Anthropology with an Attitude: Critical Essays* (Stanford, CA: Stanford University Press, 2001), p. 58.
43 Davis, *Enforcing Normalcy*, pp. 100–101.
44 Arnovick, *Written Reliquaries*, p. 245.
45 On the concept of 'Deaf Gain', see especially H-Dirksen L. Bauman and Joseph M. Murray (eds), *Deaf Gain: Raising the Stakes for Human Diversity* (Minneapolis, MN: University of Minnesota Press, 2014).
46 The resulting publication was a lightly edited transcript of a listserv discussion (ORTRAD-L). ORTRAD-L, 'Symposium, Deafness and Orality: An Electronic Conversation', *Oral Tradition*, 8 (1993), 413–437.
47 Ibid., p. 420.
48 Published under her former name, Lois Bragg, 'Visual-Kinetic Communication in Europe Before 1600: A Survey of Sign Lexicons and Finger Alphabets Prior to the Rise of Deaf Education', *Journal of*

Deaf Studies and Deaf Education, 2 (1997), 1–25, at 2. Focusing on early medieval England specifically, Nigel Barley notes that monastic 'sign systems' 'are artificial systems' rather than natural languages, 'used when other channels of communication are deliberately closed or fade into the background', 'Two Anglo-Saxon Sign Systems Compared', *Semiotica*, 12 (1974), 227–237, at 227. More recently, Scott G. Bruce has called for 'careful qualification' when applying the term 'sign language' to medieval monastic signs, which 'lacked many fundamental linguistic principles like grammar and syntax and therefore, by strict definition, did not constitute a true language in the modern sense of the word', *Silence and Sign Language in Medieval Monasticism: The Cluniac Tradition, c. 900–1200* (Cambridge: Cambridge University Press, 2010), p. 11. Further, as Foys has aptly observed in his work with the multimodal interplay of monastic signs and ringing bells, monastic sign systems did not function independently of spoken language or of sound: 'in these soft signs, mouths still work, bells still ring and the ears, ever open, still hear', 'A Sensual Philology for Anglo-Saxon England', *postmedieval: a journal of medieval cultural studies*, 5 (2014), 456–472, p. 465. Whether or not we call the monastic sign systems 'language', Sayers' larger point that they operate much differently than sign languages used as a primary mode of communication within deaf communities still stands.

49 These references to the 'Dark Past' and 'Dread and Despair' are section and chapter titles from Margret Winzer's influential history of deafness and special education, *The History of Special Education: From Isolation to Integration* (Washington, DC: Gallaudet University Press, 1993).
50 Bragg, 'Visual-Kinetic Communication', p. 3.
51 Emily Cockayne, 'Experiences of the Deaf in Early Modern England', *The Historical Journal*, 46 (2003), 493–510, at 494.
52 Jonathan Rée, *I See a Voice: Deafness, Language, and the Senses—A Philosophical History* (New York: Henry Holt and Company, 1999), p. 85.
53 Kesling, *Medical*, p. 5.
54 Christopher Krentz, *Writing Deafness: The Hearing Line in Nineteenth-Century American Literature* (Chapel Hill, NC: University of North Carolina Press, 2012), p. 2.
55 See *DOE*, s.v. *deafu*, 'deafness'.
56 Doyle provides this analogue from *Physica Plinii Bambergensis*, 9.9. For extensive discussion of the *Leechbooks* in relation to the *Physica*

Plinii, see Adams and Deegan, 'Bald's "Leechbook"'. This particular parallel is treated on p. 105.

57 Two Latin analogues for remedy 8, similarly requiring ear drops made from crushed ant eggs, do, however, mention deafness in particular: 'ad surdum uel qui grauiter audiunt' ['for those who are deaf or poorly hearing']. See Doyle, *Anglo-Saxon Medicine*, vol. 2, p. 46.
58 Doyle provides a Latin analogue from *Marcelli de medicamentis liber*, 9.66. *Anglo-Saxon Medicine*, vol. 2, p. 47.
59 Cockayne's edition abandons the literal meaning and translates as 'have a tendency to grow deaf'. Cockayne, *Leechdoms*, vol. 2, p. 41. In Cockayne's numbering, this remedy falls under item 6. Doyle translates as 'will deafen', with the following note: 'I'm not quite sure what this auxilliary is doing here. It normally indicates volition', *Anglo-Saxon Medicine*, vol. 2, p. 47, n. 54. See further Chapter 5 on the shift of *willan* from a verb of volition to a future auxiliary.
60 DOE, s.v. *adeafian*. Emphasis added.
61 Audrey Meaney, 'Variant versions of Old English medical remedies and the compilation of Bald's "Leechbook"', *Anglo-Saxon England*, 13 (1984), 235–268, at 249.
62 Meaney identifies approximately 50 remedies from the Nowell transcription and argues that both the BL Cotton Otho B.xi and *Bald's Leechbook* 'go back to a common ancestor rather than that Otho copied from Royal'. Meaney translates as 'if ears are growing deaf', 'Variant', pp. 248, 250, fn. 54.
63 It is important to note that *yfel* in medieval medical contexts does not have the moral implications of modern English *evil* and is most typically translated as 'poor' or 'ill'. Bosworth and Toller even provide a separate entry for *yfel-hæbbende* (which breaks apart literally into 'evil-having'), defined in medical usage simply as 'sick, ill'. The Old English Thesaurus project offers 'disease, infirmity, sickness' as the first entry in the noun form and 'insalubrious, injurious to health' as the first adjectival sense (https://oldenglishthesaurus.arts.gla.ac.uk/category-selection/?qsearch=yfel). Accessed 3 June 2021.
64 Interestingly, both ground ivy and ribwort continue to be recommended even today for certain ear problems. For example, extract of plantain—the family to which ribwort belongs—was recommended in the book *Tinnitus STOP*, published as recently as 2014, and Yvonne Tait offers a recipe for 'an herbal mixture which may help with Ear infection' that includes 40 ml. of ground ivy (2016, n. p.). Annette P. Price, *Tinnitus STOP! The Complete Guide on Ringing in the Ears, Natural Tinnitus Remedies, and a Holistic System for Permanent*

Tinnitus Relief (United States: Living Plus Healthy Publishing, 2014), pp. 64–65. Yvonne Tait, *Your Health, Your Vitality, Your Choice: An Interlude with an Esoteric Herbalist* (Bloomington, IN: Balboa Press, 2016. Kindle edition).

65 Cockayne, *Leechdoms*, vol. 1, p. 213.
66 Pollington, *Leechcraft*, p. 155.
67 I regret having followed this definition in my own 2017 article. 'Deaf Studies', p. 29.
68 Cockayne, vol. 1, p. 215.
69 Van Arsdall's reworking of the sentence to read 'if the ears do not work well' offers another way to retain the utilitarian aspect of the original Old English. The *Herbarium*'s analogous Latin entry describes the condition as 'aurium inutilitatem', 'unusefulness of the ears', *Medieval Herbal Remedies*, p. 194. Cf. de Vriend, *Old English Herbarium*, p. 145.
70 Entry I.iii.8 also involves the eggs of ants.
71 Jolly, *Popular*, p. 130.
72 Storms, *Anglo-Saxon Magic*, p. 117.
73 On the rarity of actual earwigs and the origins of earwig legends in classical and medieval traditions, see May R. Berenbaum, *The Earwig's Tail: A Modern Bestiary of Multi-Legged Legends* (Cambridge, MA: Harvard University Press, 2009), pp. 9–14.
74 Sounds within the ear are also indicated in other medical texts, including a remedy in the *Lacnunga* (entry 178) for 'earena swinsunge' ['song of the ears'].
75 Kristen Harmon, 'Addressing Deafness: From Hearing Loss to Deaf Gain', *Profession* (Modern Language Association, 2010), 124–130, at 125.
76 Ibid., p. 126.
77 Ibid., p. 128. The *Lacnunga* does include a remedy for *ungehyrnesse* ['unhearingness'], a rare instance of a medical condition named in terms of a lack. Notably, however, *ungehyrnesse* occurs in a very lengthy list of ailments in a recipe for a *morgendrænc* ['morning drink'] attributed to the 'wis 7 læcecræftig' ['wise and leech-crafty'] king Arestolobius, a recipe that promises healing 'wið eallum untrumnessum þe mannes lichoman iondstyriað innan oððe utan' ['against all infirmities that stir one's body, inside and out']. In short, the remedy proposed is presented as a panacea against virtually any problem one might face and would seem less reflective of more precise understandings of health and healing.
78 Irina Metzler, *Disability in Medieval Europe: Thinking About Physical Impairment in the High Middle Ages, c. 1100–c. 1400* (New

York: Routledge, 2006), p. 102. See also her discussion of congenital deafness in pre-modern periods in 'Perceptions of Deafness in the Central Middle Ages', in Cordula Nolte (ed.), *Homo debilis: Behinderte—Kranke—Versehrte in der Gesallschaft des Mittelalters* (Korb: Didymos-Verlag, 2009), pp. 79–98, at 80.

79 Brenda Jo Brueggemann, *Deaf Subjects: Between Identities and Places* (New York: New York University Press, 2009). p. 9 *et passim*.
80 Harmon, 'Addressing Deafness', p. 128.
81 Ibid., p. 128.
82 Under Æthelberht, for instance, 25 shillings could be assessed as compensation if the hearing in either ear was destroyed ('nawhit gehereð, xxv scill gebete', cap. 39), twelve shillings were incurred if hearing was only diminished when an ear was struck [*aslagen*] (cap. 40), 3 shillings if an ear was pierced [*þirel*] (cap. 41), and 6 shillings if an ear was lacerated [*sceard*] (cap. 42). Lisi Oliver explains that medical knowledge in early medieval medicine 'recognized that the external ear assists in, but is not integral to, the hearing process'. Thus 'striking off an ear, which lessens the acuteness of hearing (as it eliminates the reverse megaphone that drew in sound)' draws a lesser penalty. Similarly, under Alfred, the loss of an ear that does not severely impact hearing warrants 30 shillings (cap. 46.1), doubled to 60 shillings if the victim can no longer hear. Lisi Oliver, *The Beginnings of English Law* (Toronto: University of Toronto Press, 2002), p. 100.
83 National Association of the Deaf, 'Community and Culture: Frequently Asked Questions': www.nad.org/resources/american-sign-language/community-and-culture-frequently-asked-questions/. Accessed 5 June 2021.
84 F. Liebermann (ed.), *Die Gesetze der Angelsachsen* (Halle: Scientia Aalen, 1960), p. 398. Many thanks to Andrew Rabin for drawing my attention to this text.
85 Patrick Wormald, *The Making of English Law: King Alfred to the Twelfth Century*, vol. 1 (Oxford: Blackwell, 2001), p. 384.
86 Liebermann, *Die Gesetze*, p. 48. Attenborough translates 'or', but only with the qualifying endnote referencing Liebermann's translation as 'and'.
87 Text taken from Krapp and Dobbie, *Exeter Book*.
88 Text taken from George Philip Krapp (ed.), *The Vercelli Book*. ASPR, vol. 2 (New York: Columbia University Press, 1932).
89 Mary Clayton and Hugh Magennis (eds), *The Old English Lives of St. Margaret* (Cambridge: Cambridge University Press, 1994), pp. 118–119; pp. 128–129.

90 Ursula Schaefer, 'Twin Collocations in the Early Middle English Lives of the *Katherine Group*', in Herbert Pilch (ed.), *Orality and Literacy in Early Middle English*, ScriptOralia (Tübingen: Gunter Narr Verlag, 1996), pp. 179–198, at 187.

91 Ruth Lang-Roth notes that prior to standard infant hearing screenings, deafness and other differences in hearing were typically not recognized until at least 12 months, with diagnoses made at the median age of 20 months. 'Hearing Impairment and Language Delay in Infants: Diagnostics and Genetics', *GMS Current Topics in Otorhinolaryngology, Head and Neck Surgery*, 13 (2014), p. 1.

92 Christian Laes, 'Silent Witnesses: Deaf-Mutes in Graeco-Roman Antiquity', *Classical World*, 104 (2011), 451–473, at 472–473.

93 Oliver, *Beginnings*, p. 33.

94 Ibid., p. 35.

95 Levi Roach, 'Law Codes and Legal Norms in Later Anglo-Saxon England', *Historical Research*, 86 (2013), 465–486, at 485.

96 Matthias Ammons, '"Ge mid wedde ge mid aðe": The Functions of Oath and Pledge in Anglo-Saxon Legal Culture', *Historical Research*, 86 (2013), 515–535, at 518.

97 Quotations are from Colgrave and Mynors, *Bede's* Ecclesiastical History.

98 George Montgomery and Arthur Dimmock, *Venerable Legacy: Saint Bede and the Anglo-Celtic Contribution to Literary, Numerical and Manual Language* (Edinburgh: Edinburgh Scottish Workshop, 1998), p. 3.

99 Hannah Lewis, *Deaf Liberation Theology* (Aldershot: Ashgate, 2007), p. 71.

100 H. S. Bowden (ed.), *Miniature Lives of Saints*, vol. 2 (London: Burns and Oates, 2nd edn, 1877), p. 233.

101 Miranda Wilcox, 'Confessing the Faith in Anglo-Saxon England', *Journal of English and Germanic Philology*, 113 (2014), 308–341, at 308.

102 Irina A. Dumitrescu, 'Bede's Liberation Philology: Releasing the English Tongue', *PMLA*, 128 (2013), 40–56, at 43.

103 Lee, 'Disability', p. 27.

104 Aude de Saint-Loup, 'A History of Misunderstandings: The History of the Deaf', *Diogenes*, 44 (1996), 1–26, at 12.

105 Gwen Dalby, Keith Manchester, and Charlotte A. Roberts, 'Otosclerosis and Stapedial Footplate Fixation in Archaeological Material', *International Journal of Osteoarchaeology*, 3 (1993), 207–212, at 207.

106 Ibid., p. 207.

107 See, for instance, information available for patients experiencing otosclerosis on the National Institute on Deafness and Other Communication Disorders website: www.nidcd.nih.gov/health/hearing/pages/otosclerosis.aspx#6. Accessed 12 August 2021.
108 Dalby, Manchester, and Roberts, 'Otosclerosis', p. 207.
109 G. Drinkall and M. Foreman, *The Anglo-Saxon Cemetery at Castledyke South, Barton-on-Humber*. Sheffield Excavation Reports, vol. 6 (Sheffield: Sheffield Academic, 1998), p. 235.
110 For a complete description and inventory of grave goods, see Drinkall and Foreman, *Anglo-Saxon Cemetery*, p. 46. For a sketch of the grave in relation to those that surround it, see p. 105.
111 D. M. Hadley, 'Social and Physical Difference in and beyond the Anglo-Saxon Churchyard', in J. Buckberry and A. Cherryson (eds), *Burial in Later Anglo-Saxon England* (Oxford: Oxbow Books, 2010), pp. 101–113, at 110.
112 Mara Mills, 'Deafness', in David Novak and Matt Sakakeeny (eds), *Keywords in Sound* (Durham, NC: Duke University Press, 2015, Kindle edition).
113 The *Sage Deaf Studies Encyclopedia* entry on 'Deaf History, Northern Europe', for instance, makes the following assertion: 'Ancient medical science treated deafness as the influence of supernatural forces on the individual, so the physicians came to the conclusion that the deaf could not be rehabilitated because they were inherently evil. The low level of science available in the medieval period, especially in anatomy and physiology, did not allow consideration of the causes and consequences of being deaf'. Genie Gertz and Patrick Boudreault (eds), *The Sage Deaf Studies Encyclopedia* (Los Angeles: Sage, 2016), p. 229.
114 I count myself among those perpetuating this pattern (e.g., Lori Ann Garner, 'Medieval Voices,' *Oral Tradition*, 18.2 (2003), 216–218).

7

From remedies to riddles: hybridity of genre in an Exeter Book riddle

'Let's get you to a healer'.
'Not this time, old friend'.
(Wiglaf and Beowulf, *Beowulf*, 2007)

     'Frofre ne wene,
þæt me geoc cyme guðgewinnes ...'

['I do not expect comfort,
that relief from toil of war might come to me ...']
(Exeter Book riddle)

In Robert Zemeckis's 2007 film adaptation of *Beowulf*, as in the Old English poem, immediately after Beowulf is fatally wounded during his final battle with the dragon, the loyal Wiglaf arrives at his side. In the poem, Beowulf's injury is then described in particularly bloody terms: 'He geblodegod wearð / sawuldriore. Swat yðum weoll' ['He became bloodied with life-blood. Blood welled in waves'] (2693–2694). In the space of two lines, Beowulf's body is connected with three synonyms that all best translate as 'blood': the basic *blod* in *geblodeged* ['bloodied'] followed by *dreor*, which is particularly suggestive of 'dripping or flowing' blood, and then *swat*, referring more to blood as bodily moisture, and etymologically related to modern *sweat*.[1] Most translations, however, downplay this repetition in the description of the physical damage incurred by Beowulf,[2] as does the 2007 movie, which transfers the bloodiness from Beowulf's own death scene to the previous scene where he slays the dragon by ripping its heart out with his bare hands. Even so, in the film Wiglaf's first impulse at this moment is, quite naturally, to seek medical assistance: 'Let's get you to a healer', he says. To which Beowulf responds, 'Not this time, old friend'.

Of course, in the Old English epic, there is no mention of a doctor as Beowulf approaches death. On the contrary, Wiglaf reminds Beowulf, shortly before he receives his mortal wound, that a hero's health is in fact his own responsibility, and his alone: 'Scealt nu dædum rof, æðeling anhydig, ealle mægene, feorh ealgian' ['You, a single-minded hero famous in deeds, must now protect your life with all strength'] (2667–2669). The common addition of healers into modern adaptations could thus be dismissed easily as one of many ways that such modern renderings are 'inauthentic'.[3] Not only is there not a dedicated healer in *Beowulf*, but beyond the collections of medical texts discussed throughout the preceding chapters, references to herbal healing in Old English literature are virtually non-existent. Yet though it is clearly a departure from the Old English epic, the movie-Wiglaf's response is arguably far more logical and reasonable; his companion and leader is wounded and dying and he wants nothing more than to seek immediate help. Such departures from the Old English text in the modern imagination underscore just how strangely illogical it is that healers aren't ever seen on the battlefield in Old English poetry, how bizarre it appears that Wiglaf did not even attempt to summon healing assistance during Beowulf's final moments. It should perhaps be unsurprising, then, that the Exeter Book riddle *Anhaga*, containing one of the very few references to healers and herbal healing outside of the medical texts, points us not directly toward healers but specifically toward their absence.[4] And it is thus that we now conclude where we began, with the missing healers of *Anhaga*,[5] but now better equipped to understand what the absent healers might have signaled to audiences familiar with the wider healing tradition and how this seemingly tangential line might impact modern interpretations.

This short poem, as we saw before, begins straightforwardly enough. The long-suffering speaker elegiacally laments its tragic state as one who is all alone (l. 1) and recounts its subjection to hard, sharp blades that relentlessly strike day and night without abatement. The riddle's paradox emerges in line 6: even when describing itself as entirely *forwurðe* (l. 6)—which is usually translated in this particular context as 'destroyed' or 'ruined' but more typically means to have actually died (*DOE* sense 1)[6]—the speaker's voice cannot be silenced. If we remain at all unclear with regard to the speaker's impossible situation as simultaneously lifeless and speaking, the last line's description of repeated death-blows [*deaðslege*, l. 14] removes any doubt. And the speaker's grim fate had actually been sealed earlier in line 10: no healer can be found.[7]

At the surface level, this exiled speaker adopts the language of a heroic warrior slain in battle, and, as we shall see, the riddle's most commonly proposed solution retains the battle context but shifts the identity from an actual human hero to a material object: a *shield* that is continually being struck by the sharp implements of war. However, in recent years alternative non-military solutions have been gaining ground, most notably *whetstone* and *chopping block*. Any of these solutions successfully resolves the initial level of paradox created by a personified material object. But like the double-entendre Old English riddles that operate on multiple levels simultaneously, *Anhaga*'s full import is best realized by understanding these two kinds of solutions—military and domestic—as actually working in tandem. The discussion that follows explores these various solutions in turn and demonstrates that the multiple viable solutions offer more than simply clever alternatives. The competing solutions create—and ultimately resolve—a second layer of paradox, implicitly drawing attention to the overlap of the military sphere of the shield with the domestic sphere of the chopping block, an overlap represented in both the healing tradition and weaponry of early medieval England by the multifunctional whetstone. Though the (absent) healer's herbs are of no benefit to the shield/whetstone/chopping block, they do indeed come to the aid of readers, providing a crucial link that connects the riddle's various layers.

Building paradox through battle

The irresistible pull of the riddle genre towards the hidden answer(s) lurking beneath the surface can make it tempting to skip over the non-metaphorical, face-value reading of these playfully interactive poems. Such is especially the case with a riddle such as *Anhaga*, whose surface imagery at a first glance can seem quite unremarkable, even boring. The short poem employs conventional language that is formulaic almost to the point of being trite. Cautiously measuring formulicity as phraseology 'recur[ring] more than once elsewhere in the corpus' (and responsibly avoiding the temptation to equate oral traditional language unequivocally with oral provenance), Anita Riedinger posits a formulaic density of 'nearly 68%' for this riddle.[8] But to dismiss the surface reading as merely a necessary means to a more interesting end would be to miss a crucial aspect of the poem's insights. The riddle exploits its idiomatic language to complicate the very ideals it appears on the surface to embrace. The remaining, less conventional language offers a counter-narrative to the unflagging heroism of the epic world conveyed through the poem's otherwise traditional language of heroism and exile, presenting instead a world where wounds continue to grow, where aid (*geoc*) is desired, and—most of all—where healers and herbs are needed and expected. At a time of unendurable need, 'Næfre læcecynn on folcstede findan meahte þara þe mid wyrtum wunde gehælde' ['Never the healer kind could I find in the dwelling place, one of those who healed a wound with herbs'] (ll. 10–11). The backdrop of the intensely formulaic language of the rest of the poem has the effect, then, of thrusting these non-formulaic lines into sharp relief, and, as a complex generic hybrid, this poem thus deftly combines the motifs of elegy with the paradox of the riddle, evoking the ideals of heroic poetry and implicitly contrasting them with the human vulnerability manifest in the medical texts.

As Williamson observes, the 'basic riddlic game' involves 'hiding nonhuman creatures in human disguise',[9] the riddle's subject becoming in effect a kind of human/non-human hybrid via paradoxical language. In this case the solitary, largely conventional warrior that serves as the poem's narrative persona does indeed lead us to the anticipated paradox, and the various proposed solutions of *shield, chopping block*, and *whetstone* will each be engaged below. However, the poem's skillful subversion of expectation actually begins well before we are confronted with the poem's ambiguity, at the level of the seemingly straightforward human mask. As Patrick Murphy observes, 'there is more to the riddle than its solution',[10] and important meaning and insight can also be gleaned from what Murphy discusses as the *proposition*, 'the description to be posed',[11] represented in this poem by the warrior imagery. So before we delve into the range of possible solutions, I'd like us to first step back and forget that this poem is a riddle, imagining, if only temporarily, that the speaker is nothing more than the suffering, lonely, hopeless warrior presented to the manuscript's readers. Through that lens, the juxtaposition of conventional warrior imagery with the extremely unconventional acknowledgment of healers exposes the vulnerability of such warriors, collapses the heroic ideal in upon itself, and—most important of all—invites us to consider herbal healing as an essential and deeply collaborative endeavor.

As should be evident even from the basic summary above, the greater portion of this riddle evokes contexts of exile and warfare, and the unusually high level of formulaic language might lead us to expect a more conventional exiled warrior than we in fact get. Riedinger's analysis leaves only nine half-lines of the 14-line poem, unprecedented in Old English heroic or exile verse. While rigid divisions of any text into formulaic units can be deeply problematic, the larger patterns revealed in the nature of such language are very much worth noting. For instance, focusing especially on the traditional associations of the epithet *anhaga*,[12] a compound that occurs eleven times in Old English poetry, Riedinger observes that the speaker of this riddle aligns itself idiomatically with figures such as the famous *anhaga* of the *Wanderer* (l. 1), the imprisoned Andreas (l. 1351), and even Beowulf (l. 2368).

But despite a level of heroic-code formulicity that would seem to border on cliché, the speaker—or more properly the speaker's assumed human persona—is not the conventional warrior that the traditional language might lead us to expect. As Riedinger notes, the epithet *anhaga* powerfully indexes not only heroes in battle but also such figures as the wolf in *Maxims II* (l. 19a), who, as 'as a member of the triadic Beasts of Battle' is 'instantly associated with warfare and death'.[13] Riedinger contends that 'this was clearly a poet who knew the Old English formulaic tradition intimately: he drew on it for the basic composition of his poem, and for the thematic complication of his riddle';[14] thus, for an audience attuned to the traditional idiom, the opening of the poem conveys isolation, specifically of an exiled warrior facing imminent death.[15] Similarly, Edward B. Irving argues convincingly that riddles such as this one permit a 'certain significantly non-heroic subtext to be expressed',[16] and the speaker of *Anhaga* specifically narrates the experience of a warrior as from a purely defensive position, with all hope replaced by pain and suffering. The poem thus evokes the ethos of the warrior ideal through 'the inherited style of oral heroic tradition' only to subvert it, thereby 'challenging fundamental values of heroic behavior' as the speaker shows us nothing less than resignation and despair.[17] This paradoxical presentation of war is even more noticeable when we realize the riddle's speaker also seems to lack any support from a *comitatus*, that band of loyal retainers symbolically representative of communal social structures in the Germanic tradition and thus the antithesis of the lonely and abandoned warrior.

It is from within the gap between these two contexts of solitary exile and the heroic warrior that the speaker's vulnerability emerges most clearly, and the poem's lines that are elsewhere unprecedented—the *non*-formulaic lines—are the ones that in turn must be used to bridge that gap and point us toward the riddle's solution(s). As mentioned earlier, multiple solutions have been proposed to resolve the paradox of the speaker who continues to endure repeated attacks long after it has been slain beyond the hope of any healer, but because the formulaic language employed here more typically appears in explicitly heroic contexts, *shield* has long been the most widely accepted solution,[18] the wooden portion of the shield gashed and scarred by incessant sword strikes. Following such a line of interpretation, Murphy notes that this riddle 'displays a particular brand of transfer whereby inanimate objects are animated by the very feelings they typically arouse in those who use them in daily life', riddles in which the 'proposition reflects the life of the solution's owner',[19] in this case the shield characterized as the warrior, its bearer. For Williamson, the key to arriving at the *shield* solution is the (absent) healer:

> while the shield, like man, may sustain wounds in battle, unlike man, it may not be healed by the *læcecynn*. Still, despite the shield's particular vulnerability, it is able to sustain over a long period of time many more wounds without dying than man could ever sustain. [...]

Where the shield cannot be easily cured, it cannot also be easily killed. Its strength (wood) is also its weakness. That is the paradox of the riddle.[20]

Shield does indeed offer a satisfying resolution to the paradox, and many of the most readily available modern translations and editions accordingly provide *shield* as the primary, if not only, solution.[21]

However, while an anthropomorphized shield perhaps offers the most transparent solution, the search for a single overriding solution has not entirely squeezed out alternatives. For some, like William Sayers, *shield* is 'only one of the false bottoms to the poem', the interpretive path leading 'from one highly charged context to another one'.[22] The most well-received solution outside of *shield* has been the *chopping block*, widely accepted as interchangeable with *cutting board*.[23] As early as 1894 Moritz Trautmann proposed *chopping block* ('der Hackeklotz'),[24] a possibility that has been convincingly renewed by Anita Riedinger and subsequently accepted as an additional valid reading by Patrick Murphy[25] and Tiffany Beechy.[26] The *chopping block* solution accounts for the fact that the speaker is subject to constant cutting from blades, not just in times of battle but always, 'dagum ond nihtum' ['by day and night'] (l. 14). Further support can be found for this non-military reading in the poem's reference to edges and sharpness of iron, language that could be applied to domestic items as well as battle implements, rather than referencing specific weapons of warfare. The *bill* in line 2, for instance, is most easily translated as *sword*—the first sense provided in the *Dictionary of Old English*—but could also refer to a 'pruning hook or blade', or an 'implement for cutting wood' (sense 2 in the *DOE*).

Like the solution *shield*, the solution *chopping block* offers itself up in part through departures from traditional language, departures that tend to express vulnerability. If the heroic ideal requires an unassailable warrior, then any search for a healer—such as that implied by lines 10b–12 of the riddle—would be, at least to an extent, inherently unheroic.[27] The vulnerability suggested by the need of medical assistance therefore helps explain why physicians are so conspicuously absent from heroic verse, but this riddle cleverly challenges that heroic ideal by fracturing the construct of the selfless warrior willing to die in glory with an explicit desire not to valiantly accept defeat—but rather to heal. Riedinger notes the dissonance of lines 10b–12; where the vast majority of lines elsewhere in the poem have precedent within the heroic tradition, this line and a half 'has no traditional context',[28] and the term *læcecynn* 'is used nowhere else in Old English poetry'.[29] For Riedinger, this lack of traditionality in a poem where formulaic language dominates is key: 'This verse is invented by the poet to pose the riddle and to lead the audience accurately to the solution', an emphasis that 'leads away from "Shield" to "Cutting Board" or "Chopping Block"'.[30] The proposed solution as *cutting board* or *chopping block* therefore would depend heavily on the power of traditional language to guide interpretation towards the significance of herbal healing.

Finally, William Sayers has argued persuasively for the solution *whetstone*,[31] an answer that potentially brings together the domestic and military contexts, a view seen as plausible by Olsen as well.[32] If we view the blade as a military weapon, Sayers' solution provides a nice symmetry, with the interpretive path leading from the battlefield 'toward the smithy—and thus in roundabout fashion back to the battlefield'.[33] Equally, though, a whetstone could be used for everyday knives in hunting, food preparation, and other household tasks. Like the shield and cutting board, the whetstone's very purpose of existence is to interact with the blades of sharp objects. Sayers' analysis focuses especially on the poem's use of conventional exile motifs, most notably the speaker's identification as an *anhaga*, a solitary dweller. He argues that the speaker's self-identification as a solitary *anhaga* not only suggests a solution rarer than 'the ubiquitous shield, as common as the warrior which is the mask worn by the poem', but also 'relates to the unique status of the stone among many tools and weapons'.[34] The particular stone used for whetstones 'had of necessity to keep pace with advances in metallurgy', and Sayers suggests that *haga* in this context could evoke its meaning as *enclosure* and thus reference 'the practice of carrying a personal hone in a small case'.[35] The poem's frequent reference to injury by metal in phrases such as 'iserne wund' 'names the stone's fundamental opponent, iron, with which it enjoys an ambivalent symbiotic relationship as does the warrior with his enemy'.[36] Thus, the speaker's repeated injuries from weapons could reference 'the potentially rapid incapacitation of the wooden shield' but could also be invoking 'the more gradual but no less inevitable abrasion of an important tool in medieval craftsmanship'.[37] This solution depends upon the recognition that mortal harm need not be from a single, devastating blow but can be caused by small and endlessly repeated attacks as well.

The riddle quite cleverly, then, leaves both military and domestic solutions open through metonymic language such as the phraseology focusing on edges and blades that could refer to either context. And, as Beechy puts it, 'of course, we have no answer key, so all solutions are on the table (or, as it were, the chopping-block)'.[38] Fortunately, we do not have to force any single reading onto this multivalent text, which clearly supports multiple solutions. Such diversity of solutions is generally characteristic of riddles in performance and is therefore frequently a defining feature of oral and oral-derived riddles.[39] Building from N. F. Barley's structural analysis of spoken riddles that 'presuppose at least two parties, the poser and the solver, and constitute a dialogue between the two',[40] John Niles draws attention to the futility of insisting on a single 'right' answer, since in performance 'the "correct" answer to a riddle is whatever the poser says is right'.[41] What I want to argue going forward is that within the social and performative genre of riddles, multiple solutions aren't only possible, but, rather, are fundamental to understanding the poem in the fullest, richest way.

Resolving paradox through healing

Thus far we have examined the *Anhaga* riddle's speaker/solution paradox, through which the solution bridges the gap between persona and (personified) object. But the riddle also invites us to resolve this paradox across *multiple* solutions, military and domestic, by employing an interpretive framework akin to that which enables the double-entendre riddles, a sub-genre in which double meaning is truly a defining feature. Few would insist, for instance, that we choose the 'correct' of two or more proposed readings with regard to 'lock and key' or 'bread dough' riddles that rely heavily on double-entendre;[42] rather than being viewed as competing solutions where one must be chosen over the other, the two are typically understood as working in tandem toward a specific—in that case, humorous—effect. Similarly, in *Anhaga*, the 'competing' solutions are each fully supported by the text of the poem and potentially work together to create meaning, albeit in a different way from their double-entendre counterparts. Together the multiple solutions of *shield, cutting board* or *chopping block*, and *whetstone* form this riddle into a hybrid entity that underscores the tensions between the domestic and military spheres. Karin Olsen's analysis, which focuses especially on the speaker's identity as *anhaga*, beautifully illustrates the points of intersection across these solutions through two charts of 'inputs'.[43] The effect is to emphasize the irony we see even within the speaker's persona—the warrior described in (almost excessively) heroic terms, who nonetheless feels the fear, dread, and resignation that is typically left out of heroic verse. At every level, *Anhaga* forces us to consider the heroic military ideal in the context of everyday life and to take into account the physical and emotional trauma that the heroic ideals of battle set in motion. In lamenting the lack of healers, this riddle's speaker reminds readers that to prevent further loss of life—of warriors who are perhaps also farmers, cooks, or smiths—the heroic ideal of invulnerability must ultimately give way and open a space for healing to occur. Taking the riddle's solutions together in light of Old English medical texts thus begins to reconcile these conflicting ideals, a reminder that war's impact doesn't stay on the battlefield but can be felt sharply in the home as well.[44]

Even though *shield* is by far the most commonly accepted solution of this riddle, and *chopping block, cutting board*, and *whetstone* may feel like a greater stretch for modern readers, these 'secondary' solutions—as we shall see—may have been much more transparent to the poem's earliest audiences. And at the center of all these interpretations is the riddle's carefully crafted reference (in lines 10–12) to the unavailability of healers and their herbs in this heroic scenario, a reference that is entirely consistent with the methodologies and descriptions found in the medical remedies of early medieval England. In earlier chapters we repeatedly encountered Old English medical texts employing battle imagery and traditional heroic phraseology within a healing context. Even the dedication page of the *Herbarium* (MS Cotton Vitellius C.iii) establishes visually compelling connections between herbal healing and battle, depicting the book's recipient as not only holding a book but also armed with a spear.[45] And, as we saw in Chapter 2, numerous herbs in the English language tradition are linked to warfare, as several *Herbarium* entries include native plant names in which weapons are used as an identifier of leaf-shape, such as the obvious *sperewyrt*. Accordingly, if one thinks of the riddle's herbs themselves as weapons, then the competing solutions of *shield* and *cutting board/ chopping block* can sit together much more companionably.

In fact, the distance between *cutting board* and *shield* already becomes far more compressed if we remember that Old English *bord* has a broad semantic range and can accommodate both military and domestic contexts.[46] Niles has quite logically argued that 'whenever feasible, a riddle ought to be answered *in the language in which it is posed*',[47] and while modern English requires two separate solutions, *bord* allows for both senses in a single word, this term frequently being used to refer to shields (especially in poetic contexts) but also to tables and other such surfaces that might be used for cutting.[48] The feast scene on the Bayeux Tapestry would suggest that the overlapping senses are indeed more than purely semantic, with one shield holding a cup and bowl and a second holding a loaf and knife.[49] This notion that *Anhaga* could easily make use of both senses at once is reinforced by another riddle, *Gingra Broþor Mec Adraf* ['Younger brother drove me out'], which actually employs *bord* in these two different senses within a few lines of each other: 'bord biton' ['they bit into shields'] is followed a few lines later by a quill pen stepping out 'on stið bord' ['onto a stiff board'].[50] The *bord* onto which the quill steps could even be understood as the surface of the vellum itself, indicating that any stiff surface might be rendered as *bord*. It would seem quite possible, then, that this semantic open-endedness might allow for associative possibilities—among shields, cutting boards, chopping blocks, and perhaps even the hard surface of a flat, broad whetstone—that would far exceed those connected with our modern English terminology. And if we take into account herbal and medicinal contexts, the possible connections with *whetstone* become even more apparent. While herbs would of course more typically be chopped on a cutting board, certain remedies do indeed call for chopping herbs on a whetstone. *Lacnunga* remedy XXXVIII, for instance, calls for a healer to 'nim þon(ne) *hwetstan* bradne 7 gnid ða buteran on ðæm hwetstane mid copore þ(æt) heo beo wel' ['take then a broad *whetstone* and grind the butter on the whetstone with copper'; emphasis added]. In this context, a 'broad whetstone' would then function very much like a chopping block or cutting board.[51]

The fact that some whetstones seem to have been carved in the shape of humans collapses the distinction even further. The whetstone/scepter at Sutton Hoo is the most famous such case, with its four faces carved on each side of a stone bar,[52] but other such objects identified as whetstones have also survived, including one found at Hough-on-the-Hill in Lincolnshire and 'decorated with a terminal head and shoulders of human form in the round' whose surface indicates use 'as a percussive tool or as a grinding tool'.[53] Its deeply scarred face and torso are certainly reminiscent of the warrior speaker of *Anhaga*. In such a situation, blades would be striking the human-shaped stone, an entity not at all unlike the speaker of this riddle, the perpetual recipient of death blows from blades. A carved broad whetstone, such as that found at Lincolnshire, presumably could function as a cutting board as well, struck by knives chopping herbs and also by the herbs themselves as a prelude to their use as weapons against ailments—regardless of whether the treated maladies originated on the field of battle or in a more domestic setting.

The focus on the warrior's suffering potentially links the multiple solutions of cutting board, chopping block, shield, and whetstone and serves to highlight points of connection between military and domestic spheres through multi-use objects and multi-valent vocabulary. But we could demonstrate many more points of overlap between these contexts as well. For instance, though the warrior persona of this riddle laments that there is no healer who might heal with herbs, the herbs themselves are not stated as being absent. Medical texts frequently describe herbal preparations that are to be applied to skin, so presumably if a healer *could* have been found, the herbs likely would have been applied to the wounded skin of the repeatedly cut speaker. But just as with so many other aspects of the riddle, this image of herbs on skin becomes yet another instance of the riddle blurring boundaries between the military and the domestic when we take into account wider cultural contexts, in this case shield construction. Wooden shields of early medieval England were typically covered with leather, the function of which is in fact very much like skin, serving as 'a shock absorber against slashing blows by spreading the force of the blow across the whole of the shield and reducing the likelihood of the boards splitting or shattering under the impact of the blow'.[54] If we return to Irving's point that the riddle serves as a commentary on suffering in war, the simultaneous references to herbs on skin and weapons on shields become all the more poignant, the riddle cleverly rendering wound and remedy in a single powerful image.

Also, the healer is not the only human conspicuously absent. The person making use of the shield/chopping block/cutting board/ whetstone is never mentioned, a situation that renders the battle as one of object versus object—sword against shield, knife against whetstone, or—if we allow for the possibility that healing plants themselves are blades—herbs against wounds. Murphy notes that in the reading of the speaker as shield 'the riddle's proposition reflects the life of the solution's owner (i.e., the shield bearer)'.[55] If we understand herbs as the healer's weapon, this same observation could be seen as equally applicable for the lines on healing, the herbs reflecting the life of the healer, fighting against ailment and striking against skin in an effort to cure. Contrarily, as Wim Tigges observes, there would be 'a humorous irony' to the riddle if the *wyrtum* that cannot heal the speaker are both those that are attacking the speaker but also 'the very vegetables that are chopped on the block'.[56]

The speaker's self-identification as *anhaga* also works at both levels, in military as well as domestic/vegetative contexts. Jeff Massey and Karma DeGruy stress that the most common translations of *anhaga* as 'loner' or 'solitary one' address only one half of the compound (*an*: "one" or "lone") at the expense of the other (*haga*: "hedge" or "haw").[57] Charters of early medieval England provide numerous examples of uncompounded occurrences of *haga*, a term that in isolation most frequently refers to a hedge, composed of individual plants. Massey and DeGruy note the overlap in military and domestic contexts of the term: 'Horticulturally speaking, a hedge is composed of individual plants', which collectively serve to 'contain livestock and prevent their predation'; 'Martially speaking, a hedge is composed of individual shields', which together 'protect their allies behind them'.[58]

In all of these ways, then, the riddle *Anhaga* demonstrates how 'a poet steeped in oral traditions could compose a new poem by drawing on the Old English poetic tradition for traditional formulas and, sometimes, traditional concepts'.[59] Far from limiting meaning, semantically ambiguous language combined with seemingly out-of-place phraseology, such as the reference to absent healers in an otherwise highly formulaic exposition on warrior culture, helps open up multiple solutions as viable for this paradoxical human/non-human hybrid. But there is absolutely no ambiguity with regard to the terrible violence inflicted and harm sustained. The riddle's paradox thus goes far beyond the fact that an inanimate object speaks; its many forms of riddlic hybridity expose numerous fundamental contradictions within the larger lived experience of early medieval England—especially at the overlap between the military and domestic spheres. Healing is battle; an herb is a blade. A fearless warrior is afraid, and even the slain endure. A shield is a cutting board is a whetstone. An epic is a riddle is a charm.

Healers in the *folcstede*

Finally, it is also possible to explore this riddle's relationship to the medical texts in the other direction and use it to shed additional light on early medieval conceptions of healing and actual healing practice. Doing so allows us to return with at least a bit more clarity to the dilemma that launched our initial inquiry in the introduction—how can we understand the healing tradition with so little known about the healers themselves? The speaker's complaint of being unable to find an herbal healer in the dwelling place to heal its wounds suggests that ordinarily one *would* seek out a healer for battle wounds, that such wounds would probably be treated with herbs, and that healers could, under normal circumstances, reliably be found in the *folcstede*. The specific reference to *læcecynne* ['healer-kind']—especially when the second part of this compound term would have been unnecessary for alliterative purposes—reinforces this sense that healers should not be understood as rare individuals, but rather as integral parts within an ever-present *cynn*, a *kind* of person one could expect to find anywhere people dwell in groups.

The riddle's lines about herbal healing also draw further attention to themselves as a rarity within heroic verse, but at the same time they point us to where warriors might have expected to find healers, and suggest that the expectation of healing might be present in the heroic texts even if the healers themselves, as in the *Anhaga* riddle, are conspicuously absent. A number of scholars have previously explored the affinities that exist between *Beowulf* and Old English medicine, especially the metrical charm texts. Sara Frances Burdorff, for instance, has noted extensive parallels between language describing Grendel's mother and such figures as the female riders of *Wið færstice* and the *sigewif* of *Wið ymbe*.[60] In this construct the *guðleoð* ['battle-song'] (l. 1522) performed by Beowulf's sword becomes especially resonant with such texts as *Lacnunga* entry 26, where a healing incantation is preceded by instructions to 'sing ðis leoð'[61] ['sing this song'] into the ear of the afflicted individual.[62] Stephen Glosecki has even gone so far as to assert that Beowulf 'is subtly but indelibly marked by reflexes of Germanic shamanism', a category that in Glosecki's interpretation applies to 'respected doctors'.[63] Translators, too, have picked up on subtle links between Beowulf and healing. In Craig Williamson's translation, for example, Beowulf announces himself as a 'healer': 'I am the healer who can help Hrothgar—I bring a remedy for the sickening foe'.[64] The original text makes no explicit references to healers or sickness, aside from the word *bot* in line 281, glossed in the *Electronic Beowulf* with a fairly wide semantic range as 'relief, deliverance, remedy, help':

Ic þæs Hroðgar mæg, / þurh rumne sefan, ræd gelæran, / hu he, frod 7 god, feond oferswyðeþ – / gyf him edwendan æfre scolde, / bealuwa bisigu, bot eft cuman.

[For that, I am able, through great spirit, to teach Hrothgar counsel, how he, wise and good, will overcome the fiend – if for him the affliction of woes must ever change, a remedy to come again.]

Although 'remedy' ranks fairly low on the list of possible meanings for *bot*, there is clearly something in the text that has long led readers to see healing as a force present in *Beowulf* despite its lack of healers. Through this lens, the 2007 movie-Wiglaf becomes much more plausible, assuming a possibility of healers that *Beowulf* on the surface actively rejects, and it is this presence of healers implied by their very absence that is shared by the Exeter Book riddle *Anhaga*, which begins to bridge the noticeable gap between a warrior hero's vulnerability and traditional sources of healing.

But at the same time that this riddle demonstrates the importance of the relatively under-appreciated healing tradition for our understanding of work produced outside the medical texts themselves, it also provides a model of paradox and metaphor that parallels the larger healing tradition more closely than it might seem at first glance. As Williamson has noted, in Old English poetry the two genres of riddles and charms 'share a metaphoric world',[65] and even while broadening his discussion of these genres out to a cross-cultural level, Northrop Frye can state that '[t]he riddle is essentially a charm in reverse: it represents the revolt of the intelligence against the hypnotic power of commanding words',[66] and adopting a biological analogy in his discussion of this generic overlap, Frye discusses charms and riddles as 'generic seeds or kernels, possibilities of expression sprouting and exfoliating into new literary phenomena'.[67] And, of course, another biological metaphor is apt here as well; the duality exhibited by both the riddles and the healing remedies is wholly relatable to the idea of hybridity as it has been explored throughout this volume. Peter Clemoes, for instance, has described the tendency in the Old English riddles to combine inanimate objects with the human capacity for speech as a type of 'hybridization'.[68] But medical texts, too, become a similar type of hybrid, drawing from multiple traditions to free individuals from the constraints of physical ailments.

Though Old English poetry leaves us largely with no healers to be found, we can nonetheless learn much from their absence. Modern depictions of early medieval culture often present medieval narratives in very binary, polarizing ways—with heroes pitted against aggressively savage monsters or villains, and of course this level of violence is undeniably there in the texts that survive. But this same poetry also challenges us to accept a hero as vulnerable, to face the trauma that occurs when a domestic object becomes weaponized, and finally to recognize the need for healing in a world of incessant suffering. Indeed, when we enter the 'folc-stede' presented in the *Anhaga* riddle, we may not find healers, but we do discover a space in which shields, cutting boards, whetstones, and warriors alike should be able to seek care, in which the distance between warrior and exile, between domestic and military, even between human and non-human effectively collapse. James Paz's notion of 'nonhuman' time offers a way of thinking about these connections as far more than interpretive ambivalence or linguistic ambiguity:

> By granting a voice to mere things, and coaxing them to talk about their current and future uses, riddles do not allow us to take for granted the inertia of objects. Material artefacts that seem to be unmoving are lyrically transformed into other kinds of things as time enacts change and as processes of creation, exchange, use, decay, suffering and shape-shifting unfold.[69]

The *Anhaga* riddle and the medical texts we have seen in the preceding chapters display this same impulse, their own lyrical transformations of common elements combined into forceful healing power. Considering remedies as emergent from the same impulse as riddles opens a space to explore the relationship between our vulnerable bodies and the world around us with wonder.

It is the generic hybridity to which *Anhaga* alerts us that offers a way through the many questions the medical texts pose; it obviates the need for final resolution and offers instead empowerment, an empowerment that comes with great promise but also substantial risk. In the ultimate paradox collapsing hope and despair, *Anhaga* suggests a ubiquitous healing presence precisely through its assertion of inexplicable absence. Similarly, in the implicit riddles posed by the medical texts, we find agency and subjectivity simultaneously inside ourselves and without. In collapsing the boundaries separating human from nonhuman, disease from cure, these texts thus confront us with a type of disconnected connectedness, one that must be met with empathy and imagination, as well as an openness to uncertainty and change.

Appendix

Text and translation

Below are an edited text and translation of *Anhaga* (Riddle 3 in Williamson, *Old English Riddles*; Riddle 5 in Krapp and Dobbie (eds), *The Exeter Book*. ASPR) that reflect the underpinnings of this chapter's analysis, followed by commentary on especially pertinent choices.

Exeter Book	
Ic eom anhaga, iserne wund,	I am a solitary being, wounded by iron,
bille gebennad, beadoweorca sæd,	wounded by a *bill*, tired of battle work,
ecgum werig. Oft ic wig seo, frecne feohtan— frofre ne wene,	weary from edges. Often I see war, fierce fighting—I do not expect comfort,
þæt me geoc cyme guðgewinnes	that consolation come to me in battle-strife
ær ic mid ældum eal forwurðe;	before I, among men, perish completely;
ac mec hnossiað homera lafe, heardecg	but leavings of hammers strike me,
heoroscearp hondweorc smiþa	hard-edged, sword-sharp hand-work of smiths
bitað in burgum; ic abidan sceal	bite in the strongholds; I must endure
laþran gemotes. Næfre læcecynn	a more hateful meeting. Never healer-kind
on folcstede findan meahte,	could I find in the people-place, one of those
þara þe mid wyrtum wunde gehælde,	who healed a wound with herbs,
ac me ecga dolg eacen weorðað	but for me wounds from edges grow great
þurh deaðslege dagum ond nihtum.	through death-blows by day and by night.

l. 2: *Bill* in the *Dictionary of Old English* is defined in the first sense as 'sword', which works with the *shield* solution. The second definition, 'pruning hook or blade, implement for cutting wood' works especially well in the domestic contexts of the 'cutting board' solution. The third sense of *bill*, 'hoe, mattock, digging implement', evokes the context of the *wyrtum* ['plants'] of line 12.

l. 6: ms *forwurde*. This emendation is defended in Williamson, *Old English Riddles*, pp. 146–147.

l. 8: ms 7 *weorc*. Most editors have accepted this emendation, which resolves the line's alliteration. Muir's edition expands 7 *weorc* to *ondweorc*, noting that the form is 'for hondweorc'.[70] *And-weorc* is commonly attested as a 'material, substance (which can be shaped)' (*DOE*, s.v. *and-weorc*). Bitterli notes that this abbreviated compound with 7 for *ond* follows a similar principle to the runes that occur in compounds elsewhere in the Exeter Book riddles (e.g., *mod [wynn]* for 'heart's joy' in Riddle 91), the shortcut itself a form of riddlic play.[71]

l. 11: My literal rendering here of *cynn* in *læcecynn* as *kind* is, perhaps surprisingly, somewhat unusual. Murphy translates as 'a physician'.[72] But, as this chapter has shown, the understanding that the speaker's worldview included not just one but an entire *cynn* of healers is crucial to our understanding of what the riddle conveys about traditional herbal medicine and its practitioners.

Notes

1 *DOE*, s.v. *blod*, *dreor* (sense 1); Bosworth and Toller, s.v. *swat* (sense 1, 'sweat, perspiration'; sense 2, 'used of other moisture that comes from the body', including 'blood').

2 E.g., Seamus Heaney (trans.), *Beowulf* (London: Faber and Faber, 2000): 'Beowulf's body ran wet with his life-blood: it came welling out'. Even the generally very literal *Electronic Beowulf* renders the lines with somewhat less 'blood', glossing *swat* as 'blood' but translating it in this line as 'gore', presumably to avoid the repetition of 'blood' three times within a line and a half. Kevin Kiernan, *Electronic Beowulf 4.0* (2015), http://ebeowulf.uky.edu/ebeo4.0/CD/main.html. Accessed 4 August 2021.

3 Additional examples of this phenomenon include: the 2016 TV miniseries *Beowulf: Return to the Shieldlands*, which adds, among other invented characters, Elvina, Heorot's healer; Susan Signe Morrison's

Hybridity of genre in an Exeter Book riddle 267

Grendel's Mother: The Saga of the Wyrd-Wife (Winchester: Top Hat Books, 2015), which portrays Grendel's mother—here named Brimhild—as a healer.

4 As noted in the Introduction, I am following the title suggested in Neville's 'Modest Proposal'. This poem appears as Riddle 3 in Williamson, *Old English Riddles* and Riddle 5 in ASPR (Krapp and Dobbie).
5 A full text and translation can be found in the appendix to this chapter.
6 E.g., Anita Riedinger translates as 'destroyed', 'The Formulaic Style in the Old English Riddles', *Studia Neophilologica*, 76 (2004), 30–43. The *DOE* gives sense 1.a as 'to perish, die' (s.v. *for-weorþan*).
7 Phyllis Portnoy's structural analysis of this riddle explicitly links the demise indicated by *forwurðe* in line 6 with the lack of healers in line 10 as parallel units within the poem's ring composition. 'Laf-Craft in Five Old English Riddles (K-D 5, 20, 56, 71, 91)', *Neophilologus*, 97 (2013), 555–579, at 562.
8 Riedinger, 'Formulaic', pp. 31, 33.
9 Williamson, *Old English Riddles*, p. 147.
10 Patrick J. Murphy, *Unriddling the Exeter Riddles* (University Park, PA: Pennsylvania State University Press, 2011), p. 63.
11 Ibid., p. 35.
12 Riedinger, 'Formulaic', p. 34. See further Karin Olsen's excellent analysis of the network of meaning in this riddle's use of *anhaga*. 'Warriors and Their Battle Gear: Conceptual Blending in *Anhaga* (R.5) and *Wæpnum Awyrged* (R.20)', in Megan Cavell and Jennifer Neville (eds), *Riddles at Work in the Early Medieval Tradition: Words, Ideas, Interactions* (Manchester: Manchester University Press, 2020), pp. 111–127, esp. 115–120.
13 Riedinger, 'Formulaic', p. 33.
14 Ibid., p. 34.
15 Ibid.
16 Edward B. Irving, 'Heroic Experience in Old English Riddles', in Katherine O'Brien O'Keeffe (ed.), *Old English Shorter Poems: Basic Readings* (New York: Garland), 199–212, at 199.
17 Ibid., p. 199; p. 201.
18 Williamson credits C. Müller's 1835 *Collectanea Anglo-Saxonica* (pp. 63–64) as the first to propose this solution, which has since been accepted by most major editions, most notably Krapp and Dobbie, *Exeter Book*, p. 325 and Williamson, *Old English Riddles*, p. 146.
19 Murphy, *Unriddling*, p. 70.
20 Williamson, *Old English Riddles*, p. 147.

21 Williamson offers the unqualified description of this riddle as a 'fierce wooden warrior, the *shield*, ... the first of many weapon riddles in the Exeter collection', Craig Williamson (trans.), *A Feast of Creatures: Anglo-Saxon Riddle-Songs* (Philadelphia, PA: The University of Pennsylvania Press, 1982), p. 163. Krapp and Dobbie (*Exeter Book*, p. 325) acknowledge Trautmann's solution of *chopping block* but immediately shut down any notion of multiple possibilities, arguing that this solution is 'ruled out by ll. 3b–4a'. Delanty and Matto's list of riddle solutions offers only 'A Shield' (*Word Exchange*, p. 541), as does the widely available Oxford World's Classics edition of *The Anglo-Saxon World* (Kevin Crossley-Holland [trans], *Anglo-Saxon World* [Oxford: Oxford University Press, 2009], p. 250). *The Cambridge Old English Reader*, published in 2015, gives only 'Shield' in its table of contents (Richard Marsden, *The Cambridge Old English Reader*, 2nd ed, Cambridge: Cambridge University Press, 2015, p. vii). The Blackwell *Old and Middle English Anthology* provides *shield* as the solution in the main text and refers readers to Tigges, 'Snakes and Ladders', for an alternative, but without saying what that alternative is (Wim Tigges, 'Snakes and Ladders: Ambiguity and Coherence in the Exeter Book Riddles and Maxims', in Henk Aertsen and Rolf H. Bremmer, Jr. [eds], *Companion to Old English Poetry* [Amsterdam: VU University Press, 1994], pp. 95–118). Bradley's *Anglo-Saxon Poetry* gives only *shield*, p. 372. Moritz Trautmann, 'Die Auflösungen der altenglischen Rätsel', *Anglia Beiblatt*, 5 (1894), 46–51. Elaine Treharne (ed.), *Old and Middle English c. 890–c. 1400: An Anthology* (Oxford: Blackwell Publishing, 2nd edn, 2004), p. 66.
22 William Sayers, 'Exeter Book Riddle No. 5: Whetstone?', *Neuphilologische Mitteilungen*, 97 (1996), 387–392, at 388.
23 E.g., Riedinger, 'Formulaic', 34; Olsen, 'Warriors', 119.
24 Trautmann, 'Auflösungen', p. 48.
25 Murphy, *Unriddling*, pp. 68–70.
26 Tiffany Beechy, *The Poetics of Old English* (Burlington, VT: Ashgate Publishing, 2010), p. 91.
27 Cf. Irving, 'Heroic'.
28 Riedinger, 'Formulaic', p. 34.
29 Ibid., p. 34.
30 Ibid.
31 Sayers, 'Exeter Book Riddle', p. 388.
32 Olsen, 'Warriors', p. 119.
33 Sayers, 'Exeter Book Riddle', p. 388.
34 Ibid.

35 Ibid.
36 Ibid.
37 Ibid.
38 Beechy, *Poetics*, p. 91.
39 Exploring the Old English riddles as oral-derived of course in no way denies their status as 'carefully crafted literary riddles' with a 'clear debt to a rich Anglo-Latin tradition', Murphy, *Unriddling*, p. 48.
40 Nigel F. Barley, 'Structural Aspects of the Anglo-Saxon Riddle', *Semiotica*, 10 (1974), 143–175, at 143–144.
41 John D. Niles, *Old English Enigmatic Poems and the Play of the Texts* (Turnhout: Brepols, 2006), pp. 23–24. As an example, he offers the riddle 'What is black and white and red all over?', which supports multiple 'right' answers, depending on the riddle poser, such as newspaper, blushing zebra, skunk with diaper rash, among others.
42 On the popular 'Riddle Ages' site, for instance, Megan Cavell observes that for *Wrætlic Hongað bi Weres þeo* ['A wonder hangs by a man's thigh'], ASPR Riddle 44 (solved 'key and lock' or 'phallus'), 'all the basics of a nudge-nudge joke are there for even the most sheltered of individuals to catch'. Even in a forum designed with non-specialists in mind, the doubleness is deemed too obvious to require any further explanation. For texts, translations, and commentary of these and all of the Exeter Book riddles, see https://theriddleages.com/riddles/collection/the-exeter-book/. Accessed 7 June 2021.
43 Olsen, 'Warriors', pp. 116–117.
44 This doubleness can of course be felt by readers regardless of the poet's intent.
45 On this dedication page, see Linda Ehrsam Voigts, 'A New Look at a Manuscript Containing the Old English Translation of the *Herbarium Apulei*', *Manuscripta*, 21 (1976), 40–60. In the same way, the *Medicina Antiqua* produced in thirteenth-century Italy (Vienna Österreichische Nationalbibliothek, Cod. Vind. 93) includes an illustration of a man attacking a snake with a spear in his right hand and a plant in his left (f. 23v). Similar illustrations of men armed against ailments with a combination of weapons and plants appear on folios 68v, 74v, and 78v. See Peter Murray Jones' beautiful facsimile: *Medicina Antiqua* (London: Harvey Miller Publishers, 1999), descriptions pp. 34, 43, 45–46. Many thanks to Jack Niles for drawing this manuscript to my attention.
46 *DOE*, s.v. *shield*. Sense 1 is 'shield'; sense 3 is 'table'. On this possible wordplay, see also Murphy, *Unriddling*, 69–70.
47 Niles, *Old English Enigmatic*, p. 103.

48 On the importance of considering possibilities within Old English vocabulary in solving riddles, see further Corinne Dale, *The Natural World in the Exeter Book Riddles* (Woodbridge: D. S. Brewer, 2017), p. 126. Though Niles himself offers *scild* as the solution to this riddle, the suggestion of *bord* would seem to be in keeping with his larger point and to accommodate a wider range of the poem's multiple meanings. Niles, *Old English Enigmatic*, p. 141.
49 Gale R. Owen-Crocker, 'Stylistic Variation and Roman Influence in the Bayeux Tapestry', *Peregrinations: Journal of Medieval Art and Architecture*, 2.4 (2009), 51–96, at 70.
50 Williamson, *Old English Riddles*, pp. 89, 24, 31. ASPR Riddle 93.
51 Archeological evidence shows that whetstones could be quite large, such as a stone of 17.5 cm found in Linford, Essex, believed to be a 'flat building stone reused for sharpening'. Vera I. Evison 'Pagan Saxon Whetstones', *The Antiquaries Journal*, 55 (1975), 70–85, at 74.
52 Sidney Cohen suggests that a stone such as this might have functioned to sharpen knives used in a ritual context. Sidney L. Cohen, 'The Sutton Hoo Whetstone', *Speculum*, 41 (1966), 466–470, at 469. Debate does, however, continue as to the function of the stone. See, for instance, Paul Mortimer and Stephen Pollington, *Remaking the Sutton Hoo Stone: The Ansell-Roper Replica and its Context* (Cambridgeshire: Anglo-Saxon Books, 2013).
53 Description in *The Corpus of Anglo-Saxon Stone Sculpture, 5: Lincolnshire*, https://chacklepie.com/ascorpus/catvol5.php?pageNum_urls=171&totalRows_urls=369. Accessed 1 June 2021.
54 I. P. Stephenson, *The Anglo-Saxon Shield* (Stroud: Tempus. 2004), p. 41.
55 Murphy, *Unriddling*, p. 70.
56 Tigges, 'Snakes and Ladders', p. 100. The effect of the chopped victim becoming aligned with the chopping antagonist is perhaps similar to that found in *Deor*, where the victimized Weland of the first stanza is implicitly conveyed as Beaduhild's rapist in the second.
57 Jeff Massey and Karma DeGruy, 'Riddling Meaning from Old English -*haga* Compounds', *Studies in Philology*, 112 (2015), 24–38, at 24.
58 Ibid.
59 Riedinger, 'Formulaic', p. 30.
60 Burdorff, 'Re-Reading Grendel's Mother, pp. 95–96 and 99.
61 On the nuances of *leoð* in relation to words with overlapping meanings, such as *spel*, see Beechy, *Poetics*, pp. 34–36.
62 This resonance is especially significant, given the common depiction of healing herbs in terms of battle gear, as discussed in Chapters 2 and 3.

Hybridity of genre in an Exeter Book riddle 271

63 Stephen O. Glosecki, 'Wolf of the Bees: Germanic Shamanism and the Bear Hero', *Journal of Ritual Studies*, 2.1 (1988), 31–53, at 36.
64 Craig Williamson (trans.), *The Complete Old English Poems* (Philadelphia, PA: University of Pennsylvania Press, 2017), p. 614.
65 Williamson, *Feast*, p. 34.
66 Northrop Frye, *Spiritus Mundi: Essays on Literature, Myth, and Society* (Bloomington, IN: Indiana University Press, 1976), p. 137. On further connections between charms and riddles in Old English, particularly with regard to form, see Beechy, *Poetics*, Ch. 3 'Bind and Loose: Poetics and the Word in Old English Law, Charm, and Riddle', esp. p. 93.
67 Frye, *Spiritus*, p. 123. In a discussion of 'applied myth as charm', Calvert Watkins notes shared Indo-European patterns in 'an Old English dragon-slaying narrative' that are manifest in both *Beowulf* and the 'Nine Herbs Charm', *How to Kill a Dragon: Aspects of Indo-European Poetics* (Oxford: Oxford University Press, 1995), p. 424. Also seeing cross-genre connections, Megan Cavell has argued for a link between early medieval medicine and an Exeter Book riddle: 'Powerful Patens in the Anglo-Saxon Medical Tradition and Exeter Book Riddle 48, *Neophilologus*, 101 (2017), 129–138.
68 Peter Clemoes, *Interactions of Thought and Language in Old English Poetry* (Cambridge: Cambridge University Press, 1995), p. 98.
69 Paz, *Nonhuman Voices*, p. 61.
70 Bernard Muir (ed.), *The Exeter Anthology of Old English Poetry*, 2 vols. (Liverpool: Liverpool University Press, 2000).
71 Dieter Bitterli, *Say What I am Called: The Old English Riddles of the Exeter Book and the Anglo-Latin Riddle Tradition* (Toronto: University of Toronto Press, 2009).
72 Murphy, *Unriddling*, p. 68.

Conclusion: with empathy and imagination—hybridity in the field

> Ðeos wyrt þe man pedem leonis 7 oðrum naman leonfot nemneð, heo bið cenned on feldon 7 on dicon 7 on hreodbeddon.
>
> [This plant which some call *pedem leonis* and others lionfoot, it is known in fields and in ditches and in reedbeds.]
> (Old English *Herbarium*, Cotton Vitellius C.iii f. 24v)
>
> … that I might knock on others' doors and learn how to listen to the conversations going on among my fellow scholars in other fields and disciplines.
> (Donna Beth Ellard *Anglo-Saxon(ist) Pasts, postSaxon Futures*)[1]

Old English medical texts such as the *Herbarium* frequently direct practitioners to find healing herbs, such as *leonfot* above, 'in fields' ['on feldon']. Though *feld* has since come to refer to cultivated land 'devoted to a particular crop', the Old English word had a sense of wildness about it: 'open country', 'land unencumbered by obstruction'.[2] It was the Old English word *æcer* (as in the *Æcerbot* land remedy) that more specifically denoted prescribed boundaries and cultivation.[3] But it was in the open, untamed fields that hybridity might abound and new healing resources might be discovered. And in turn it is in correspondingly open academic fields where the complex texts from early medieval England can be most fully understood.

Across these past chapters I hope to have shown the need for 'hybrid' approaches to meet the hybridity of culture and form as manifested in surviving Old English remedies and medical texts. And I also hope that in these pages there can be felt an urgency for greater openness to the variation and variability inherent in these multivalent texts—texts that can still hold important meanings today. Most of all, I hope through this series of close explorations to have conveyed the importance of understanding each individual remedy as emerging in its own unique way from diverse influences within a dynamic, living tradition of healing practice and lore. The biological basis of hybridity implies new life and new forms of being, and so to better understand the subtleties and limits of the metaphor, I have proposed that we return both literally and metaphorically to the spaces where plants are found and hybridized: in the field. Like the lion's foot sought in ditches and reedbeds as well as in open fields, answers are not always easy to find, sometimes requiring us to wade into unfamiliar terrain—in Donna Beth Ellard's words, to 'knock on others' doors and learn how to listen'.

One reason to revisit the medical texts today, remedy by remedy, is that the era in which the now standard editions were created, and upon which many accepted translations are now based, was not especially open to such listening. I'll share here one brief but illustrative example. In 1922, significantly after Thomas Oswald Cockayne's *Leechdoms* and Felix Grendon's 1909 edition of *Anglo-Saxon Charms* but still well before Godfrid Storms' *Anglo-Saxon Magic* in 1948, gardener and herbalist Eleanour Sinclair Rohde offered a sharp critique in *The Old English Herbals* of scholars who 'miss all that is most worth learning in old books through regarding anything in them that is unfamiliar as merely quaint, if not ridiculous'. 'This attitude', she wrote, 'seals a book as effectually and as permanently as it seals a sensitive human being'.[4] In contrast to the tendency in her time—a tendency that eventually became a long-established norm—to dismiss 'superstition' or 'folklore' in these texts, she suggested simply that 'we try to read them with understanding', to approach medieval remedies not with disdain but with 'sympathy and imagination'.[5] Though she worked closely with Charles Singer—whose work on Old English medicine influenced the field for decades to come[6]—her work was little appreciated in scholarly circles, largely on the basis of its multidisciplinary goals. Archivist Hilary Jenkinson, for instance, argued that 'we can imagine the horticulturist saying that it is a book which may interest historians with a turn for gardening, and historians dismissing it as one which will appeal to gardeners who have a smattering of history'.⁷ George Sarton's 1923 review likewise harshly critiqued her 'unusual combination of popular writing and learning'.⁸ Rather than appreciating her efforts to share the medical texts with a wider readership, he berated her for being 'terribly afraid of scaring the "general reader"', described her 'whole attitude' as 'one of revolt against scientific methods', and saw her 'three learned appendixes' as 'unkind' for having been wasted on non-specialist readers.⁹ Rohde's experience here is indicative of the climate in which the earliest editions of Old English medical texts—many of which are still widely used today—were produced. The largely unexamined acceptance of this tendency to close off open and empathetic engagement with the texts goes far in explaining why there are so many assumptions, misleading translations, and questionable emendations that remain, to this day, unchallenged and uncorrected. The emendation noted in Chapter 2 where a spear is erroneously added to protective gear in a poem for travelers effectively masks an essential element of that text's meaning, and the removal of a phrase—*hand ofer heafod* ['hand over head']—for its presumed redundancy in the same poem risks omitting an essential part of a ritual involving repetition and bodily movement. Similarly, ever-so-slight but ultimately unnecessary syntactical changes to the *Leechbook* entries on hearing, discussed in Chapter 6, pull the modern translation into alignment with modern medical models but obscure the diversity of sensory experience actually conveyed through the Old English wording. These are only a very few of a vast number of instances where even a small amount of imagination might offer a way to see and understand the texts on their own terms. And, as the extensive work cited in this volume has shown, the field of medieval studies today is moving toward much greater support of such diverse scholarship, something perhaps akin to a biologically 'hybrid zone',¹⁰ now far more ready to engage the diverse body of medical texts with the empathy and imagination they deserve.

It is in this spirit of creative engagement, then, that, rather than a conventional summative conclusion, I want to bring the analyses of the previous chapters together, in a type of final hybridity, with the various threads from previous analyses repeatedly crossing in the hopes of demonstrating wider application of the approach and of identifying core components underlying Old English healing practice and lore. One of the unavoidable limits of the present book is that the close engagement renders any kind of comprehensive treatment impossible. What I want to offer instead is a reading practice that can unlock meanings easily missed in virtually any remedy or medical text. To this end, we'll first look closely at a single brief remedy through the lens of each chapter's approach in turn. Following this up-close strategy, we will then pan back out to examine how the analyses in the preceding chapters intersect with and inform one another.

Small seeds in large fields: locating hybridity in an everyday remedy

Alchemilla vulgaris, the scientific name for lion's foot (also known as lady's mantle) is widespread across Europe today and would have been common in medieval England as well. Its entry in the *Herbarium* is correspondingly ordinary, a brief remedy that is fairly typical within the larger corpus, with rather unremarkable instructions for medicinal use. Yet, if examined closely, an impulse towards diversity and hybridity can be seen in even this most unassuming of early medieval medical texts. To illustrate the intricate connections that become transparent across the medical texts with a hybrid approach, I thus want to employ this unassuming entry for lion's foot, quoted in full below (and formatted to highlight structural and rhetorical patterns), to demonstrate how several of the concepts from previous chapters can effectively draw out new insights and, in some cases, correct long-standing assumptions and misconceptions. As simple as it is, the remedy supports and rewards such close engagement.

    Leonfot[11]
    þeos wyrt þe man pedem leonis 7 oðrum naman leonfot nemneð, heo bið on feldon 7 on dicon 7 on hreodbeddon.
        Hyf hwa on þære untrumnysse sy þæt he sy cis, þonne meaht ðu hine unbindan,
            genim þysse wyrte þe we[12] leonfot nemdon fif ðyfelas butan wyrttruman,
            seoð on wætere on wanwægendum monan

⁊ ðweah hine þærmid
⁊ læd ut of þam huse onforan nihte
⁊ ster hyne mid þære wyrte þe man aristolochiam nemneð,
⁊ þonne he ut ga ne beseo he hyne na onbæc;
þus ðu hine meaht of þære untrumnysse unbindan.

Lionfoot
[This plant which some call *pedem leonis* and others lionfoot, it is known in fields and in ditches and in reed-beds.

If someone is in illness such that he is nauseated,[13] then you might unbind him.
Take five of this plant, which we call lionfoot, except for the roots.
Simmer in water during a waning moon
and wash him with it,
and lead him out of the house in the early night
and cleanse him with the plant which one calls *aristolochia*,
and when he goes out, let him not look back;
thus you might unbind him from the illness.]

To begin, Chapter 1 brought the concepts of biological and cultural hybridity into direct conversation, demonstrating the metaphor's relevance (and limits) beyond the common understanding of 'hybrid' texts as reflective of mere cultural syncretism, and such hybridity underpins virtually every aspect of this simple entry for lion's foot. At even its most literal level, lion's foot manifests the power of hybridity, hybridization having been posited as one of the 'major modes of speciation' for *alchemilla vulgaris*.[14] As adaptive mechanisms, cultural and biological hybridity go hand in hand; transmission and adaptation of the stories and traditions connected to an herb can parallel the biological adaptation of plants in new geographical environments. And as we shall see, the biological hybridity contained within the lion's foot plant itself is indeed mirrored by the culturally hybridized impulse toward diversity exhibited within its brief medical text entry.

Bringing methodologies from archaeology to bear on literary texts, Chapter 2 underscored connections linking the healing tradition to material culture. The plant-names *astula regia* and *sperewyrt* (king's spear and spear-plant respectively), for instance, reflect a very literal understanding of plants as weapons against pain. *Leonfot* can be seen to operate on a similar principle. Based on Latin *pes leonis* and literally meaning 'lion's foot', this is one of many plant names identified as 'hybrid formations' deriving from both English and Latin elements, the Latin *leonis* retained while *pes* is translated into English *fot*.[15] It is quite possible, though, that this name, which could be understood simply as a mnemonic based on the plant's shape, had further significance for an audience sensitive to traditional associations. Archaeological evidence suggests that lions were unsurprisingly understood as generally threatening and dangerous creatures in early medieval England, but they were more specifically employed through a common motif where they were depicted as guardians of hell.[16] The English nomenclature *leonfot* thus implicitly brings into the healing process not only the lion's power but also something of its fearsome and alien nature. As we have seen throughout this volume, the healing tradition frequently incurs risk, drawing power from even those things most feared.

Chapter 3's analysis of *Wið færstice* drew from performance theory and military history to better interpret the poem's grammatical and narrative ambiguities, in particular within its language rendering the tactics of the disease-bearing forces as indistinguishable from those of the healing practitioners. *Wið færstice* offers an especially pronounced reminder that Old English healing was frequently envisioned as a physical battle taking place, where any simple or reductive boundaries at the sites of conquest become blurry at best. Such is the case for *leonfot* as well, albeit in perhaps more subtle ways. For an audience attuned to the lion's liminal status as guardian of dangerous spaces, the portion of the ritual requiring the suffering individual to leave the space where lion's foot has been simmering would take on added dimension, the ritual not only getting the patient to fresh air but also enacting an exit from a threat—away from the plant that carries the potential for both health and danger. The directive to 'ne beseo he hyne na onbæc' ['let him not look back'] then amplifies the sense of danger.[17] Chapter 3 also employed ethnopoetic techniques for editing and translating *Wið færstice*, an approach that can also benefit the lion's foot entry (or, really, any entry). Through the addition of simple line breaks and indentations such as those given above, the introduction on harvesting lion's foot becomes more clearly a component separate from the ritual, which is framed by parallel language, repeating the problem *untrumnysse* ['illness'] and the goal *unbindan* ['to unbind']. Such structuring is obscured by standard conventions in modern print, and I would argue that nearly every remedy might become better understood through this type of ethnopoetic rendering.

Chapter 4's approach of linking rhetoric with oral theory revealed patterns of sentience attributed to healing plants and the deeply collaborative relationship between healer and medicinal herbs. Though the *leonfot* remedy does not prescribe direct speech to this plant, it does employ language implying that such speech has perhaps taken place at some earlier point. Twice the entry reminds the practitioner of the need to 'unbind'. As Tiffany Beechy has observed, 'the act of poetic creation is also described with the lexicon of binding', the spoken word and verbal performance intricately tied to release of ailment.[18] In this construct, words can bind, and words can loose.[19] The possibility that the plant is responsive to the spoken word lends heightened significance to the directive to leave the roots ('butam wyrttruman'), which is not only practical for future use but also demonstrates respect for the plant's continuing life.

Bringing plant philosophy to bear on manuscript variants of the *Herbarium*'s mandrake entry, Chapter 5 argued that the admittedly rare personification seen in the *mandragora* illustrations and verbal descriptions reflects a much more widespread, though subtle, acceptance of plants' agency and subjectivity. Likely named for a lion's paw due to its large lobed leaves, *leonfot* evokes a practical hybrid animal/plant identity.[20] And, as with the mandrake, awareness of this function in facilitating identification and harvesting helps break down false distinctions we have seen between science and so-called superstition. Additionally, in Chapter 5 we saw that between the Cotton Vitellius C.iii and the later Harley 6258B, changes in the *mandragora* entry moved ever so slightly in the direction of what was later to be accepted as objective science. The *leonfot* entry also exhibits that same perspectival shift; while the earlier manuscripts employ the more intimate first person (*we* leonfot nemdon' ['*we* call lion-foot']), the familiar *we* is rendered in the twelfth-century manuscript through the much more detached *Engle* [English]. The patterns represented by the mandrake's hybridity thus embody similar patterns across the tradition more widely.

In Chapter 6, a hybrid methodology drawing from Deaf studies and oral theory exposed long-standing biases that privilege hearing as a default. Far from assuming hearing as a monolithic experience shared by all, the remedies in *Bald's Leechbook* suggest a wide spectrum of auditory possibilities. Close attention to the grammar of the Old English *leonfot* entry in relation to its closest Latin analogue reveals a similar pattern. The oldest extant Latin analogue of the *Herbarium*[21] prescribes *herba leontipodium* (lionfoot) 'si quis devotus defixusque fuerit' ['if one is accursed and fixed'].[22] The adjectives *devotus* and *defixus*, however, are rendered quite differently in the Old English *Herbarium*: 'Hyf hwa on þære untrumnysse sy þæt he sy cis' ['If one is in illness such that he is nauseated']. At the level of syntax, the dative 'untrumnysse' implies not a trait or identity marker of the afflicted individual, but a state that one temporarily inhabits. The Old English therefore conveys an individual as occupying a space '*in* illness' rather than holding an identity as one who is 'ill' or even 'accursed'. Sentence structure matters. But this is not all that is changed. Just as standard translations of *Leechbook* entry I.iii for hearing, discussed in Chapter 6, have often medicalized hearing in a way that stigmatizes deafness, so too have standard modern translations overlooked the literal Old English vocabulary in favor of Latin analogues that mystify and stigmatize illness and pain. In addition to changing the dative in the Old English *leonfot* entry, modern translations also tend to render *cis* as 'being under an evil spell', even though its default definition in both de Vriend's edition of the *Herbarium* and the *Dictionary of Old English* is medical, implying gastrointestinal problems.[23]

In Chapter 7, we saw how the *Anhaga* riddle of the Exeter Book implies the presence of medics and healing herbs in communities, the overlap of domestic and military spheres, and the need to ease suffering from war and battle. These insights, too, resonate powerfully with the *leonfot* entry. As noted above, *leonfot*, is said twice to 'unbind', *unbindan*, language paralleled within the riddle tradition. Much like *Anhaga*, Exeter Book riddle *Holt Hweorfende* links suffering with binding, specifically suffering from battle: the riddle's subject (typically solved as loom or lathe) experiences woe (*weo*, l. 5) from battle-wounds (*heapoglemma*, l. 3) as it is bound fast (*fæste gebunden*, l. 6). In the riddles as in remedies like that for *leonfot*, unbinding is the means by which suffering can be eased. Healing is a force to be unlocked, to unbind in much the same way that a riddle's mystery is solved.

Collectively, these insights emerging from various disciplines and methodologies reveal a remedy far more fraught with meaning and potential healing power than might seem to be the case at first glance. Some aspects of the remedy, such as its requirement that plants be simmered in water specifically during a waning phase of the moon ('wanwægendum monan'), might lead one to dismiss its healing approach. But doing so means overlooking the nature of the remedy as a medical/ritual hybrid. For instance, the prescription to leave the room after inhaling steam from the plant and being bathed with it could serve as a preventive measure against side effects, and even today lion's foot is sometimes recommended for gastrointestinal problems;[24] however, the remedy's practical physical value need not negate the additional possibility of psychological comfort from powerful symbolism. In this ritual, the afflicted individual is called upon to walk out of the enclosed space of suffering, to move literally through and away from adversity, with the hope that suffering will end with the waning moon and that change will arrive with new light.[25]

Again, it is important that we recognize such hybridity as more than just a simple combining or juxtaposition of disparate elements and instead understand the metaphor in terms of its biological reality involving new entities from diverse crossings—new narratives, new poetic forms, new rituals, fundamentally new ways of thinking. But it is equally important to recognize the significance of more common instances of hybridity, the subtle shifts and changes that are sometimes apparent only against the backdrop of more extreme occurrences. Without an acceptance of the hybrid nature of the entire healing tradition—as opposed to the more obvious examples such as the mandrake within that tradition—established misconceptions, unnecessary emendations, and misleading translations might continue to persist unchallenged. In a hybrid reading, the simple *leonfot* becomes more than just a practical medicinal herb; rather it assumes a complex identity as an instrument of both power and danger, a link between Latin and English, a force with the strength to unlock painful bonds, and, most of all, a source of healing hope.

To this point, I have, for the most part, resisted the impulse to draw broad overarching conclusions based on the small selection of remedies treated in these chapters. It is, after all, in the individual instances that meaning is generated rather than the other way around. But here at the close it might perhaps still be generative to think through a few prominent tendencies shared across these early medieval texts, ones that become more readily apparent through the hybrid approaches explored throughout this volume.

Variation, life, and empathy in a hybrid model of healing

As early as Chapter 1 we saw that some of the most problematic elements of the hybridity model are precisely what make the framework most relevant to the study of medieval medical texts in the first place. As useful as it has proven in many ways, the hybridity metaphor remains one that must be approached with the same caution and respect as the powerful remedies themselves. When pushed to its extreme, the metaphor of hybridity exposes the dangers of romanticizing, colonizing tendencies, and reminds us that claims of cultural hybridity can mask a darker cultural appropriation, in biological terms a 'swamping' or even extinction. At the same time, the remedies themselves put on full display a strong belief in the power of a hybridized form of healing, with the medical texts blending, merging, and juxtaposing a vast range of linguistic, generic, cultural, and religious modes of signification. Sites of hybridity are inherently sites of contest, not all traits emerging in any single hybridized form and not all hybrids successful. There is risk. But the underlying logic inherent across the healing texts aims to overcome this risk through the unceasing employment of three specific elements: an openness and flexibility that accommodates variation and change; an aliveness that goes beyond any single practitioner and depends upon a deeply collaborative enterprise of healing belief; and a profound empathy that extends beyond the immediate subject of healing to encompass the plant and material worlds alongside the human, and even enfold the seeming external enemy within one's immediate community. These are the checks and balances offered by a model of hybrid healing.

Variation and variability

Although each chapter of this volume focused on a different text or grouping of remedies and employed a different set of analytical approaches, the importance of variation as a vital element of healing power emerges as a constant. The texts analyzed in Chapter 2 witness medicinal herbs in roles connected simultaneously with battle and healing; and an increased awareness of how such metaphors function, in turn, enabled us to see multiple viable readings of an enigmatic poem for a journey in the margins of CCCC 41, with the encircling *gyrde* evoking a range of senses as plant-shoot, walking stick, or ritual staff. In Chapter 3 variation was evident in terms of mode, the incantation that narrates a battle in *Wið færstice* in effect serving as a verbal variant of the accompanying herbal preparation. And in Chapter 4 we saw variation in speech toward plants, as the plant-persuading incantations of the Harley 585 manuscript's medical texts manifest both Latin and Germanic rhetorical traditions. The manuscript variation across the Harley 6258B and the earlier Cotton Vitellius C.iii noted in Chapter 5 then allowed us to see subtle but meaningful changes in medieval understandings of the mandrake and the healing power it represented, while the remedies of *Bald's Leechbook* discussed in Chapter 6 revealed an openness to variation of ability and sensory experience inherent in the early medieval texts and extending into many aspects of daily life. Finally, in Chapter 7 we found that allowing the Exeter Book's *Anhaga* riddle to draw our attention to a network of variant solutions—shield, cutting board, chopping block, and whetstone—led to a much richer understanding of material culture as reflected in poetry.

Aliveness

The medical texts analyzed across these chapters also reveal an element of vibrancy and aliveness that is not always readily apparent within a modern medical model of healing. *Ic me on þisse gyrde beluce*, examined in Chapter 2, metaphorically transforms material weapons—specifically those that would have been owned and used by the highest social classes—into human gospel authors, and when we accept the more medievally appropriate notion of plants as living beings, the interpretive gap between plant-shoot and rod collapses in this text, as even the speaker becomes akin to an encircled plant, metaphorically harvested into God's own hand. And in the metaphorical battle narrated by *Wið færstice* and investigated in Chapter 3, the practitioner is pitted against causes of pain that are personified as living and formidable foes attacking with weapons comparable to the healer's own, while the plants of the *Lacnunga*'s 'Nine Herbs Charm' and the periwinkle and *ricinum* plants of the Old English *Herbarium*, all discussed in Chapter 4, are alive in the fullest sense, with sentience, subjectivity, and an ability to make choices in how (and if) they will provide healing aid. The remedies for hearing in *Bald's Leechbook*, discussed in Chapter 6, show us a model of hearing much more dynamic than in the modern medical model, one where ears have independent agency, with the ability to deafen, ring, and din, not as a fault but as a matter of course, reflecting the range of possibilities inherent in the faculty of hearing. And of course the mandrake of the Old English *Herbarium*, examined in Chapter 5 and unforgettably illustrated as a plant/human hybrid in the Cotton Vitellius C.iii, is described as a living being with its own subjectivity and its own volition, its own powerful capacity to harm or heal. Nowhere, however, is the trait of aliveness more apparent and profound than in the riddles, such as the *Anhaga* text treated in Chapter 7, where the inanimate speaker and subject—be it a shield, cutting board, chopping block, or whetstone—not only speaks in the first person (as is typical of many riddles) but expresses terribly painful bodily experiences and emotion.

Empathy

Finally, because a hybrid approach allows each individual remedy to be analyzed more fully on its own terms through a combination of methodologies, it correspondingly reveals a consistent capacity for empathy and sensitivity to suffering that is not always readily apparent in broader, more comprehensive treatments of the medical texts collectively. With such perspective, the poem for protection during a journey—inscribed in the margins of CCCC 41—clearly conveys the real and metaphorical dangers facing early medieval travelers while also forging a close connection with the beings called upon for assistance, imagined there in the familiar terms of heroic warriors from the epic tradition. In *Wið færstice*, not only is the individual suffering severe pain met with empathy, but empathy is implicitly directed, too, towards the cause of the pain itself, adversity caused not by monstrous villains but by heroic opponents using weapons forged by able smiths. And we saw that the plants of Harley 585's *Lacnunga* and *Herbarium* are similarly addressed as equals—or even superiors—capable of compassion and understanding; even the mandrake—reputed for centuries as deceptive and dangerous—is portrayed with a degree of empathy, invested with its own fears and desires, particularly its poignant yet ineffectual wish to flee and evade capture. And rather than portraying differences in the faculty of hearing simply as flaws, *Bald's Leechbook* presents a wide and shifting range of hearing experience, a tendency reflected in the period's archaeological record, historical texts, and law codes as well. Lastly, with no healer to be found, the endlessly suffering speaker of the riddle *Anhaga* elicits deep empathy for its trauma, both the pain of endless attacks and also the excruciating loneliness of a solitary warrior.

Collectively these analyses have shown both the payoff and the limits of this close-reading approach, and before closing I want to acknowledge explicitly and directly that this 'conclusion' is in no way conclusive. It would be impossible in any single monograph to treat all of the medieval English medical texts with the same care, and there are many lines of inquiry I wish I could have pursued. For instance, Christina Lee's interdisciplinary work with textiles and medical texts promises fascinating possibilities for future endeavors.[26] And even though much attention was given in these pages to the *Herbarium*, its manuscript companion, the *Medicina de Quadrupedibus* was barely touched upon, even though its treatment of animals offers limitless space for investigating hybridity. Similarly, historical shifts in the early medieval healing tradition as it adapted across the Norman Conquest and even into the Early Modern period offer countless more opportunities for examination of hybridized developments in literature and culture alike. I hope that the ideas and approaches in this book might provide some helpful insights for others in future endeavors as the field continues to grow and reshape itself.

Like the concept of hybridity itself, Old English remedies are frequently the very embodiment of contradiction. Ever amorphous and far from predictable, early medieval medical texts show us a world where the capacity for healing is frequently infused with violence and vice versa; these deeply complex texts confront us with brutality even in the portrayal of medicinal herbs. But at the same time, medicinal remedies, as paradoxical as they are powerful, invite compassion, not only for those suffering but also for less likely recipients—for implements of battle, for bearers of harm, and even for disease itself. Such is the paradox of hybridity with which we first began in Chapter 1. Sometimes hybridity brings other than anticipated results, and of course not every remedy lives up to its promise that 'bið sona sel' ['it will soon be well']. But, at its best, the hybridity of the medical corpus opens up a space for fierce compassion, one in which healing, acceptance, and change have the potential to take root and thrive. In the process, the performance arena of Old English healing becomes one filled with boundless hope and significant risk, but, above all, endless wonder.

Notes

1 Ellard, *Anglo-Saxon(ist) Pasts*, p. 341.
2 *AHD*, s.v. field, sense 1.c; *OED*, s.v. field.
3 'a plot of land', 'specifically of cultivated land', *DOE*, s.v. *æcer*, sense 1.a.
4 Eleanour Sinclair Rohde, *The Old English Herbals* (London: Longmans, Green, and Co., 1922), p. 4.
5 Ibid., p. 4. Though her respect for the healing tradition is admirable, I do not wish to overstate the strengths of Rohde's book. Her desire to connect personally with a 'Saxon' past is deeply problematic at best, and even her most supportive contemporary critic writing in 1925 admitted that her 'pride in the Saxon ancestry has got the best of her'. M. Gaster, Review of *The Old English Herbals* by Eleanour Sinclair Rohde, *Folklore*, 33.4 (1922), 415–420, at 418.

6 On Singer's role 'as the fount of a long tradition', see Hall, *Elves*, p. 6. Particularly influential was his statement for the British Academy, 'Early English Magic and Medicine', *Proceedings of the British Academy*, 9 (1919–20), 341–374. See also Grattan and Singer, *Anglo-Saxon Magic*.

7 Hilary Jenkinson, Review of *The Old English Herbals* by Eleanour Sinclair Rohde, *The English Historical Review*, 38 (1923), 587–588, at 587.

8 G. Sarton, Review of *The Old English Herbals* by Eleanour Sinclair Rohde, *Isis*, 5.2 (1923), 457–461, at 457–458.

9 Ibid., p. 458.

10 As early as the 1940s, biologists had recognized that the landscape itself must be accommodating for the diversification of hybridity to thrive. Edgar Anderson wrote that 'if anything beyond the first generation is to pull through, we must have habitats not only that are intermediate but also that present all possible recombinations of the contrasting differences.... Only by a hybridization of the habitat can the hybrid recombinations be preserved in nature', Edgar Anderson, *Introgressive Hybridization* (New York: John Wylie and Sons, Inc., 1940), p. 17. See further Grant's discussion of hybridized habitats in *Plant Speciation*, p. 201.

11 This header and the text that follows are taken from the Cotton Vitellius C.iii. The Harley 6258B heads the entry with the Latin *Pes Leonis* and indexes the remedy 'Gif man si cis' ['If one is nauseated'] in the marginal gloss.

12 The Harley 6258B replaces 'we' with 'Engle' ['English'].

13 *DOE*, s.v. *cis*: 'fastidious, squeamish (in eating), nauseated'.

14 Syed Mudassir Jeelani, Santosh Kumari, and Raghbir Chand Gupta, 'Meiotic Studies in some Selected Angiosperms from the Kashmir Himalayas', *Journal of Systematics and Evolution*, 50.3 (2012), 244–257, at 251.

15 C. P. Biggam, 'An Introduction to Anglo-Saxon Plant-Name Studies and to this Special Issue', *Leeds Studies in English*, 44 (2013), 1–9, at 6. Cf. Latin/Old English hybrids *cisir-beam* (deriving from Latin *ceras(i) us* ['cherry'] and Old English *beam* ['tree']) and *candel-wyrt* (Latin *candela* ['candle'] and Old English *wyrt* ['plant']). See further Sauer, 'Morphology', p. 171.

16 Catherine Karkov, *Text and Picture in Anglo-Saxon England* (Cambridge University Press, 2001), p. 61.

17 This line could even be seen as evocative of the folkloric motif 'travelers to other world must not look back' seen in such tales as Orpheus

and Eurydice. Motif C331.2 in S. Thompson, *Motif Index of Folk Literature* (Bloomington, IN: Indiana University Press, 1955–58).
18 Beechy, *Poetics*, p. 85.
19 See *DOE*, s. v. *bindan*, sense D.6, which notes that in ecclesiastical use 'binding' is associated with condemnation and 'loosing' with absolution, both of which could involve speech acts.
20 The *DOEPN* gives the etymology as a 'loan translation of L PES LEONIOS referring to the lobed leaves'.
21 MS Vo. eiden, Bibliotheek der Rijksuniversiteit, Vossianus Latinus Q9, as cited in de Vriend, *Old English Herbarium*, p. xlviii. *Leonfot* analogue, p. 53.
22 *Dictionary of Medieval Latin from British Sources*, ed. Richard Ashdowne et al. (London: Oxford University Press for the British Academy, 1975–2013), s.v. *devotus*. 'Accursed' here seems to be an extension of 'devoted', attached against one's will; s.v. *defixus*, translated by some as 'bewitched' or 'enchanted' following the sense of Charlton Thomas's early *Latin Dictionary* (New York: Harpers', 1907), p. 530, sense II.B.2.b.
23 Van Arsdall, for instance, translates *cis* as 'the condition of being under an evil spell', noting that *cis* is offered as an Old English translation of *defixus*, which can be translated as 'bewitched', *Medieval*, p. 151. However, the *DOE* defines *cis* as 'fastidious, squeamish (in eating), nauseated', offering examples from *Bald's Leechbook*. It is also worth noting that Bosworth and Toller define *untrumness* as 'weakness, sickness, illness, infirmity', with no hint of supernatural intervention.
24 E.g., WebMD notes that the tannins in alchemilla (known by many names including lion's foot) 'might help diarrhea' (www.webmd.com/vitamins/ai/ingredientmono-654/alchemilla, accessed 17 August 2021). Grieve's *Modern Herbal* also notes the herb's use in treatments for vomiting and other stomach ailments. M. Grieve, *A Modern Herbal*, vol. 2 (New York: Dover, 1971; orig., 1931), p. 463.
25 Some, such as Sinead Spearing, see remedies connected to the moon's cycle as a form of sympathetic healing, a ritual during a waning moon followed in the hopes that suffering 'would diminish and wane with the lunar cycle', *Old English Remedies* (Barnsley: Pen and Sword History, 2018), p. 44.
26 Christina Lee, 'Threads and Needles: The Use of Textiles for Medical Purposes', in Maren Clegg Hyer and Jill Frederick (eds), *Textiles, Text, Intertext: Essays in Honour of Gale R. Owen-Crocker*, (Woodbridge: Boydell and Brewer, 2016), pp. 103–117.

Bibliography

Acevedo, Eulalia Sosa, 'Exploring Semantic and Syntactic Relations within the Old English Verbs of Hearing', in M. Brito and M. Martín González (eds), *Insights and Bearings: Festschrift for Dr. Juan Sebastián Amador Bedford* (La Laguna: Universidad de La Laguna, 2007), pp. 317–330.

Adams, J. N., and Marilyn Deegan, 'Bald's "Leechbook" and the "Physica Plinii"', *Anglo-Saxon England*, 21 (1992), 87–114.

Alexander, Michael, *A History of Old English Literature* (Peterborough, ON: Broadview Press, 2002).

American Heritage Dictionary (AHD), ed. Joseph P. Pickett et al. (Boston: Houghton Mifflin Harcourt, 5th edn, 2011).

Ammons, Matthias, '"Ge mid wedde ge mid aðe": The Functions of Oath and Pledge in Anglo-Saxon Legal Culture', *Historical Research*, 86 (2013), 515–535.

Amodio, Mark C. (ed.), *John Miles Foley's World of Oralities: Text, Tradition, and Contemporary Oral Theory* (Leeds: ARC Humanities Press, 2020).

Amodio, Mark C., *Writing the Oral Tradition: Oral Poetics and Literate Culture in Medieval England* (Notre Dame, IN: University of Notre Dame Press, 2004).

Anderson, Edgar, *Introgressive Hybridization* (New York: John Wylie and Sons, Inc., 1940).

Applequist, Wendy L., and Daniel E. Moerman, 'Yarrow (*Achillea millefolium* L.): A Neglected Panacea? A Review of Ethnobotany, Bioactivity, and Biomedical Research', *Economic Botany*, 65 (2011), 209–225.

Arnovick, Leslie K., *Written Reliquaries: The Resonance of Orality in Medieval English Texts* (Philadelphia, PA: John Benjamins Publishing, 2006).

Arthur, Ciaran, *'Charms', Liturgies, and Secret Rites in Early Medieval England* (Woodbridge: Boydell Press, 2018).

Arthur, Ciaran, 'Ploughing through Cotton Caligula A. VII: Reading the Sacred Words of the "Heliand" and the "Æcerbot"', *Review of English Studies*, 65 (2014), 1–17.

Ashcroft, Bill, Gareth Griffiths, and Helen Tiffin, *Post-Colonial Studies: The Key Concepts* (London: Routledge, 2000).

Attebery, Brian, *Stories about Stories: Fantasy and the Remaking of Myth* (Oxford: Oxford University Press, 2014).

Attenborough, F. L. (ed. and trans.), *The Laws of the Earliest English Kings* (New York: Russell and Russell, Inc., 1963).

Bakhtin, M. M., *The Dialogic Imagination: Four Essays*, ed. Michael Holquist, trans. Caryl Emerson and Michael Holquist (Austin, TX: University of Texas Press, 1982).

Banham, Debby, 'England Joins the Medical Mainstream: New Texts in Eleventh-Century Manuscripts', in Hans Sauer and Joanna Story (eds), *Anglo-Saxon England and the Continent*. MRTS Essays in Anglo-Saxon Studies, 3. Tempe: ACMRS (2011), 341–350.

Banham, Debby, 'A Millennium in Medicine? New Medical Texts and Ideas in England in the Eleventh Century', in Simon Keynes and Alfred P. Smyth (eds), *Anglo-Saxons: Studies Presented to Cyril Roy Hart* (Dublin: Four Courts Press, 2006), pp. 230–242.

Banham, Debby, and Rosamond Faith, *Anglo-Saxon Farms and Farming* (Oxford: Oxford University Press, 2014).

Baranwal, Vinay Kumar et al., 'Heterosis: Emerging Ideas about Hybrid Vigour', *Journal of Experimental Botany*, 63.18 (2012), 6309–6314.

Barley, Nigel F, 'Structural Aspects of the Anglo-Saxon Riddle', *Semiotica*, 10 (1974), 143–175.

Barley, Nigel F, 'Two Anglo-Saxon Sign Systems Compared', *Semiotica*, 12 (1974), 227–237.

Batten, Caroline, and Mark Williams, '*Erce* in the Old English *Æcerbot* Charm: An Irish Solution', *Notes and Queries*, 67.2 (2020), 168–172.

Bauman, H-Dirksen, 'Introduction: Listening to Deaf Studies', in H-Dirksen L. Bauman (ed.), *Open Your Eyes: Deaf Studies Talking* (Minneapolis, MN: University of Minnesota Press, 2008), pp. 1–34.

Bauman, H-Dirksen L., and Joseph M. Murray (eds), *Deaf Gain: Raising the Stakes for Human Diversity* (Minneapolis, MN: University of Minnesota Press, 2014).

Bede, *Libri II De Arte Metrica et De Schematibus et Tropis: The Art of Poetry and Rhetoric*, ed. and trans. Calvin B. Kendall (Saarbrücken: AQ-Verlag, 1991).

Beechy, Tiffany, *The Poetics of Old English* (Burlington, VT: Ashgate Publishing, 2010).

Berberich, Hugo, *Das Herbarium Apuleii nach einer früh-mittelenglischen Fassung* (Heidelberg: Carl Winter's Universitätsbuchhandlung, 1902).

Berenbaum, May R., *The Earwig's Tail: A Modern Bestiary of Multi-Legged Legends* (Cambridge, MA: Harvard University Press, 2009).

Bhabha, Homi, *The Location of Culture* (London: Routledge, 1994).

Biggam, C. P., 'An Introduction to Anglo-Saxon Plant-Name Studies and to this Special Issue', *Leeds Studies in English*, 44 (2013), pp. 1–9.

Birchler, James et al., 'Heterosis', *The Plant Cell*, 22 (2010), 2105–2112.

Birchler, James A., Hong Yao, and Sivanandan Chudalayandi, 'Unraveling the Genetic Basis of Hybrid Vigor', *Proceedings of the National Academy of Sciences in the United States of America, [PNAS]*, 103.35 (2006), 12957–12958.

Bishop, Louise, M., *Words, Stones, and Herbs: The Healing Word in Medieval and Early Modern England* (Syracuse: Syracuse University Press, 2007).

Bitterli, Dieter, *Say What I am Called: The Old English Riddles of the Exeter Book and the Anglo-Latin Riddle Tradition* (Toronto: University of Toronto Press, 2009).

Bjork, Robert (ed. and trans.), *Old English Shorter Poems, Vol. II: Wisdom and Lyric*. Dumbarton Oaks Medieval Library 32. (Cambridge, MA: Harvard University Press, 2014).

Bliss, A. J., 'Single-Half-Lines in Old English Poetry', *Notes and Queries*, 18.12 (1971), 442–449.

Bowden, H. S. (ed.), *Miniature Lives of Saints*, vol. 2 (London: Burns and Oates, 2nd edn, 1877).

Bosworth, Joseph, *An Anglo-Saxon Dictionary*, ed. and enlarged T. Northcote Toller (Oxford: Oxford University Press, 1898; suppl. 1921). Online edition available at www.bosworthtoller.com. Accessed 1 July 2021.

Bradley, S. A. J. (ed. and trans.), *Anglo-Saxon Poetry* (London: J. M. Dent, 1982).

Bradshaw, Paul, 'Difficulties in Doing Liturgical Theology', *Pacifica*, 11 (1998), 181–194.

Brady, Lindy, *Writing the Welsh Borderlands in Anglo-Saxon England* (Manchester: Manchester University Press, 2019).

Bragg, Lois, 'The Modes of the Old English Metrical Charms', *Comparatist*, 16 (1992), 3–23.

Bragg, Lois, 'Visual-Kinetic Communication in Europe Before 1600: A Survey of Sign Lexicons and Finger Alphabets Prior to the Rise of Deaf Education', *Journal of Deaf Studies and Deaf Education*, 2 (1997), 1–25.

Brooks, Nicholas, 'Arms and Armour', in M. Lapidge, J. Blair, and D. Scragg (eds), *The Blackwell Encyclopedia of Anglo-Saxon England* (Oxford: Blackwell Publishers, 1999), pp. 45–47.

Brooks, Nicholas, 'Weapons and Armour', in Donald Scragg (ed.), *The Battle of Maldon, A.D. 991* (Oxford: Basil Blackwell, in association with the Manchester Centre for Anglo-Saxon Studies, 1991), pp. 208–219.

Bruce, Scott G., *Silence and Sign Language in Medieval Monasticism: The Cluniac Tradition*, c. *900–1200* (Cambridge: Cambridge University Press, 2010).
Brueggemann, Brenda Jo, *Deaf Subjects: Between Identities and Places* (New York: New York University Press, 2009).
Brueggemann, Brenda Jo, *Lend Me Your Ear: Rhetorical Constructions of Deafness* (Washington, DC: Gallaudet University Press, 1999).
Burdorff, Sara Frances, 'Re-Reading Grendel's Mother: *Beowulf* and the Anglo-Saxon Metrical Charms', *Comitatus: A Journal of Medieval and Renaissance Studies*, 45 (2014), 91–103.
Camargo, Martin, 'Defining Medieval Rhetoric', in Constant J. Mews, Cary J. Nederman, and Rodney M. Thomson (eds), *Rhetoric and Renewal in the Latin West 1100–1540*. Disputatio 2. (Turnhout: Brepols, 2007), pp. 21–34.
Camargo, Martin (ed. and intro.), *Poetria Nova*, by Geoffrey of Vinsauf, trans. Margaret F. Nims (Toronto: Pontifical Institute of Mediaeval Studies, rev. edn, 2010).
Cameron, M. L, *Anglo-Saxon Medicine* (Cambridge: Cambridge University Press, 1993).
Cameron, M. L. 'Bald's "Leechbook" and Cultural Interactions in Anglo-Saxon England', *Anglo-Saxon England*, 19 (1990), 5–12.
Campbell, Jackson J., 'Learned Rhetoric in Old English Poetry', *Modern Philology*, 63 (1966), 189–201.
Campbell, Jackson J., 'Rhetoric in Old English Literature: Adaptation of Classical Rhetoric in Old English Literature', in James J. Murphy (ed.), *Medieval Eloquence: Studies in the Theory and Practice of Medieval Rhetoric* (Berkeley, CA: University of California Press, 1978), pp. 173–197.
Caplan, Harry (ed. and trans.), *Rhetorica ad Herennium*, LCL 403 (Cambridge, MA: Harvard University Press, 1954).
Cavell, Megan, 'Powerful Patens in the Anglo-Saxon Medical Tradition and Exeter Book Riddle 48', *Neophilologus*, 101 (2017), 129–138.
Cech, Richo, 'Growing Mandrake—Beyond the Basics', https://blog.strictlymedicinalseeds.com/growing-mandrake-beyond-the-basics/. Accessed 26 July 2021.
Chen, Z. Jeffrey, 'Molecular Mechanisms of Polyploidy and Hybrid Vigor', *Trans Plant Sci.*, 15.2 (2010), 57–71.
Chickering, Howell, 'The Literary Magic of *Wið Færstice*', *Viator*, 2 (1971), 83–104.
Clair, Colin, *Of Herbs and Spices* (London: Abelard, 1961).
Clayton, Mary, and Hugh Magennis (eds), *The Old English Lives of St. Margaret* (Cambridge: Cambridge University Press, 1994).
Clemoes, Peter, *Interactions of Thought and Language in Old English Poetry* (Cambridge: Cambridge University Press, 1995).

Cockayne, Emily, 'Experiences of the Deaf in Early Modern England', *The Historical Journal*, 46 (2003), 493–510.

Cockayne, Thomas Oswald (ed.), *Leechdoms, Wortcunning, and Starcraft of Early England*, 3 vols (London: Rerum Britannicarum Medii Aevi Scriptores, 1864–66. Reprint 1965).

Cohen, Jeffrey Jerome (ed.), *Animal, Vegetable, Mineral: Ethics and Objects* (Santa Barbara, CA: Punctum Books, 2012).

Cohen, Jeffrey Jerome, *Hybridity, Identity, and Monstrosity in Medieval Britain: On Difficult Middles* (New York: Palgrave Macmillan, 2006).

Cohen, Sidney, L. 'The Sutton Hoo Whetstone', *Speculum*, 41 (1966), 466–470.

Colebrook, Claire, *Death of the Posthuman. Essays on Extinction*, vol. 1, Critical Climate Change series (London: Open Humanities Press, 2014).

Colgrave, Bertram, and R. A. B. Mynors (eds), *Bede's* Ecclesiastical History, Oxford Medieval Texts (Oxford: Clarendon Press, 1969).

Conrad, David C. (trans.), *Sunjata: A West African Epic of the Mande Peoples*, narrated by Djanka Tassey Condé (Indianapolis: Hackett Publishing Company, 2014).

Crossley-Holland, Kevin (trans), *The Anglo-Saxon World* (Oxford: Oxford University Press, 2009).

Crow, James F., '90 Years Ago: The Beginning of Hybrid Maize', *Genetics*, 148 (1998), 923–928.

Dalby, Gwen, Keith Manchester, and Charlotte A. Roberts, 'Otosclerosis and Stapedial Footplate Fixation in Archaeological Material', *International Journal of Osteoarchaeology*, 3 (1993), 207–212.

Dale, Corinne, *The Natural World in the Exeter Book Riddles* (Woodbridge: D. S. Brewer, 2017).

D'Aronco, Maria Amalia, 'Anglo-Saxon Medical and Botanical Texts, Glosses and Glossaries after the Norman Conquest: Continuations and Beginnings. An Overview', in Patrizia Lendinara, Loredana Lazzari, and Claudia Di Sciacca (eds), *Rethinking and Recontextualizing Glosses: New Perspectives in the Study of Late Anglo-Saxon Glossography* (Turnhout: Brepols, 2012), pp. 228–248.

D'Aronco, Maria Amalia, 'Anglo-Saxon Plant Pharmacy and the Latin Medical Tradition', in C. P. Biggam (ed.), *From Earth to Art: The Many Aspects of the Plant-World in Anglo-Saxon England* (Amsterdam and New York: Rodopi, 2003), pp. 133–151.

D'Aronco, Maria Amalia, 'Gardens on Vellum: Plants and Herbs in Anglo-Saxon Manuscripts', in Peter Dendle and Alain Touwaide (eds), *Health and Healing from the Medieval Garden* (Woodbridge: Boydell Press, 2008), pp. 101–127.

Darwin, Charles, *The Effects of Cross and Self Fertilisation in the Vegetable Kingdom* (London: John Murray, 1876).

Darwin, Charles, *Life and Letters of Charles Darwin*, vol. 2, ed. Francis Darwin (London: John Murray, 1887).

Davis, Lennard J, *Enforcing Normalcy: Disability, Deafness, and the Body* (London: New Left Books, 1995).

Delanty, Greg, and Michael Matto (eds), *The Word Exchange: Anglo-Saxon Poems in Translation* (New York: Norton, 2012).

Demaitre, Luke E., 'The Art and Science of Prognostication in Early University Medicine', *Bulletin of the History of Medicine*, 77 (2003), 765–788.

Dendle, Peter, 'Plants in the Early Medieval Cosmos: Herbs, Divine Potency, and the *Scala natura*', in Peter Dendle and Alain Touwaide (eds), *Health and Healing from the Medieval Garden* (Woodbridge: Boydell Press, 2008), 47–59.

de Saint-Loup, Aude, 'A History of Misunderstandings: The History of the Deaf', *Diogenes*, 44 (1996), 1–26.

de Vriend, Hubert Jan (ed.), *The Old English Herbarium and Medicina de Quadrupedibus* (Oxford: Oxford University Press, 1984).

Dictionary of Medieval Latin from British Sources, ed. Richard Ashdowne et al. (London: Oxford University Press for the British Academy, 1975–2013).

Dictionary of Old English (DOE), ed. Antonette diPaolo Healey et al., Pontifical Institute of Mediaeval Studies, online edition, http://doe.utoronto.ca. Accessed 15 July 2021.

Dictionary of Old English Plant Names (DOEPN), ed. Peter Bierbaumer and Hans Sauer with Helmut W. Klug and Ulrike Krischke. 2007–2009. http://oldenglish-plantnames.org. Accessed 15 July 2021.

Discenza, Nicole Guenther, *Inhabited Spaces: Anglo-Saxon Constructions of Place* (Toronto: University of Toronto Press, 2017).

Doane, A. N, 'Editing Old English Oral/Written Texts: Problems of Method (With an Illustrated Edition of Charm 4, *Wiþ Færstice*)', in Donald G. Scragg and Paul E. Szarmach (eds), *The Editing of Old English: Papers from the 1990 Manchester Conference* (Cambridge: D. S. Brewer, 1994), pp. 125–145.

Dobbie, Elliott Van Kirk (ed.), *The Anglo-Saxon Minor Poems*. Anglo-Saxon Poetic Records, vol. 6 (New York: Columbia University Press, 1942).

Donoghue, Daniel, *How the Anglo-Saxons Read Their Poems* (Philadelphia, PA: University of Pennsylvania Press, 2018).

Doskow, Minna, 'Poetic Structure and the Problem of the Smiths in *Wið Færstice*', *Papers on Language and Literature*, 12 (1979), 321–326.

Doyle, Conan (ed.), *Anglo-Saxon Medicine and Disease: A Semantic Approach*, 2 vols (doctoral thesis, University of Cambridge, 2017).

Drinkall, G., and M. Foreman, *The Anglo-Saxon Cemetery at Castledyke South, Barton-on-Humber. Sheffield Excavation Reports*, vol. 6 (Sheffield: Sheffield Academic Press, 1998).

Drout, Michael, *Tradition and Influence in Anglo-Saxon Literature: An Evolutionary, Cognitivist Approach* (London: Palgrave Macmillan, 2013).

Duckert, Audrey, 'Erce and Other Possibly Keltic Elements in the Old English Charm for Unfruitful Land', *Names*, 20.2 (1972), 83–90.

Dumitrescu, Irina A., 'Bede's Liberation Philology: Releasing the English Tongue', *PMLA*, 128 (2013), 40–56.

Einarsson, Stefán, 'Old English *Beot* and Old Icelandic *Heitstrenging*', *PMLA*, 49 (1934), 975–993.

Ellard, Donna Beth, *Anglo-Saxon(ist) Pasts, postSaxon Futures* (Santa Barbara, CA: Punctum Books, 2019).

Esposito, Anthony, 'Medieval Plant-Names in the *Oxford English Dictionary*', in C. P. Biggam (ed.), *From Earth to Art: The Many Aspects of the Plant-World in Anglo-Saxon England* (Amsterdam and New York: Rodopi, 2003), pp. 231–248.

Evison, Vera I., 'Pagan Saxon Whetstones', *The Antiquaries Journal*, 55 (1975), 70–85.

Fabian, Johannes, *Anthropology with an Attitude: Critical Essays* (Stanford, CA: Stanford University Press, 2001).

Faivre, Bruno et al., 'Morphological Variation and the Recent Evolution of Wing Length in the Icterine Warbler: A Case of Unidirectional Introgression?', *Journal of Avian Biology*, 30.2 (1999), 152–158.

Fay, Jacqueline, 'The Farmacy: Wild and Cultivated Plants in Early Medieval England', *ISLE: Interdisciplinary Studies in Literature and Environment*, 28.1 (2021), 186–206.

Foley, John Miles, 'Genre(s) in the Making: Diction, Audience and Text in the Old English *Seafarer*', *Poetics Today*, 4.4 (1983), 683–706.

Foley, John Miles, 'How Genres Leak in Traditional Verse', in Mark C. Amodio and Katherine O'Brien O'Keeffe (eds), *Unlocking the Wordhord* (Toronto: University of Toronto Press, 2003), 76–108.

Foley, John Miles, *How to Read an Oral Poem* (Urbana, IL: University of Illinois Press, 2002).

Foley, John Miles, 'Hybrid Prosody and Single Half-lines in Old English and Serbo-Croatian Poetry', *Neophilologus*, 64 (1990), 284–289.

Foley, John Miles, *Immanent Art: From Structure to Meaning in Traditional Oral Epic* (Bloomington, IN: Indiana University Press, 1991).

Foley, John Miles, 'Læcedom and Bajanje: A Comparative Study of Old English and Serbo-Croatian Charms', *Centerpoint*, 4 (1981), 33–41.

Foley, John Miles, *Oral Tradition and the Internet: Pathways of the Mind* (Urbana, IL: University of Illinois Press, 2012).

Foley, John Miles, *The Singer of Tales in Performance* (Bloomington, IN: Indiana University Press, 1995).

Foley, John Miles, *Traditional Oral Epic: The Odyssey, Beowulf, and the Serbo-Croatian Return Song* (Berkeley, CA: University of California Press, 1993).
Foley, John Miles (ed. and trans.) *The Wedding of Mustajbey's Son Bećirbey as performed by Halil Bajgorić*, Folklore Fellows Communications 283 (Helsinki: Academia Scientiarum Fennica, 2004).
Foys, Martin K., 'A Sensual Philology for Anglo-Saxon England', *postmedieval: a journal of medieval cultural studies*, 5 (2014), 456–472.
Frye, Northrop, *Spiritus Mundi: Essays on Literature, Myth, and Society* (Bloomington, IN: Indiana University Press, 1976).
Fulk, R. D., Robert E. Bjork, and John D. Niles, *Klaeber's* Beowulf (Toronto: University of Toronto Press, 4th edn, 2008).
Gale, David A., 'The Seax', in Sonia Chadwick Hawkes (ed.), *Weapons and Warfare in Anglo-Saxon England* (Oxford: Oxford University Committee for Archaeology, 1989), pp. 71–84.
Garner, Lori Ann, 'Deaf Studies, Oral Tradition, and Old English Texts', *Exemplaria*, 29.1 (2017), 21–40.
Garner, Lori Ann, 'Medieval Voices', *Oral Tradition*, 18.2 (2003), 216–218.
Garner, Lori Ann, 'Rhetoric and Remedies; or, How to Persuade a Plant in Anglo-Saxon England', in Georgiana Donovan and Denise Stodola (eds), *Public Declamations: Essays on Medieval Rhetoric, Education, and Letters in Honor of Martin Camargo* (Turnhout: Brepols, 2015), pp. 155–168.
Garner, Lori Ann, and Kayla M. Miller, '"A Swarm in July": Beekeeping Perspectives on the Old English *Wið Ymbe* Charm', *Oral Tradition*, 26.2 (2012), 355–376.
Garner, R. Scott, 'Annotated Bibliography of Works by John Miles Foley', Special Issue: Festschrift for John Miles Foley, *Oral Tradition*, 26.2 (2011), 677–724.
Gaster, M., Review of *The Old English Herbals* by Eleanour Sinclair Rohde, *Folklore*, 33.4 (1922), 415–420.
Gertz, Genie, and Patrick Boudreault (eds), *The Sage Deaf Studies Encyclopedia* (Los Angeles: Sage, 2016).
Glickman, Neil, 'The Development of Culturally Deaf Identities', in Neil S. Glickman and Michael A. Harvey (eds), *Culturally Affirmative Psychotherapy with Deaf Persons* (New York: Routledge, 1996), pp. 115–154.
Glosecki, Stephen O., *Shamanism and Old English Poetry*, Albert Bates Lord Studies in Oral Tradition 2 (Shrewsbury, MA: Garland, 1989).
Glosecki, Stephen O., 'Wolf of the Bees: Germanic Shamanism and the Bear Hero', *Journal of Ritual Studies*, 2.1 (1988), 31–53.
Gordon, R. K., *Anglo-Saxon Poetry* (London: Everyman, 1954).

Grant, Verne, *Plant Speciation* (New York: Columbia University Press, 2nd edn, 1981).

Grattan, J. H., and Charles Singer, *Anglo-Saxon Magic and Medicine* (Oxford: Oxford University Press, 1952).

Grendon, Felix (ed. and trans.), 'The Anglo-Saxon Charms', *Journal of American Folklore*, 22 (1909), 105–237.

Grieve, M., *A Modern Herbal*, vol. 2 (New York: Dover, 1971; orig., 1931).

Griffiths, Bill, *Aspects of Anglo-Saxon Magic* (Norfolk: Anglo-Saxon Books, 1996).

Grimm, J., *Deutsche Mythologie* (Berlin: F. Dümmler, 1875).

Gunther, Robert T. (ed.), *The Greek Herbal of Dioscorides* (New York: Hafner Publishing, 1968).

Hadley, D. M., 'Social and Physical Difference in and beyond the Anglo-Saxon Churchyard', in J. Buckberry and A. Cherryson (eds), *Burial in Later Anglo-Saxon England* (Oxford: Oxbow Books, 2010), pp. 101–113.

Hall, Alaric, *Elves in Anglo-Saxon England: Matters of Belief, Health, Gender, and Identity* (Woodbridge: Boydell Press, 2007).

Hall, Matthew, *Plants as Persons: A Philosophical Botany* (New York: SUNY Press, 2011).

Halpern, Barbara Kerewsky, and John Miles Foley, 'The Power of the Word: Healing Charms as an Oral Genre', *Journal of American Folklore*, 92 (1978), 903–924.

Hamerow, Helena et al., 'Feeding Anglo-Saxon England: The Bioarchaeology of an Agricultural Revolution', *Antiquity*, 93 (2019), 1–4.

Härke, Heinrich, 'Circulation of Weapons in Anglo-Saxon Society', in Frans Theuws and Janet L. Nelson (eds), *Rituals of Power*, ed. (Leiden: Brill, 2000), pp. 377–399.

Härke, Heinrich, 'Early Saxon Weapon Burials: Frequencies, Distributions and Weapon Combinations', in Sonia Chadwick Hawkes (ed.), *Weapons and Warfare in Anglo-Saxon England* (Oxford: Oxford University Committee for Archaeology, 1989), 49–61.

Härke, Heinrich, '"Warrior Graves"? The Background of the Anglo-Saxon Weapon Burial Rite', *Past and Present*, 126 (1990), 22–43.

Harmon, Kristen, 'Addressing Deafness: From Hearing Loss to Deaf Gain', *Profession* (Modern Language Association, 2010), 124–130.

Harmon, Kristen, '"If there are Greek epics, there should be Deaf epics": How Protest Became Poetry', in H-Dirksen L. Bauman, Jennifer L. Nelson, and Heidi M. Rose (eds), *Signing the Body Poetic: Essays on American Sign Language Literature* (Berkeley, CA: University of California Press, 2006), pp. 169–194.

Haycock, Dean A., Zenobia C. Cofer, and Emily Jane Willingham, 'Dissociative Fugue', in Brigham Narins (ed), *The Gale Encyclopedia of*

Mental Health, vol. 2 (Farmington Hills, MI: Gale Publishing, 4th edn, 2019).

Heaney, Seamus (trans.), *Beowulf* (London: Faber and Faber, 2000).

Hegarty, Matthew J., and Simon J. Hiscock, 'Hybrid Speciation in Plants: New Insights from Molecular Studies', *New Phytologist*, 165.2 (2004), 411–423.

Henvey, Megan, 'Crossing Borders: Re-Assessing the "Need to Group" the High Crosses in Ireland', in Cynthia Thickpenny, Katherine Forsyth, J. Geddes, and Kate Mathis (eds), *Peopling Insular Art: Practice, Performance, Perception: Proceedings of the Eighth International Conference on Insular Art, Glasgow 2017* (Oxford: Oxbow Books, 2020), pp. 179–187.

Hermann, John P., *Allegories of War: Language and Violence in Old English Poetry* (Ann Arbor, MI: University of Michigan Press, 1989).

Hill, Thomas D., 'The "Æcerbot" Charm and its Christian User', *Anglo-Saxon England*, 6 (1977), 213–221.

Hill, Thomas D., 'Invocation of the Trinity and the Tradition of the Lorica in Old English Poetry', *Speculum*, 56 (1981), 259–267.

Hill, Thomas D., 'The Rod of Protection and the Witches' Ride: Christian and Germanic Syncretism in Two Old English Metrical Charms', *Journal of English and Germanic Philology*, 111 (2012), 145–168.

Hines, John, 'The Military Context of *Adventus Saxonum*: Some Continental Evidence', in Sonia Chadwick Hawkes (ed.), *Weapons and Warfare in Anglo-Saxon England* (Oxford: Oxford University Committee for Archaeology, 1989), pp. 25–48.

Holcomb, Thomas K., *Introduction to American Deaf Culture* (Oxford: Oxford University Press, 2013).

Hollis, Stephanie, 'Anglo-Saxon Secular Learning and the Vernacular: An Overview', in László Sándor Chardonnens and Bryan Carella [who now publishes under the name Kristen Carella] (eds), *Secular Learning in Anglo-Saxon England* (Amsterdam: Rodopi, 2012), pp. 1–43.

Holthausen, F., 'Zu Altenglischen Dichtungen', *Beiblatt zur Anglia XXXI*, 31 (1920), 25–32.

Hudson, Martyn, *Visualizing Worlds: World Making and Social Theory* (Abingdon and New York: Taylor and Francis, 2021).

Hunger, Friedrich Wilhelm (ed.), *The Herbal of Pseudo-Apuleius from the ninth-century manuscript in the abbey of Monte Cassino (Codex Casinensis 97) together with the first printed edition of Joh. Phil. de Lignamine (Editio princeps Romae 1481)* (Leiden: Brill, 1935).

Hymes, Del, *'In vain I tried to tell you': Essays in Native American Ethnopoetics*, with new preface by the author (Lincoln, NE: University of Nebraska Press, 2004. Orig. publ. 1981).

Irving, Edward B., 'Heroic Experience in Old English Riddles', in Katherine O'Brien O'Keeffe (ed.), *The Old English Shorter Poems: Basic Readings* (New York: Garland), 199–212.

Jeelani, Syed Mudassir, Santosh Kumari, and Raghbir Chand Gupta, 'Meiotic Studies in some Selected Angiosperms from the Kashmir Himalayas', *Journal of Systematics and Evolution*, 50.3 (2012), 244–257.

Jenkinson, Hilary, Review of *The Old English Herbals* by Eleanour Sinclair Rohde, *The English Historical Review*, 38 (1923), 587–588.

Jolly, Karen Louise, 'On the Margins of Orthodoxy: Devotional Formulas and Protective Prayers in Cambridge, Corpus Christi College MS 41', in Sarah Larratt Keefer and Rolf H. Bremmer, Jr. (eds), *Signs on the Edge: Space, Text and Margin in Medieval Manuscripts* (Leuven: Peeters, 2007), pp. 135–183.

Jolly, Karen Louise, *Popular Religion in Late Saxon England: Elf Charms in Context* (Chapel Hill, NC: University of North Carolina Press, 1996).

Jolly, Karen Louise, 'Prayers from the Field: Practical Protection and Demonic Defense in Anglo-Saxon England', *Traditio*, 61 (2006), 95–147.

Jones, Peter Murray (ed.), *Medicina Antiqua* (London: Harvey Miller Publishers, 1999).

Josephus, *Works*, trans. William Whiston (London, 1737), http://penelope.uchicago.edu/josephus/. Accessed 18 July 2021.

Kapchan, Deborah A., and Pauline Turner Strong, 'Theorizing the Hybrid', *Journal of American Folklore*, 112 (1999), 239–253.

Kaplan, Zdenek, and Judith Fehrer, 'Molecular Evidence for a Natural Primary Triple Hybrid in Plants Revealed from Direct Sequencing', *Annals of Botany*, 99 (2007), 1213–1222.

Karkov, Catherine, *Text and Picture in Anglo-Saxon England* (Cambridge: Cambridge University Press, 2001),

Karshner, Edward, 'Thought, Utterance, Power: Toward a Rhetoric of Magic', *Philosophy and Rhetoric*, 44 (2011), 52–71.

Katzman, Shoshanna, *Qigong for Staying Young* (New York: Penguin, 2003).

Keefer, Sarah Larratt, 'Margin as Archive: The Liturgical Marginalia of a Manuscript of the Old English Bede', *Traditio*, 51 (1996), 147–177.

Keefer, Sarah Larratt, 'Ðonne se cirlisca man ordales weddigeð: The Anglo-Saxon Lay Ordeal', in Stephen Baxter, Catherine Karkov, Janet L. Nelson, and David Pelteret (eds), *Early Medieval Studies in Memory of Patrick Wormald* (London: Ashgate, 2009), pp. 353–367.

Ker, Neil R., *Catalogue of Manuscripts Containing Anglo-Saxon* (Oxford: Clarendon Press, 1957).

Kesling, Emily, *Medical Texts in Anglo-Saxon Literary Culture* (Woodbridge: D. S. Brewer, 2020).
Kiernan, Kevin, *Electronic Beowulf 4.0* (2015), http://ebeowulf.uky.edu/ebeo4.0/CD/main.html. Accessed 4 August 2021.
Kinoshita, Sharon (trans.), *Marco Polo: The Description of the World* (Cambridge: Hackett Publishing, 2016).
Kinoshita, Sharon, 'Traveling Texts: De-Orientalizing Marco Polo's *Le Devisement du monde*', in Gesa Mackenthun, Andrea Nicolas, and Stephanie Wodianka (eds), *Travel, Agency, and the Circulation of Knowledge* (Waldkirchen: Waxmann, 2017), pp. 223–246.
Klaeber, Fr., '*Belucan* in dem altenglischen Reisesegen', *Beiblatt zur Anglia*, 40 (1929), 283–284.
Klinck, Anne, *The Old English Elegies: A Critical Edition and Genre Study* (Montreal: McGill-Queen's University Press, 1992).
Knappe, Gabriele, 'Classical Rhetoric in Anglo-Saxon England', *Anglo-Saxon England*, 27 (1998), 5–29.
Knoepflmacher, U. C., 'Editor's Preface: Hybrid Forms and Cultural Anxiety', *Studies in English Literature: 1500–1900*, 48.4 (2008), 745–754.
Koutserimpas, Christos, Kalliopi Alpantaki, and George Samonis, 'Trauma Management in Homer's *Iliad*', *International Wound Journal*, 14.4 (2017), 682–684.
Kramer, Johanna, *Between Earth and Heaven: Liminality and the Ascension of Christ in Anglo-Saxon Literature* (Manchester: Manchester University Press, 2014).
Krapp, George Philip (ed.), *The Vercelli Book*. The Anglo-Saxon Poetic Records, vol. 2 (New York: Columbia University Press, 1932).
Krapp, George Philip, and Elliott Van Kirk Dobbie (eds), *The Exeter Book*. The Anglo-Saxon Poetic Records, vol. 3 (New York: Columbia University Press, 1936).
Krentz, Christopher B., 'The Camera as Printing Press: How Film Has Influenced ASL Literature', in H-Dirksen L. Bauman, Jennifer L. Nelson, and Heidi M. Rose (eds), *Signing the Body Poetic: Essays on American Sign Language Literature* (Berkeley, CA: University of California Press, 2006), pp. 51–70.
Krentz, Christopher, *Writing Deafness: The Hearing Line in Nineteenth-Century American Literature* (Chapel Hill, NC: University of North Carolina Press, 2012).
Laes, Christian, 'Silent Witnesses: Deaf-Mutes in Graeco-Roman Antiquity', *Classical World*, 104 (2011), 451–473.
Lang-Roth, Ruth, 'Hearing Impairment and Language Delay in Infants: Diagnostics and Genetics', *GMS Current Topics in Otorhinolaryngology, Head and Neck Surgery*, 13 (2014), https://doi.org/10.3205/cto000108.

Lapidge, Michael, and Michael Herren (eds), *Aldhelm: The Prose Works* (Woodbridge: D. S. Brewer, 1979).

Leahy, Kevin, 'Anglo-Saxon Crafts', in Helena Hamerow, David A. Hinton, and Sally Crawford (eds), *The Oxford Handbook of Anglo-Saxon Archaeology* (Oxford: Oxford University Press, 2011), pp. 440–459.

Lee, Christina, 'Disability', in Jacqueline Stodnick and Renée R. Trilling (eds), *A Handbook of Anglo-Saxon Studies* (London: Wiley-Blackwell, 2012), pp. 23–38.

Lee, Christina, 'Threads and Needles: The Use of Textiles for Medical Purposes', in Maren Clegg Hyer and Jill Frederick (eds), *Textiles, Text, Intertext: Essays in Honour of Gale R. Owen-Crocker* (Woodbridge: Boydell and Brewer, 2016), pp. 103–117.

Leslie, R. F. (ed.), *The Wanderer* (Manchester: Manchester University Press, 1966).

Lewis, Hannah, *Deaf Liberation Theology* (Aldershot: Ashgate, 2007).

Li, Lanzhi et al., 'Dominance, Overdominance and Epistasis Condition the Heterosis in Two Heterotic Rice Hybrids', *Genetics*, 180.3 (2008), 1725–1742.

Liebermann, F. (ed.), *Die Gesetze der Angelsachsen* (Halle: Scientia Aalen, 1960).

Liis, Kasari et al., 'Hybrid ecosystems can contribute to local biodiversity conservation', *Biodiversity and Conservation*, 25.14 (2016), pp. 3023–3041.

Lindsay, W. M. (ed.), *Isidori Hispalensis Episcopi Etymologiarum Sive Originum*, vol. 1 (Oxford: Oxford University Press, 1911).

Linett, Maren Tova, *Bodies of Modernism in Transatlantic Modernist Literature* (Ann Arbor, MI: University of Michigan Press, 2017).

Lippman, Zachary, and Dani Zamir, 'Heterosis: Revisiting the Magic', *Trends in Genetics*, 23.2 (2006), 60–66.

Liu, Tianjun (ed. and trans.), *Chinese Medical Qigong* (London: Singing Dragon, 2010).

Liuzza, Roy (trans.), *Beowulf* (Toronto: Broadview Press, 2nd edn, 2012).

McClintock, Barbara, 'The Significance of Responses of the Genome to Challenge', *Science*, 226 (1984), 792–801.

McGillivray, Murray, *Old English Reader* (Toronto: Broadview Press, 2011).

Maion, Danielle, 'London, British Library, Harley 6258B Medical Treatises', in Orietta Da Rold, Takako Kato, Mary Swan, and Elaine Treharne (eds), *The Production and Use of English Manuscripts 1060–1220* (University of Leicester, 2010–13), www.le.ac.uk/english/em1060to1220/mss/EM.BL.Harl.6258B.htm#EM.BL.Harl.6258B-history-10. Accessed 8 May 2021.

Manley, J., 'The Archer and the Army in the Late Saxon Period', *Anglo-Saxon Studies in Archaeology and History*, 4 (1985), 223–235.
Marder, Michael, *Plant Thinking: A Philosophy of Vegetal Life* (New York: Columbia University Press, 2013).
Maring, Heather, *Signs that Sing: Hybrid Poetics in Old English Verse* (Gainesville, FL: University Press of Florida, 2017).
Marsden, Richard, 'Biblical Literature: The New Testament', in Malcolm Godden and Michael Lapidge (eds), *The Cambridge Companion to Old English Literature* (Cambridge: Cambridge University Press, 2013), pp. 234–250.
Marsden, Richard, *The Cambridge Old English Reader*, 2nd ed (Cambridge: Cambridge University Press, 2015).
Massey, Jeff, and Karma DeGruy, 'Riddling Meaning from Old English -haga Compounds', *Studies in Philology*, 112 (2015), 24–38.
Meaney, Audrey, 'Variant Versions of Old English Medical Remedies and the Compilation of Bald's "Leechbook"', *Anglo-Saxon England*, 13 (1984), 235–268.
Metzler, Irina, *Disability in Medieval Europe: Thinking About Physical Impairment in the High Middle Ages, c. 1100–c. 1400* (New York: Routledge, 2006).
Metzler, Irina, 'Perceptions of Deafness in the Central Middle Ages', in Cordula Nolte (ed.), *Homo debilis: Behinderte—Kranke—Versehrte in der Gesallschaft des Mittelalters* (Korb: Didymos-Verlag, 2009), pp. 79–98.
Miller, Thomas (ed. and trans.), *The Old English Version of Bede's Ecclesiastical History of the English People* (London: Early English Text Society, 1890).
Mills, Mara, 'Deafness', in David Novak and Matt Sakakeeny (eds), *Keywords in Sound* (Durham, NC: Duke University Press, 2015, Kindle edition).
Mittman, Asa Simon, *Maps and Monsters in Medieval England* (New York: Routledge, 2006).
Moffett, Lisa, 'Food Plants on Archaeological Sites', in Helena Hamerow et al. (eds), *The Oxford Handbook of Anglo-Saxon Archaeology* (Oxford: Oxford University Press, 2011), pp. 346–360.
Mongillo, John F., and Linda Zierdt-Warshaw, *Encyclopedia of Environmental Science* (Rochester, NY: University of Rochester Press, 2000).
Montgomery, George, and Arthur Dimmock, *Venerable Legacy: Saint Bede and the Anglo-Celtic Contribution to Literary, Numerical and Manual Language* (Edinburgh: Edinburgh Scottish Workshop Publications, 1998).
Morrison, Susan Signe, *Grendel's Mother: The Saga of the Wyrd-Wife* (Winchester: Top Hat Books, 2015).

Mortimer, Paul, and Stephen Pollington, *Remaking the Sutton Hoo Stone: The Ansell-Roper Replica and its Context* (Cambridgeshire: Anglo-Saxon Books, 2013).

Moses, Marya, and Toby C. S. Langen, 'Reading Martha Lamont's Crow Story Today', *Oral Tradition*, 13.1 (1998), 92–129.

Mount, Toni, *Everyday Life in Medieval London: From the Anglo-Saxons to the Tudors* (Gloucestershire: Amberley Publishing, 2014).

Mullally, Erin, 'The Cross-Gendered Gift: Weaponry in the Old English *Judith*', *Exemplaria*, 17 (2013), 255–284.

Muir, Bernard (ed.), *The Exeter Anthology of Old English Poetry*, 2 vols. (Liverpool: Liverpool University Press, 2000).

Murphy, Patrick J., *Unriddling the Exeter Riddles* (University Park, PA: Pennsylvania State University Press, 2011).

Nagy, Joseph Falaky, 'Orality in Medieval Irish Narrative: An Overview', *Oral Tradition*, 1 (1986), 272–301.

Nedo, Almudena, 'In the Form of a Man: Grendel's Changing Form in Film Adaptations', in Frank Jacob and Verena Bernardi (eds), *All Around Monstrous: Monster Media in Their Historical Contexts* (Wilmington, DE: Vernon Press, 2019), 97–126.

Negus, Tina, 'Medieval Foliate Heads: A Photographic Study of Green Men and Green Beasts in Britain', *Folklore*, 114.2 (2003), 247–261.

Nelson, Marie, and Caroline Dennis, 'Nine Herbs Charm', *Germanic Notes and Reviews*, 38 (2007), 5–10.

Neri, Jordana, et al., 'Natural Hybridization and Genetic and Morphological Variation Between Two Epiphytic Bromeliads', *Annals of Botany (AoB) Plants* 10.1 (2018), 1c+.

Neville, Jennifer, 'A Modest Proposal: Titles for the *Exeter Book* Riddles', *Medium Ævum*, 88.1 (2019), 116–123.

Neville, Jennifer, and Megan Cavell (eds), *Riddles at Work in the Early Medieval Tradition* (Manchester: Manchester University Press, 2020).

The New Oxford Annotated Bible: New Revised Standard Version, with the Apocrypha, ed. Michael Coogan (Oxford: Oxford University Press, 4th edn, 2010).

Nie, Jing-Bao et al., 'No More Militaristic and Violent Language in Medicine: Response to Open Peer Commentaries on "Healing without Waging War": Beyond Military Metaphors and HIV Cure Research', *The American Journal of Bioethics*, 16 (2016), 3–11.

Niles, John D. 'The *Æcerbot* Ritual in Context', in John D. Niles (ed.), *Old English Literature in Context* (Cambridge: D. S. Brewer, 1980), pp. 44–56.

Niles, John D., *Old English Enigmatic Poems and the Play of the Texts* (Turnhout: Brepols, 2006).

O'Brien O'Keeffe, Katherine, 'Literacy', in Michael Lapidge, John Blair, Simon Keynes, and Donald Scragg (eds), *The Blackwell Encyclopedia of Anglo-Saxon England* (Oxford: Wiley-Blackwell, 1999), pp. 289–90.
OED (Oxford English Dictionary) Online (Oxford: Oxford University Press), www.oed.com.
Oliver, Lisi, *The Beginnings of English Law* (Toronto: University of Toronto Press, 2002).
Oliver, Lisi, and Maria Mahoney, 'Episcopal Anatomies of the Early Middle Ages', in Jennifer Vaught (ed.), *Rhetorics of Bodily Disease and Health in Medieval and Early Modern England* (Farnham: Ashgate, 2010), pp. 25–41.
Olsan, Lea, 'The Inscription of Charms in Anglo-Saxon Manuscripts', *Oral Tradition*, 14 (1999), 401–419.
Olsan, Lea, 'The Marginality of Charms in Medieval England', in James Kapaló, Éva Pócs, and William Ryan (eds), *The Power of Words: Studies on Charms and Charming in Europe* (Budapest: Central European University Press, 2013), pp. 135–164.
Olsen, Karin, 'Warriors and Their Battle Gear: Conceptual Blending in *Anhaga* (R.5) and *Wæpnum Awyrged* (R.20)', in Megan Cavell and Jennifer Neville (eds), *Riddles at Work in the Early Medieval Tradition: Words, Ideas, Interactions* (Manchester: Manchester University Press, 2020), pp. 111–127.
Ong, Walter, *Orality and Literacy: The Technologizing of the Word* (London: Routledge, 1982).
ORTRAD-L, 'Symposium, Deafness and Orality: An Electronic Conversation', *Oral Tradition*, 8 (1993), 413–437.
Oswald, Dana, *Monsters, Gender and Sexuality in Medieval English Literature* (Woodbridge: D. S. Brewer, 2010).
Owen-Crocker, Gale R., 'Dress and Identity', in David A. Hinton, Sally Crawford, and Helena Hamerow (eds), *The Oxford Handbook of Anglo-Saxon Archaeology* (Oxford: Oxford University Press, 2012), pp. 91–118.
Owen-Crocker, Gale R., '"Seldom ... does the deadly spear rest for long": Weapons and Armour', in Maren Clegg Hyer and Gale R. Owen-Crocker (eds), *The Material Culture of Daily Living in the Anglo-Saxon World* (Liverpool: Liverpool University Press, 2011), pp. 201–230.
Owen-Crocker, Gale R., 'Stylistic Variation and Roman Influence in the Bayeux Tapestry', *Peregrinations: Journal of Medieval Art and Architecture*, 2.4 (2009), 51–96.
Pasternack, Carol Braun, 'Post-Structuralist Theories: The Subject and the Text', in Katherine O'Brien O'Keeffe (ed.), *Reading Old English Texts* (Cambridge: Cambridge University Press, 1997), pp. 170–191.

Paxson, James J., *The Poetics of Personification* (Cambridge: Cambridge University Press, 1994).

Paz, James, *Nonhuman Voices in Anglo-Saxon Literature and Material Culture* (Manchester: Manchester University Press, 2017).

Pearman, Tory, *Women and Disability in Medieval Literature* (New York: Palgrave Macmillan, 2010).

Penick, Douglas J., *The Warrior Song of King Gesar* (Minneapolis, MN: Mill City Press, 2009).

Pettit, Edward (ed. and trans.), *Anglo-Saxon Remedies, Charms, and Prayers from British Library MS Harley 585: The Lacnunga*, 2 vols (Lewiston: Edwin Mellen Press, 2001).

Pliny, *Natural History* VII, libri XXIV–XXVII, ed. T. E. Page, trans. W. H. S. Jones, Loeb Classical Library (Cambridge, MA: Harvard University Press, 1966).

Pollington, Stephen (trans.) *Leechcraft: Early English Charms, Plantlore, and Healing* (Cambridgeshire: Anglo-Saxon Books, 2000).

Portnoy, Phyllis, 'Laf-Craft in Five Old English Riddles (K-D 5, 20, 56, 71, 91)', *Neophilologus*, 97 (2013), 555–579.

Pound, Ezra, *The Cantos of Ezra Pound* (New York: New Directions Books, 1934).

Price, Annette P., *Tinnitus STOP! The Complete Guide on Ringing in the Ears, Natural Tinnitus Remedies, and a Holistic System for Permanent Tinnitus Relief* (United States: Living Plus Healthy Publishing, 2014).

Price, Neil et al., 'Viking Warrior Women? Reassessing Birka Chamber Grave Bj.581', *Antiquity*, 93 (2019), 181–198.

Proops, Leanne, Faith Burden, and Britta Osthaus, 'Mule Cognition: A Case of Hybrid Vigour?', *Animal Cognition*, 12 (2009), 75–84.

Rabin, Andrew, 'The Wolf's Testimony to the English: Law and the Witness in the "Sermo Lupi ad Anglos"', *Journal of English and Germanic Philology*, 15.3 (2006), 388–414.

Raffel, Burton (trans), *Beowulf* (New York: Penguin, 1963).

Rambaran-Olm, Mary, 'History Bites: Resources on the Problematic term "Anglo-Saxon"', parts 1–3 (2020), https://mrambaranolm.medium.com/history-bites-resources-on-the-problematic-term-anglo-saxon-part-1-9320b6a09eb7. Accessed 7 July 2021.

Ramsey, Justin, Alexander Robertson, and Brian Husband, 'Rapid Adaptive Divergence in New World *Achillea*, an Autopoloyploid Complex of Ecological Races, *Evolution*, 62.3 (2008), pp. 639–653.

Randolph, Charles Brewster, 'The Mandragora of the Ancients in Folk-Lore and Medicine', *Proceedings of the American Academy of Arts and Sciences*, 4.12 (1905), 487–537.

Rée, Jonathan, *I See a Voice: Deafness, Language, and the Senses—A Philosophical History* (New York: Henry Holt and Company, 1999).

Reinsma, Luke M., 'Rhetoric, Grammar, and Literature in England and Ireland before the Norman Conquest: A Select Bibliography', *Rhetoric Society Quarterly*, 8 (1978), 29–48.
Reynolds, Andrew, *Anglo-Saxon Deviant Burial Customs* (Oxford: Oxford University Press, 2009).
Richardson, Peter R., 'Making Thanes: Literature, Rhetoric and State Formation in Anglo-Saxon England', *Philological Quarterly*, 78 (1999), 215–232.
Riddle, John M., *Dioscorides on Pharmacy and Medicine* (Austin, TX: University of Texas Press, 1985).
Riddle, John M., 'Theory and Practice in Medieval Medicine', *Viator: Medieval and Renaissance Studies*, 5 (1974), 157–184.
Riedinger, Anita, 'The Formulaic Style in the Old English Riddles', *Studia Neophilologica*, 76 (2004), 30–43.
Rieger, R., A. Michaelis, and M. M. Green, *A Glossary of Genetics and Cytogenetics: Classical and Molecular* (Springer Science and Business Media, 2013).
Roach, Levi, 'Law Codes and Legal Norms in Later Anglo-Saxon England', *Historical Research*, 86 (2013), 465–486.
Rodrigues, Louis J. (ed. and trans.), *Anglo-Saxon Verse Charms, Maxims and Heroic Legends* (Middlesex: Anglo-Saxon Books, 1993).
Rohde, Eleanour Sinclair, *The Old English Herbals* (London: Longmans, Green, and Co., 1922).
Roper, Jonathan, 'Towards a Poetics, Rhetorics, and Proxemics of Verbal Charms', *Folklore*, 24 (2003), 7–49.
Rosenberg, Bruce A., 'The Meaning of Æcerbot', *Journal of American Folklore*, 79 (1966), 428–436.
Rowling, J. K., *Harry Potter and the Chamber of Secrets* (New York: Scholastic, 1998).
Rupp, Katrin, 'The Anxiety of Writing: A Reading of the Old English Journey Charm', *Oral Tradition*, 23 (2008), 255–266.
Rusche, Philip G., 'Dioscorides' *De materia medica*', in C. P. Biggam (ed.), *From Earth to Art: The Many Aspects of the Plant-World in Anglo-Saxon England* (Amsterdam and New York: Rodopi, 2003), pp. 181–194.
Saleh, G. B., D. Abdullah, and A. R. Anuar, 'Performance, Heterosis and Heritability in Selected Tropical Maize Single, Double and Three-Way Cross Hybrids', *Journal of Agricultural Science*, 138 (2002), 21–28.
Sanborn, Linda, 'An Edition of British Library MS. Harley 6258B: Peri Didaxeon' (unpublished doctoral thesis, University of Ottawa, 1983).
Sarton, G., Review of *The Old English Herbals* by Eleanour Sinclair Rohde, *Isis*, 5.2 (1923), 457–461.
Sauer, Hans, 'The Morphology of Old English Plant-Names', in C. P. Biggam (ed.), *From Earth to Art: The Many Aspects of the Plant-World*

in *Anglo-Saxon England* (Amsterdam and New York: Rodopi, 2003), pp. 161–179.

Sauer, Hans, and Elisabeth Kubaschewski, *Planting the Seeds of Knowledge: An Inventory of Old English Plant Names* (Munich: Herbert Utz Verlag, 2018).

Sayers, William, 'Exeter Book Riddle No. 5: Whetstone?', *Neuphilologische Mitteilungen*, 97 (1996), 387–392.

Schaefer, Ursula, 'Rhetoric and Style', in Robert E. Bjork and John D. Niles (eds), *A Beowulf Handbook* (Lincoln, NE: University of Nebraska Press, 1997), pp. 105–124.

Schaefer, Ursula, 'Twin Collocations in the Early Middle English Lives of the *Katherine Group*', in Herbert Pilch (ed.), *Orality and Literacy in Early Middle English*, ScriptOralia (Tübingen: Gunter Narr Verlag, 1996), pp. 179–198.

Scheil, Andrew P., *The Footsteps of Israel: Understanding Jews in Anglo-Saxon England* (Ann Arbor, MI: University of Michigan Press, 2004).

Scholfield, A. F. (trans.), *Aelian: On the Characteristics of Animals*, vol. 3, Books XII–XVII (Cambridge, MA: Harvard University Press, 1959).

Scudder, Bernard (trans.), *Egil's Saga* (New York: Penguin, 1997).

Sellerberg, U., and H. Glasl, 'Pharmacognostical Examination Concerning the Hemostyptic Effect of *Achillea millefolium* Aggregat', *Scientia Pharmaceutica*, 68 (2000), 201–206.

Shull, G. H., 'The Composition of a Field of Maize', *Journal of Heredity*, 4 (1908), 296–301.

Siewers, Alf, *Strange Beauty: Ecocritical Approaches to Early Medieval Landscape* (New York: Palgrave, 2009).

Singer, Charles, 'Early English Magic and Medicine', *Proceedings of the British Academy*, 9 (1919–20), 341–374.

Singer, Natasha, 'Teaching in the Pandemic: "This is Not Sustainable"', *New York Times*, 30 November 2020.

Siraisi, Nancy G., 'Oratory and Rhetoric in Renaissance Medicine', *Journal of the History of Ideas*, 65 (2004), 191–211.

Skemp, A. R., 'The Old English Charms', *Modern Language Review*, 6 (1911), 289–301.

Spearing, Sinead, *Old English Remedies* (Barnsley: Pen and Sword History, 2018).

Steen, Janie, *Verse and Virtuosity: The Adaptation of Latin Rhetoric in Old English Poetry* (Toronto: University of Toronto Press, 2008).

Stephenson, I. P., *The Anglo-Saxon Shield* (Stroud: Tempus, 2004).

Storms, Godfrid (ed. and trans.), *Anglo-Saxon Magic* (New York: Gordon Press, 1974. Orig. published 1948).

Stross, Brian, 'The Hybrid Metaphor: From Biology to Culture', *Journal of American Folklore*, 112 (1999), 254–267.

Stuart, Heather, "'Ic me on þisse gyrde beluce'": The Structure and Meaning of the Old English "Journey Charm"', *Medium Ævum*, 50 (1981), 259–273.

Swanton, M. J., *The Spearheads of the Anglo-Saxon Settlements* (London: The Royal Archaeological Institute, 1973).

Sweany, Erin, 'Unsettling Comparisons: Ethical Considerations of Comparative Approaches to the Old English Medical Corpus', special issue *Indigenous Futures and Medieval Pasts* (edited by Tarren Andrews and Tiffany Beechy), *English Language Notes*, 58.2 (2020), 83–100.

Swearingen, C. Jan, and Edward Schiappa, 'Historical and Comparative Rhetorical Studies: Revisionist Methods and New Directions', in Andrea A. Lunsford et al. (eds), *The Sage Handbook of Rhetorical Studies* (Newbury Park: Sage, 2009), pp. 1–12.

Sweet, Henry, *An Anglo-Saxon Reader* (Oxford: Clarendon Press, 4th edn, 1884).

Sweet, Henry (ed.), *King Alfred's West-Saxon Version of Gregory's Pastoral Care*, vol. 2 (London: Early English Text Society, 1871).

Tacitus, *Agricola and Germania*, trans. H. Mattingly; rev. S. A. Handford (New York: Penguin, 1970).

Tait, Yvonne, *Your Health, Your Vitality, Your Choice: An Interlude with an Esoteric Herbalist* (Bloomington, IN: Balboa Press, 2016. Kindle edition).

Tangherlini, Timothy R., '"Oral Tradition" in a Technologically Advanced World', *Oral Tradition*, 18 (2003), 136–138.

Thomas, Charlton, *Latin Dictionary* (New York: Harpers, 1907).

Thompson, C. J. S., *The Mystic Mandrake* (New Hyde Park: University Books, 1934).

Thompson, Logan, *Ancient Weapons in Britain* (Barnsley: Pen and Sword Military, 2005).

Thompson, S., *Motif Index of Folk Literature* (Bloomington, IN: Indiana University Press, 1955–58).

Thorpe, Benjamin (ed. and trans.), *The Homilies of the Anglo-Saxon Church*, vol. 1 (London: Richard and John Taylor, 1844).

Tigges, Wim, 'Snakes and Ladders: Ambiguity and Coherence in the Exeter Book Riddles and Maxims', in Henk Aertsen and Rolf H. Bremmer, Jr. (eds), *Companion to Old English Poetry* (Amsterdam: VU University Press, 1994), pp. 95–118.

Todesco, Marco et al., 'Hybridization and Extinction', *Evolutionary Applications*, 9 (2016), 892–908.

Toelken, Barre, *The Dynamics of Folklore* (Logan, UT: Utah State University Press, 1996).

Trautmann, Moritz, 'Die Auflösungen der altenglischen Rätsel', *Anglia Beiblatt*, 5 (1894), 46–51.

Treharne, Elaine, *Living Through Conquest: The Politics of Early English, 1020–1220*, Oxford Textual Perspectives (Oxford: Oxford University Press, 2012).

Treharne, Elaine (ed.), *Old and Middle English c. 890–c. 1400: An Anthology* (Oxford: Blackwell Publishing, 2nd edn, 2004).

Trilling, Renée, *The Aesthetics of Nostalgia: Historical Representation in Old English Verse* (Toronto: University of Toronto Press, 2009).

Trilling, Renée, 'Health and Healing in the Anglo-Saxon World', *Studies in Medieval and Renaissance History*, 13 (2016), 41–69.

Troyer, A. Forrest, 'Adaptedness and Heterosis in Corn and Mule Hybrids', *Crop Sci.*, 46 (2006), 528–543.

Tupper, Frederick, 'Notes on Old English Poems', *Journal of English and Germanic Philology*, 11 (1912), 82–103.

Underwood, Richard, *Anglo-Saxon Weapons and Warfare* (Stroud: Tempus, 1999).

Van Arsdall, Anne, 'Exploring What was Understood by "Mandragora" in Anglo-Saxon England', in Peter Bierbaumer and Helmut W. Klug (eds), *Old Names—New Growth: Proceedings of the 2nd ASPNS Conference* (Bern: Peter Lang, 2009), pp. 57–74.

Van Arsdall, Anne, *Medieval Herbal Remedies: The Old English Herbarium and Anglo-Saxon Medicine* (New York: Routledge, 2002).

Van Arsdall, Anne, 'Reading Medieval Medical Texts with an Open Mind', in Elizabeth Lane Furdell (ed.), *Textual Healing: Essays on Medieval and Early Modern Medicine* (Leiden: Brill, 2005), pp. 9–29.

Van Arsdall, Anne, Helmut W. Klug, and Paul Blanz, 'The Mandrake Plant and its Legend', in Peter Bierbaumer and Helmut W. Klug (eds), *Old Names—New Growth: Proceedings of the 2nd ASPNS Conference* (Bern: Peter Lang, 2009), pp. 285–346.

Van der Walt, A. G. P., 'Early Medieval Stylistic Rhetoric', *Literator*, 2.3 (1981), 48–61.

Van Meter, David C., 'The Ritualized Presentation of Weapons and the Ideology of Nobility in *Beowulf*', *Journal of English and Germanic Philology*, 95 (1996), 175–189.

van Tienderen, P. H., 'Hybridization in Nature: Lessons for the Introgression of Transgenes into Wild Relatives', in Hans C. M. den Nijs, Detlef Bartsch, and Jeremy Sweet (eds), *Introgression from Genetically Modified Plants into Wild Relatives* (Centre for Agriculture and Bioscience International [CABI] Publishing, 2004), 7–26.

Vaughan-Sterling, Judith A., 'The Anglo-Saxon *Metrical Charms*: Poetry as Ritual', *Journal of English and Germanic Philology*, 82 (1983), 186–200.

Vaught, Jennifer (ed.), *Rhetorics of Bodily Disease and Health in Medieval and Early Modern England* (Farnham: Ashgate, 2010).

Voigts, Linda E., 'Anglo-Saxon Plant Remedies and the Anglo-Saxons', *Isis*, 70 (1979), 250–268.
Voigts, Linda E., 'A New Look at a Manuscript Containing the Old English Translation of the *Herbarium Apulei*', *Manuscripta*, 21 (1976), 40–60.
Waiko, John D., '"Head" and "Tail": The Shaping of Oral Traditions among the Binandere in Papua New Guinea', *Oral Tradition*, 5 (1990), 334–353.
Warren, Minton, 'On the Etymology of Hybrid (Lat. Hybrida)', *The American Journal of Philology*, 5 (1884), 501–502.
Watkins, Calvert, *How to Kill a Dragon: Aspects of Indo-European Poetics* (Oxford: Oxford University Press, 1995).
Watt, Diane, *Women, Writing and Religion in England and Beyond, 650–1100* (London: Bloomsbury, 2020).
Wayne, Peter M., with Mark L. Fuerst, *The Harvard Medical School Guide to Tai Chi* (Boston: Shambhala Publications, Inc., 2013).
Wilcox, Miranda, 'Confessing the Faith in Anglo-Saxon England', *Journal of English and Germanic Philology*, 113 (2014), 308–341.
Williamson, Craig (trans.) *A Feast of Creatures: Anglo-Saxon Riddle-Songs* (Philadelphia, PA: The University of Pennsylvania Press, 1982).
Williamson, Craig (ed.) *The Old English Riddles of the 'Exeter Book'* (Chapel Hill, NC: University of North Carolina Press, 1977).
Williamson, Craig (trans.), *The Complete Old English Poems* (Philadelphia, PA: University of Pennsylvania Press, 2017).
Winzer, Margret A., *The History of Special Education: From Isolation to Integration* (Washington, DC: Gallaudet University Press, 1993).
Wormald, Patrick, *The Making of English Law: King Alfred to the Twelfth Century*, vol. 1 (Oxford: Blackwell, 2001).
Young, Robert J. C., *Colonial Desire: Hybridity in Theory, Culture and Race* (New York: Routledge, 1995).
Zemeckis, Robert (dir.), *Beowulf* (Paramount Pictures, 2007).

Index

Notes: 'n.' after a page reference indicates the number of a note (or notes) on that page; page numbers in *italic* refer to figures.

Achillea millefolium see yarrow
Achilles 11, 51, 53–55, 67, 111, 148
Æcerbot (field remedy) 10, 24–28, 36, 206, 272
Ælfric 66, 73, 151
  Lives 212
Aelian
  On the Characteristics of Animals 179, 201n.55
Æthelberht 245n.82
agency
  of ears 222–227, 283
  of plants 129, 151, 152, 184–188, 190, 191–194, 222–223, 283
Alchemilla vulgaris see leonfot
Aldhelm 7
Alfred 149, 212, 229–231, 234, 245n.82
Alpantaki, Kalliopi 126n.49
Ammons, Matthias 232
anaphora 130, 137, 143–148
Andreas 252
Anhaga riddle 17n.3, 237, 248–266, 267n.6–7, 268n.21, 270n.56, 279, 282

and absence of healers 1–2, 15, 237, 249, 257, 259–262, 267n.7, 284
exile imagery in 15, 250–253, 255
personification in 1, 250–257, 259, 261
possible solutions for 1, 15, 250–251, 253–261, 266, 267n.18, 268n.21, 270n.48, 282–283
warfare and weapons in 1, 15, 249–257, 259–263, 266, 279, 284
anthropomorphization 114–116, 254
  of *gorgonion* 174, *175*, 176
  of mandrake 13–14, 31, 160, 162, *163*, 164, 177–178, 180, 184, 187, 190, 203n.94, 206, 278, 283–284
  of other plants 5, 12–14, 31, 140, 158n.44, 176
  see also agency; memory: ascribed to plants; personification; sentience (of plants)
apostrophe 130, 137, 139–143, 145, 156n.28, 157n.34

Index

Applequist, Wendy 52, 54
armor 54–55, 111, 114–115
  in graves 72–73
  in *Ic me on þisse gyrde beluce*
    11, 48–49, 71–76, 78, 80–81,
    92n.77, 93n.96
  see also helmets; mailcoats;
    shields; warfare
Arnovick, Leslie 20n.29, 71, 78,
  216
arrows 29, 54–55, 57, 60, 89n.38,
  97, 100–102, 123n.12
  in *Wið færstice* 12, 101–104,
    106, 109, *110*, 117, 121
  see also warfare; weapons
artemisia see mugwort (*mugwyrt,
  artemisia*)
Arthur, Ciaran 25, 26, 65
Ashcroft, Bill 30, 43n.29
astula regia (woodruff) 11, 57–58,
  59, 88n.33, 276
Athelstan 73
Attebery, Brian 19n.20
Attenborough, F. L. 245n.86
attorlaðe 13, 133, 139–140, 145,
  150, 155n.16, 158n.48
audism 15, 208, 215–217, 237
  see also deafness

Bakhtin, Mikhail 33, 45n.47
Bald's Leechbook 8, 14, 29, 57,
  60–61, 88n.24, 95n.115, 148,
  209, 223, 239n.13, 243n.62,
  282, 283
  deafness in 14, 207–210,
    217–219, 220, 221–230,
    239n.16–17, 243n.57–59,
    244n.77, 274, 279, 283–284
Banham, Debby 24, 170
Barley, Nigel 241n.48, 256
battle imagery *see* armor; warfare;
  weapons
Battle of Maldon 56, 97, 100–101

Bauman, H-Dirksen 213
Bayeux Tapestry 258
Bayless, Martha 107, 125n.37
Bede
  De schematibus et tropis 143
  Historia ecclesiastica 4, 7–8, 11,
    19n.24, 48, 60, 63–64, 65–67
    70, 81, 117, 232–234
Beechy, Tiffany 254, 256, 278
bees *see* swarm charm
Beowulf 9, 99, 125n.38, 125n.41,
  153n.6, 157n.40, 208, 215,
  237, 248–249, 252, 262–263,
  270n.62, 271n.67
  Grendel's depiction in 5, 16,
    127n.60, 206, 209, 238n.2–3
  weapons and warfare in 56–57,
    61, 90n.42, 106–108,
    113–117
  see also epic
Beowulf (2007 movie) 248–249,
  263
Berberich, Hugo 168, 204n.119
Bhabha, Homi 18n.9
Bishop, Louise 132, 158n.45
Bitterli, Dieter 266
Bjork, Robert 123n.13
Blanz, Paul 180, 181, 193, 201n.58
Bliss, A. J. 105
Bodleian Library, MS Hatton 76 8,
  165, 167, 170, 173, 185–186,
  199n.21, 209
  Herbarium's mandrake entry
    162, 183, 188, 191
Bosworth, Joseph 67, 91n.72, 191,
  224, 243n.63, 287n.23
Bradley, S. A. J. 93n.96, 268n.21
Bradshaw, Paul 80
Brady, Lindy 43n.30
Bragg, Lois 93n.96
British Deaf History Society 233
British Library, MS Cotton
  Caligula A.vii 24, 26

British Library, MS Cotton Otho
  B.xi 223, 224, 243n.62
British Library, MS Cotton
  Vitellius C.iii 8, 48, 50, *50*,
  59, 88n.33, 135–136, *136*,
  152n.1, 166–168, 170–174,
  198n.3–4, 199n.21, 209, 258,
  272, 282, 286n.11
  as *Herbarium* base text 13,
    162–166, 168, 170, 172–173,
    185, 195
  Herbarium's gorgonion entry
    174–176, *175*, 184
  Herbarium's mandrake entry 5,
    160, 162, *163*, 175, 177, 179,
    183–197, 278, 283
British Library, MS Harley 585
  8, 13, 19n.19, 29, 129, 130,
  132–52, *135*, 165, 167–168,
  170, 173, 185–186, 199n.22,
  209, 282, 284
  Herbarium's mandrake entry
    162, 183, 188, 191
  Wið færstice 12, 97, 98, *104*
British Library, MS Harley 6258B
  8, 135–136, 162, 164–174,
  184, 198n.1, 198n.4, 199n.22,
  209, 239n.13, 282, 286n.11
  alphabetization in 165, 171–172,
    200n.39
  and *Herbarium*'s entry for
    mandrake 13, 160, *161*, 162,
    164–165, 171–172, 174–175,
    177–178, 182–193, 195–197,
    278
  omissions within 167–168, 170,
    173–174, 176–178, 187–191,
    193–194
British Library, MS Royal 12
  D.xvii 8, 209, 218, *220*,
  239n.13, 243n.62
Brooks, Nicholas 60, 89n.38, 100
Bruce, Scott G. 241n.48

Brueggemann, Brenda Jo 214, 228
Burdorff, Sara Frances 106, 262
burial practices 19n.20, 124n.31,
  210, 228, 235–236
  and weapons 58, 72, 87n.17,
    92n.80, 124n.31

Caedmon's Hymn 4, 33–35
Camargo, Martin 131
Cambridge College Corpus Christi
  MS 41 8, 19n.19, 43n.34, 48,
  62–63, 65–67, 69, 73, 82,
  95n.115, 97, 104, 148
Cambridge College Corpus Christi
  MS 190 43n.34
Cameron, M. L. 85n.6, 107, 109,
  126n.44
Campbell, Jackson 156n.24
Cavell, Megan 20n.32, 269n.42,
  271n.67
Cech, Richo 183
charms
  defined 20n.29, 64
  see also g(e)aldor; *individual
    remedies*; metrical charms
Chen, Z. Jeffrey 33, 45n.48
chiasmus 130, 137, 143, 145
Chickering, Howell 122n.4
chopping block 259
  as possible solution to *Anhaga*
    riddle 1, 250–251, 254–261,
    268n.21, 282–283
  see also cutting board
Christianity 4–7, 10, 19n.20, 28,
  30, 35, 38, 41, 60, 80, 138,
  233–234
  in *Æcerbot* 25–28
  in *Ic me on þisse gyrde beluce*
    12, 48–49, 71–79, 80–84,
    92n.77, 283
  and lost cattle remedy 6, 30–31
  and 'Nine Herbs Charm' 34, 38,
    133, 142, 148, 158n.43

and views toward *g(e)aldor*
  65–66, 151
and *Wið færstice* 125n.41
see also hybridity: religious;
  liturgy
Christ Lyric VIII 28
Clair, Colin 183
Clemoes, Peter 263
Cnut 70, 230
Cockayne, Emily 217
Cockayne, Thomas Oswald
  153n.5, 165, 166, 168, 170,
  173, 219, 221, 224–225,
  239n.16, 243n.59, 273
Cohen, Jeffrey Jerome 40, 194
Cohen, Sidney 270n.52
Colebrook, Claire 185
Collier, Michael 119, 123n.13
comitatus 115, 157n.40, 158n.44,
  192, 253
critical plant studies 185–186, 190
Crow, James 33
Cuthbert 66, 70, 73
cutting board 259, 264
  as possible solution to *Anhaga*
    riddle 1, 254–261, 265,
    282–283
  see also chopping block

Daniel, Book of 60, 89n.36
D'Aronco, Maria Amalia 149,
  152n.19, 157n.38, 166–169
Darwin, Charles 32–33
Davis, Lennard 208, 216
deafness 246n.91, 279
  in *Bald's Leeechbook* 14,
    207–210, 217–219, 220,
    221–230, 239n.16–17,
    243n.57–59, 244n.77, 274,
    279, 283–284
  causes of 15, 210, 222, 226–229,
    231–233, 235, 239n.17,
    245n.82

congenital 227–228, 229
and issues of orality 206–208,
  211, 214–216, 231–233,
  236–237, 241n.37
and law codes 14, 208–210,
  228–232, 234, 235, 245n.82,
  284
and legal access 229–232, 236,
  245n.82
medieval perspectives on 14–15,
  208–213, 216–217, 223–237,
  242n.49, 244n.77, 245n.82,
  247n.113
as problematic metaphor 14–15,
  213, 215–216, 228, 236
as a range of experienced
  conditions 14–15, 209–213,
  217, 221, 223–231, 235–237,
  245n.82, 274, 279, 283–284
in religious contexts 232–234
see also 'dumb ond/oððe deaf';
  monastic sign language
Deaf studies 212–217
  as neglected by other disciplines
    14, 210–211, 214–217
  and use of oral theory 14–15,
    207–208, 214–216, 236–237,
    279
DeGruy, Karma 260
Delanty, Greg 93n.96, 268n.21
Dendle, Peter 117, 141
Deor 270n.56
de Saint-Loup, Aude 234
de Vriend, Hubert Jan 88n.33,
  153n.5, 159n.63, 169, 170,
  171, 173, 174, 204n.120, 224,
  279
Dioscorides 52
  De materia medica 178, 200n.50
  see also Pseudo-Dioscorides
direct address (of plants) 13, 117,
  129–137, 139–150, 158n.44,
  206, 278, 282, 284

disability 39, 212–214, 217, 228, 234
Discenza, Nicole Guenther 4–5, 18n.13, 29
Doane, A. N. 105
Dobbie, Elliott Van Kirk 75, 76, 82, 93n.96, 96n.133, 104, 128n.66, 267n.18, 268n.21
Donoghue, Daniel 5
Doskow, Minna 103
Doyle, Conan 219, 221, 239n.16–17, 242n.56, 243n.58–59
Dream of the Rood 5
Drout, Michael 43 n.35
'dumb ond/oððe deaf' 217, 229–234
Dumitrescu, Irina 234

Eastman, Gilbert 214
ebulus see *Herbarium*: snakebite remedy
Egil's Saga 93n.97, 94n.112
elegies 4, 10, 35, 77, 251
  see also *Wanderer, The*
elf charms 4, 29
Ellard, Donna Beth 272, 273
ellenwyrt see *Herbarium*: snakebite remedy
emendation, textual 9, 130, 152, 152n.2, 266, 274, 280
  in *Ic me on þisse gyrde beluce* 12, 63, 74–81, 93n.96, 94n.104, 94n.106, 104, 274
  in *Wið færstice* 104–105, 122, 123n.21
empathy 16, 165, 178, 184, 191, 264, 274, 281, 283–285
Ephesians, Epistle to the 71–72
epic 9, 35, 61, 90n.42, 106, 208, 214–215, 249, 251

and reciprocity with healing tradition 49, 56–57, 71, 106–117, 125n.41, 126n.46–47, 126n.49, 127n.60, 261–263, 284
  see also *Beowulf*
erysipelas 68, 112
ethnopoetics 12, 99, 118–119, 122n.6, 277–278
Exeter Book 1–2, 15, 17n.3, 70, 237, 271n.67
  see also *Anhaga* riddle
Exodus (Old English) 56

Fay, Jacqueline 189, 194
Feis Tighe Chonáin 212–213
Foley, John Miles 28, 42n.21, 56, 77, 99, 112–113, 131, 147, 214, 238n.7
Foys, Martin 241n.48
Frye, Northrop 263

Gale, David A. 61
g(e)aldor 20n.30, 91n.57, 150
  and *Ic me on þisse gyrde beluce* 48–49, 65–66, 68, 81, 82
Genesis (Old English) 70
genomic shock 38–39
genre 9, 15, 45n.47, 56, 130, 147, 180, 250
  hybridity of 11, 26–27, 35, 39, 56–57, 63, 97, 207, 251–252, 262–264, 272
  and *Ic me on þisse gyrde beluce* 48–49, 62–68, 71, 74, 90n.49
  reciprocity among types of 10, 48–49, 71, 106–117, 125n.41, 126n.46–47, 126n.49, 127n.60, 261–264, 271n.67, 284
  see also *individual genres*
Geoffrey of Vinsauf
  Poetria Nova 156n.28

Index 315

Gesar epic 111, 126n.47
Gingra Broþor Mec Adraf (riddle) 258
Glickman, Neil 214
Glosecki, Stephen 98, 103, 105, 119, 127n.60, 262
gorgonion 174–177, 175, 181, 184–185, 194
Grant, Verne 25, 42n.8
Grattan, J. H. 90n.49
graves *see* burial practices
Gray, Asa 32
Gregory I, Pope
 Pastoral Rule 212
Grendon, Felix 20n.30, 62, 76, 94n.104, 95n.117, 104, 273
Grieve, M. 287n.24
Griffiths, Bill 77
Griffiths, Gareth 30, 43n.29
gyrd(e) 48, 67–70, 78–80, 82, 96n.137, 282

Hadley, D. M. 235
Hall, Alaric 98, 102, 119, 123n.13
Hall, Matthew 14, 185–186, 191, 192
Härke, Heinrich 87n.17
Harmon, Kristen 214–215, 227, 228
Harry Potter and the Chamber of Secrets 203n.111
harvesting rituals 69, 152, 155n.19, 179, 201n.55
 in *Æcerbot* 25
 for *gorgonion* 175–176
 in *Ic me on þisse gyrde beluce* 68–70, 283
 for *leonfot* 277, 278
 for mandrake 69, 162, 164, 175–180, 182–184, 187–191, 193, 201n.52, 278
 for *peruica* 134

 for *proserpinaca* 152, 182
 and *wælwyrt* 129
healers 54, 170
 as heroic warriors 51, 53–57, 60, 71, 73–74, 81, 108–109, 111, 148–149
 literary references to 1–2, 7–8, 15, 248–254, 257, 259–262, 267n.7, 284
 in modern media 15, 248–249, 263, 266n.3
 and relationship to ailments 4, 28, 98, 104, 108–109, 116, 131
 and relationship with herbs 13–14, 17, 69–70, 131, 140–143, 145–146, 149–150, 152, 158n.44, 189–193, 278
 and use of British Library, MS Harley 6258B 172–173, 177
hearing *see* deafness
Heliand 26
helmets 72–73, 76
 in *Ic me on þisse gyrde beluce* 11, 71–73, 80–81, 83, 84, 95n.113
 see also armor; warfare
Herbarium 5, 8, 13–14, 48, 81, 85n.6, 88n.24, 130, 132–134, 138, 142, 148–149, 152, 154n.13, 155n.19, 157n.39, 159n.63, 162, 165–168, 170, 186, 194, 198n.2–4, 199n.21–22, 209, 223, 284
 entry for *astula regia* 57–58, 59
 entry for *dictamnus* (dittany) 173–174
 entry for *eorðyfig* (earth-ivy) 223–224, 244n.69
 entry for *gorgonion* 174–177, 175, 181, 184–185, 194
 entry for *hæwenhudela* (*brittanica*) 171

Herbarium (cont.)
  entry for *leonfot* 15, 272, 275–280, 286n.17, 287n.23
  entry for mandrake (*mandragora*) 5, 13–14, 17, 31, 69, 160, *161*, *163*, 164–165, 171–172, 174–179, 181–193, 195–197, 207, 278
  entry for *merce* (march, wild celery) 171–172
  entry for *peruica* (periwinkle) 5, 130, 133–137, *135*, *136*, 138–141, 146–147, 149–150, 155n.20, 283
  entry for *polion* 174
  entry for *proserpinaca* (*unfortrædde*) 69, 152, 182
  entry for *ribbe* (ribwort) 224, 244n.69
  entry for *ricinum* 5, 13, 129, 130, 133–137, *135*, 138–141, 145–146, 148, 149–150, 155n.20, 156n.29, 283
  entry for *temolum* (*singrene*) 172, 200n.39
  entry for yarrow 11, 49–55, *50*, 67, 111
  snakebite remedy 129, 131, 151, 153n.5
  warfare and weapons in 49, 54, 57–58, 88n.33, 258
  see also Bodleian Library, MS Hatton 76; British Library, MS Cotton Vitellius C.iii; British Library, MS Harley 585; British Library, MS Harley 6258B
Herbarium of Pseudo-Apuleius 149, 179–180
Hermann, John 92n.77
heterosis 33–35, 37, 44n.45, 45n.57
Hill, Thomas 25, 62, 76, 90n.49, 98, 123n.13, 124n.30
Hines, John 92n.80
Hollis, Stephanie 166
Holthausen, F. 75
Holt Hweorfende 279–280
hybridity
  biological 3, 5, 10, 22–27, 30–39, 41n.4–5, 42n.8, 44n.38, 44n.43, 44n.45, 45n.48, 45n.57, 46n.58, 52, 207, 251, 263, 272–273, 276, 278, 280, 284
  bodily 28–30, 31–32, 43n.30, 152, 162, 164, 177–178, 190, 193, 209, 261
  and colonization 4, 35, 43n.29
  cultural 3, 6–7, 10, 13, 19n.22, 25, 30–31, 33–41, 43n.29–30, 51–52, 73–75, 78–80, 81, 130, 133, 138–139, 237, 257, 272, 276, 284
  defined 3, 18n.5, 18n.9, 22, 32, 44n.38, 45n.47
  and genre 11, 26–27, 35, 39, 56–57, 63, 97, 207, 251–252, 262–264, 272
  linguistic 5, 19n.19, 24–26, 138–139, 172, 195, 277
  as metaphor 3, 7, 10–11, 17, 22–23, 27–40, 45n.53, 47n.85, 207, 273, 276, 280, 281
  poetic 5, 9, 28, 33–36, 51–52, 66, 77–78, 81, 97–98
  religious 4, 6–7, 12, 19n.20, 25–28, 30–31, 33–34, 38, 41, 49, 73–75, 78, 133
  risks and limitations of 3, 7, 10, 22–24, 30–32, 37–41, 43n.30–31, 43n.35, 281
hybrid sterility 23, 25, 36
hybrid swamping 23, 37–38, 281
hybrid swarming 37–38
hybrid vigor 5, 23, 33–37, 44n.45

Index

hybrid zones 37–38, 274
Hymes, Del 99, 122n.6

Ic me on þisse gyrde beluce 11–12, 20n.30, 34, 62–84, 90n.43, 91n.72, 92n.77, 95n.117, 97, 148, 206, 282–284
  and encirclement 67–70, 78–80, 96n.137, 283
  as *g(e)aldor* 48–49, 65–66, 68
  and genre 48–49, 62–68, 71, 74, 90n.49
  seraphim in 75–76, 93n.96, 94n.104
  and textual emendation 12, 63, 74–81, 93n.96, 94n.104, 94n.106, 104, 274
  weapons and warfare in 11, 34, 48–49, 63–64, 68, 69–81, 84, 90n.43, 92n.77, 93n.96, 94n.104, 116–117, 282–284
  see also gyrd(e)
Iliad 111, 126n.49
incantations 8, 9, 12, 29, 38, 49, 61–62, 68–69, 129, 131, 137–138, 146–147, 149, 151, 154n.13, 176, 211
  in *Æcerbot* 24–27, 28, 36
  as form of time keeping 107, 125n.37
  in *Herbarium*'s entry for *peruica* 134–141, 148, 149
  in *Herbarium*'s entry for *ricinum* 134–141, 145–146, 148, 149
  in *Ic me on þisse gyrde beluce* 63–84
  in lost cattle remedy 6
  in 'Nine Herbs Charm' 133, 138–150, 157n.38, 158n.44, 159n.50
  in the swarm charm 183
  in *Wið færstice* 12, 97–109, *110*, 118–121, 122n.4, 282

Irving, Edward B. 253, 260
Isidore of Seville
  Etymologiae 86n.13

javelins *see* spears
Jenkinson, Hilary 273
John of Beverley 8, 19n.24, 232–234
John of Hexham 233
Jolly, Karen Louise 4, 6–7, 62–63, 66–67, 73, 82, 85n.4, 93n.91, 95n.115, 96n.133, 119, 123n.13, 124n.30, 226
Josephus, Flavius
  Jewish War 179
'Journey Charm' *see Ic me on þisse gyrde beluce*
Judith (Old English) 56, 101, 102

Kapchan, Deborah 40
Karshner, Edward 153n.6
Keefer, Sarah Larratt 63
Ker, Neil 168
Kerewsky-Halpern, Barbara 127n.53
Kesling, Emily 19n.22, 157n.39, 218
Kinoshita, Sharon 180–181
Klaeber, F. 95n.124
Klinck, Anne 77–78
Klug, Helmut 180, 181, 193, 201n.58
knives 54, 81, 89n.36, 89n.38, 258, 259, 270n.52
  in *Anhaga* riddle 255–256, 259–260
  in epic 61, 90n.42, 106
  in graves 124n.31, 235
  in healing rituals 11, 54, 55, 60–62, 109
  in *Lacnunga* 61–62

knives (cont.)
  seax 60–62, 81, 89n.38, 90n.42, 97–98, 104–106, 108–109, *110*, 117, 120, 122, 125n.42, 126n.44
  in Wið færstice 97–98, 103–106, 108–109, *110*, 117, 122, 125n.42, 125n.44
  see also swords; warfare; weapons
Knoepflmacher, U. C. 30
Koutserimpas, Christos 126n.49
Kramer, Johanna 26
Krapp, George Philip 267n.18, 268n.21
Krentz, Christopher 206, 215, 241n.37
Kubaschewski, Elisabeth 154n.15, 200n.40

Lacnunga 8, 13, 29, 68–69, 88n.24, 90n.49, 95n.115, *104*, 130, 133, 138, 151, 199n.22, 206, 209, 244n.77, 259, 262, 270n.62, 284
  weapons and warfare in 12, 57, 61–62, 81
  see also British Library, MS Harley 585; *individual herbs and remedies*
Laes, Christian 231
Langen, Toby 119
Lang-Roth, Ruth 246n.91
law codes 70, 230
  and deafness 14, 208–210, 228–232, 234, 235, 245n.82, 284
Leahy, Kevin 89n.36
Lee, Christina 212, 214, 234, 284
Leechbook III 8, 88n.24, 95n.115, 209, 239n.13
  warfare and weapons in 57, 60–62

leonfot 15, 272–273, 275–280, 287n.24
Lewis, Hannah 233
Li, Lanzhi 34
Liebermann, F. 230, 245n.86
Linett, Maren Tova 208
lion's foot see *leonfot*
Lippman, Zachary 34
liturgy 4, 28, 41, 60, 73–74, 80, 95n.115, 125n.37
  and *Ic me on þisse gyrde beluce* 12, 34, 63, 66–67, 71, 74–75, 80
  see also Christianity
Liu, Tianjun 79
loricae 49, 62, 71, 90n.49
lost cattle remedy 6, 9, 29–31

McClintock, Barbara 38
McGillivray, Murray 123n.21, 128n.66
mægðe (maythe) 13, 133, 139, 142, 144–145
Mahoney, Maria 132
mailcoats 73, 90n.42, 115
  in *Ic me on þisse gyrde beluce* 11, 71–73, 80–81, 84
  see also armor; warfare
Maion, Danielle 166
mandrake (*mandragora*) 5, 13, 17, 152, 160, *161*, *163*, 164–165, 171–172, 174–197, 201n.58, 202n.75, 207, 278, 282
  anthropomorphized 13–14, 31, 160, 162, *163*, 164, 177–178, 180, 184, 187, 190, 203n.94, 206, 278, 283–284
  as described by Dioscorides 178, 200n.50
  harvesting ritual for 69, 162, 164, 175–180, 182–184, 187–191, 193, 201n.52, 278
Manley, John 60, 102

manuscripts *see* Bodleian Library, MS Hatton 76; British Library, MS Cotton Caligula A.vii; British Library, MS Cotton Otho B.xi; British Library, MS Cotton Vitellius C.iii; British Library, MS Harley 585; British Library, MS Harley 6258B; British Library, MS Royal 12 D.xvii; Cambridge College Corpus Christi MS 41; Cambridge College Corpus Christi MS 190
Marcelli de medicamentis liber 243n.58
Marco Polo
  Description of the World, The 5, 29, 180–181
Marder, Michael 14, 185, 186–188, 190, 202n.85
Margery Kempe 39
Maring, Heather 5, 28
Marsden, Richard 62, 92n.77, 93n.96
Massey, Jeff 260
Matto, Michael 93n.96, 268n.21
Maxims I 76–78
Maxims II 55–56, 252
Meaney, Audrey 223, 243n.62
Medicina de Quadrupedibus 154n.13, 162, 198n.2, 199n.22, 284
memory 138, 141, 148, 212–213
  ascribed to plants 5, 139, 141
metonymy 52, 74, 105, 122, 123n.9, 130, 131, 137, 146–149, 159n.49, 181, 256
metrical charms 8, 9, 26, 30, 81, 123n.21, 133, 262
  see also g(e)aldor; *individual remedies*
Metzler, Irina 227
Moerman, Daniel 52, 54

monastic sign language 216, 233, 241n.48
Moses, Mariah 119
Mount, Toni 19n.20
mugwort (*mugwyrt, artemisia*) 13, 57, 129, 133, 139, 142, 144–145, 148–149, 154n.14, 159n.50, 174
Muir, Bernard 266
Müller, C. 267n.18
Murphy, Patrick 251–252, 253, 254, 260, 266

Nagy, Joseph Falaky 212
National Association of the Deaf 229
Neville, Jennifer 20n.32, 267n.4
Nie, Jing-Bao 128n.63
Niles, John 256, 258, 269n.41, 270n.48
'Nine Herbs Charm' 4, 5, 13, 57, 129, 130, 133, 137, 158n.48, 159n.50, 271n.67, 283
  Christian elements within 34, 38, 133, 142, 148, 158n.43
  incantation in 133, 138–150, 157n.38, 158n.44, 159n.50
  ritual and herbal preparation in 133, 150
Nowell, Lawrence 223, 224, 243n.62

Oliver, Lisi 132, 231–232, 245n.82
Olsan, Lea 31, 64, 73
Olsen, Karin 255, 257
Ong, Walter 200n.34
oral theory 11, 278
  and Deaf studies 14–15, 207–208, 214–216, 236–237, 279
orans posture 79
Oswald, Dana 5
Owen-Crocker, Gale R. 56, 75, 124n.31

Pasternack, Carol Braun 80
Paxson, James J. 157n.34
Paz, James 70, 264
Pearman, Tory 39, 212, 213
Penick, Douglas 126n.47
performance arena 28, 42n.21, 56, 285
Peri didaxeon 168, 198n.2, 199n.22
personification 130, 137, 139–141, 143, 156n.28, 156n.32, 158n.44, 178, 184, 191, 194, 206, 278, 283
  in *Anhaga* riddle 1, 250–257, 259, 261
  see also anthropomorphization
peruica (periwinkle) 5, 13, 130, 133–137, *135*, *136*, 138–141, 146–147, 149–150, 155n.20, 200n.40, 283
Pettit, Edward 102, 105, 145, 158n.48
Philippe de Thaon
  Bestiary 193
Physica Plinii 242n.56
Pliny
  Natural History 51–54, 85n.6, 86n.12, 167, 178–179
Pollington, Stephen 119, 123n.13, 153n.5, 204n.125, 224
Portnoy, Phyllis 267n.7
Pound, Ezra
  Cantos 111
prayers 49, 62–63, 71, 95n.115, 125n.37, 141, 155n.19
proserpinaca (*unfortrædde*) 69, 152, 182
prosopopoeia 130, 137, 139, 140, 157n.34
Pseudo-Dioscorides
  Curae herbarum 155n.20
  Liber medicinae ex herbis femininis 155n.20

Rabin, Andrew 70, 91n.73
Rée, Jonathan 217
rhetoric 12, 38, 73, 118, 130–133, 137–152, 153n.6, 154n.12, 156n.24, 156n.28, 157n.34–35, 158n.45, 159n.49, 207, 214, *218*, *275*, *278*, *282*
  directed toward plants 13, *110*, 131–133, 136–152, 153n.6, 278, 282
  see also individual devices
Rhetorica ad Herennium 140, 141, 157n.35, 159n.49
ribwort 224, 243n.64
ricinum 5, 13, 129, 130, 133–137, *135*, 138–141, 145–146, 148, 149–150, 155n.20, 156n.29, 283
Riddle, John 156n.27
riddles 2, 35, 70, 140, 250–253, 256–258, 263, 269n.41, 271n.67, 279–280, 283
  and issues of orality 256, 261, 269n.39
  nomenclature for 20n.32
  see also Anhaga riddle; *Gingra Broþor Mec Adraf*; *Holt Hweorfende*
Riedinger, Anita 251, 252, 254, 255, 267n.6
Roach, Levi 232
Rodrigues, Louis J. 119, 123n.13
Rohde, Eleanour Sinclair 273–274, 285n.5
Roper, Jonathan 153n.6

St. Bede's Centre for Deaf People in London 233
St. Margaret, Old English Life of 231
Samonis, George 126n.49
Sanborn, Linda 167
Sarton, George 274

Sauer, Hans 149, 154n.15, 155n.16, 200n.40
Sayers, Edna Edith 216–217, 241n.48
Sayers, William 254, 255
Schaefer, Ursula 153n.6, 231
Scheil, Andrew 28
Schiappa, Edward 154n.12
seax *see* knives: seax
sentience (of plants) 12, 131, 139–152, 158n.44, 184–185, 187–188, 191–194, 203n.94, 278, 283
Shakespeare, William
  Romeo and Juliet 160
shields 56, 87n.18, 97, 258, 260, 264
  in epic 100, 114–115
  in graves 72, 87n.17, 124n.31
  in *Ic me on þisse gyrde beluce* 11, 67, 71–72, 79–81, 85
  as possible solution to *Anhaga* riddle 1, 250–251, 253–261, 265, 267n.18, 268n.21, 270n.48, 282–283
  in *Wið færstice* 100–101, 110, 114, 121, 123n.9
  see also armor; warfare
Shull, George 33, 44n.43
Siewers, Alf 5
Singer, Charles 90n.49, 226, 273, 286n.6
Siraisi, Nancy G. 137
Sirr, Peter 93n.96
Skemp, A. R. 125n.42
snakebite remedy *see Herbarium*: snakebite remedy
'Soul and Body I' 231
Spearing, Sinead 287n.25
spears 12, 29, 53, 54–58, 59, 60–61, 76, 81, 88n.33, 89n.38, 93n.97, 100–102, 106, 114–115, 123n.12, 258, 269n.45
  in *Ic me on þisse gyrde beluce* 75–76, 93n.96, 274
  in *Wið færstice* 102–104, 106–107, 109, 110, 117, 123n.13, 148
  see also warfare; weapons
sperewyrt 11, 49, 57, 258, 276
Steen, Janie 138, 157n.35
Storms, Godfrid 20n.30, 62, 77, 78, 82, 96n.133, 96n.135, 103, 125n.41, 126n.44, 226, 273
Strong, Pauline Turner 40
Stross, Brian 31, 39, 45n.53
Stuart, Heather 76, 93n.96
Sunjata 111
Sutton Hoo 72, 202n.76, 259
Swanton, M. J. 58, 75
swarm charm 29, 57, 87n.22, 148, 183
Swearingen, C. Jan 154n.12
Swerian 230
swords 55, 56, 61, 75–76, 89n.38, 93n.97, 126n.45, 179, 262
  in *Anhaga* riddle 253–256, 260, 265
  in graves 72, 124n.31
  as healing implements 53–55
  in *Ic me on þisse gyrde beluce* 11, 71–73, 75–76, 80–81, 84
  in *Wið færstice* 105–106, 115, 122
  see also knives; warfare; weapons

Tacitus
  Germania 60
Tait, Yvonne 243n.64
Textus Roffensis 125n.37
Theophrastus 201n.52
Thompson, C. J. S. 201n.58
Thompson, Logan 19n.20
Tiffin, Helen 30, 43n.29
Tigges, Wim 260

Toelken, Barre 37
Toller, T. Northcote 67, 91n.72, 191, 224, 243n.63, 287n.23
Trautmann, Moritz 254, 268n.21
Treharne, Elaine 3, 169
Trilling, Renée 4, 35, 176–177
Troyer, A. Forrest 45n.57
Tupper, Frederick 77, 78, 95n.113

Underhill, Richard 183
Underwood, Richard 60, 102

Van Arsdall, Anne 138, 149, 153n.5, 168, 180, 181, 182–183, 193, 198n.3, 201n.55, 201n.58, 204n.124, 244n.69, 287n.23
Vaughan-Sterling, Judith 93n.96, 148
violence *see* warfare; weapons
volition *see* agency

wælwyrt 129, 131
  see also Herbarium: snakebite remedy
Wanderer, The 78, 156n.24, 252
warfare 55–56, 61, 98, 100–102, 128n.63, 257
  in *Anhaga* riddle 249–257, 259–263, 279, 284
  in *Beowulf* 56–57, 61, 90n.42, 106–108, 113–117
  in the *Herbarium* 49, 54, 57–58, 88n.33, 258
  in *Ic me on þisse gyrde beluce* 34, 68, 69–81, 84, 94n.104, 116–117, 282, 284
  in *Lacnunga* 12, 57
  as metaphor for healing 11–12, 34, 40–41, 49, 54–57, 61, 69–81, 97–117, 129
  in riddles 1–2, 15, 249–257, 259–263, 279–280
  in *Wið færstice* 97–109, *110*, 113–117, 206, 277, 282–283
  see also armor; helmets; knives; mailcoats; shields; spears; swords; weapons
Warren, Minton 32
Watkins, Calvert 271n.67
waybroad *see wegbrade*
weapons 11–12, 55–56, 57, 61, 89n.38, 93n.97, 98, 100–101
  in *Anhaga* riddle 249–250, 253–256, 259–260
  in *Bald's Leechbook* 57, 60–62
  in epic 61, 90n.42, 106
  gendered use of 61, 90n.42, 106, 124n.31
  in graves 58, 72, 87n.17, 92n.80, 124n.31
  as healing implements 11, 49, 53–56, 60–62, 109
  in the *Herbarium* 57–58, 88n.33, 258
  herbs as 11, 40–41, 49, 54–55, 57–58, 60, 62, 109, 126n.45, 258, 260–261, 270n.62, 276
  in *Ic me on þisse gyrde beluce* 11, 63–64, 71–76, 78, 80–81, 90n.43, 93n.96, 116–117, 274, 282–283
  in *Lacnunga* 12, 57, 61–62, 81
  and status 61, 72–76, 78, 81, 92n.80, 105–106, 117, 124n.31
  in *Wið færstice* 12, 97–99, 101–109, *110*, 115, 117, 121, 123n.13, 125n.42, 126n.44, 148, 283–284
  see also arrows; knives; spears; swords; warfare

wegbrade (waybroad) 13, 120, 133, 139, 144, 154n.15, 158n.44, 159n.50
whetstones 1, 250–251, 255–261, 264, 270n.51–52, 282–283
Widsið 102
Wilcox, Miranda 233
Williamson, Craig 251, 253, 262, 263, 267n.18
Winzer, Margaret 242n.49
Wið færstice 12, 81, 97–122, *104*, 128n.66, 148, 262, 277, 284
  incantation in 12, 97–109, *110*, 118–121, 122n.4, 282
  ritual and herbal preparation in 97–99, 101–103, 105, 107–109, *110*, 118–121, 125n.42, 126n.44
  shields in 100–101, *110*, 114, 121, 123n.9
  smiths in 12, 97, 103–106, 109, 121
  and textual emendation 104–105, 122, 123n.21

weapons and warfare in 12, 97–109, *110*, 113–117, 119, 121, 122, 123n.13, 125n.42, 126n.44, 148, 206, 277, 282–284
Woden 4, 19n.20, 34, 38, 133, 142, 148
Wonders of the East see Marco Polo: *Description of the World, The*
woodruff *see astula regia* (woodruff)
Wulfstan 73

yarrow 11, 49–55, *50*, 67, 86n.9, 86n.11–12, 111, 148–149
Young, Robert 40

Zamir, Dani 34
Zemeckis, Robert 248

EU authorised representative for GPSR:
Easy Access System Europe, Mustamäe tee 50,
10621 Tallinn, Estonia
gpsr.requests@easproject.com

www.ingramcontent.com/pod-product-compliance
Ingram Content Group UK Ltd.
Pitfield, Milton Keynes, MK11 3LW, UK
UKHW021830210426